TOTAL
BEAUTY

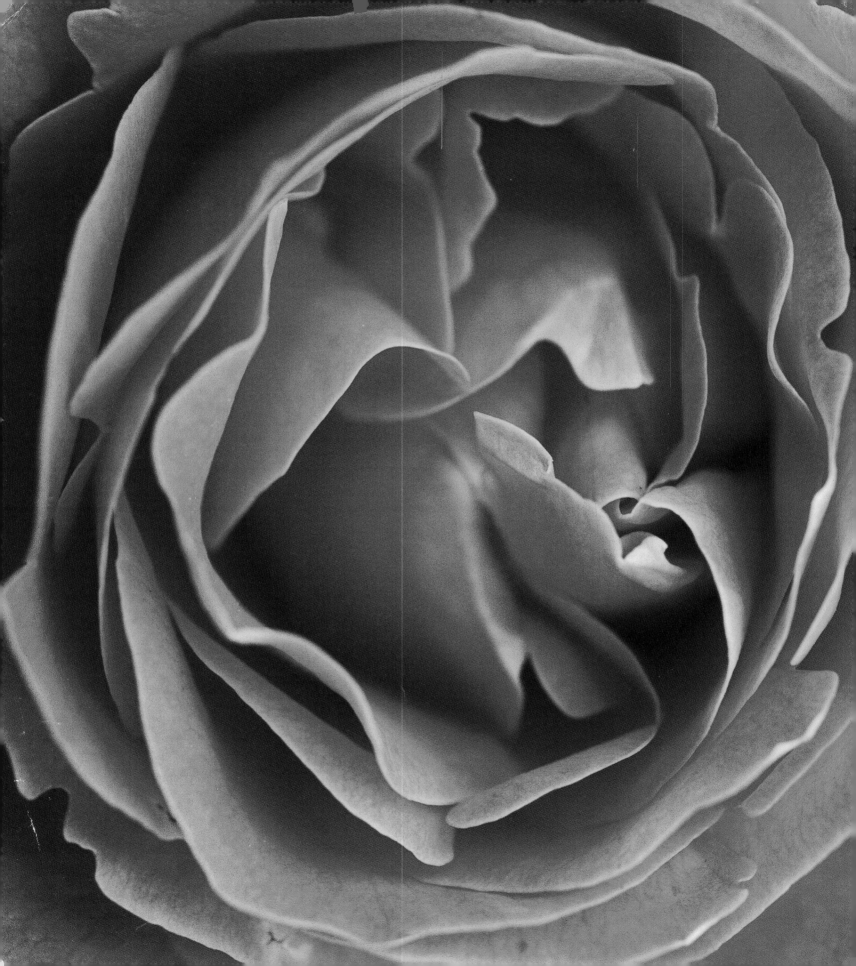

TOTAL BEAUTY

SARAH STACEY & JOSEPHINE FAIRLEY

Sterling Publishing Co., Inc.
New York

This book is dedicated to Kay McCauley – our friend, agent and the most gorgeous woman we know

Library of Congress Cataloging-in-Publication Data Available

2 4 6 8 10 9 7 5 3 1

Publishing in the U.S. in 2004 by Sterling Publishing Co., Inc.
387 Park Avenue South, New York, NY 10016

Distributed in Canada by Sterling Publishing
c/o Canadian Manda Group, 165 Dufferin Street
Toronto, Ontario, Canada M6K 3H6

Sterling ISBN: 1-4027-1776-8

First published in Great Britain in 2002 by
Kyle Cathie Limited

Copyright © 2002, 2004 by Sarah Stacey and Josephine Fairley
Illustrations © David Downton

Project manager: Grapevine Publishing
Editor: Gill Paul
Design: Mark Latter at Vivid Design
Picture research: Josephine Thompson
Special photography: Francesca Yorke

Production: Lorraine Baird & Sha Huxtable
Color origination: Colourscan, Singapore
Printed and bound in Singapore by Tien-Wah Press

Contents

INTRODUCTION

It's a beauty jungle out there. Thousands of products and procedures. Endless extravagant claims. Scientific gobbledegook – and tons of feel-good "natural" hype. In real life, though, how many women have time to read the blurb – or sample the mountains of miracle creams, mascaras, lip-plumpers and skin-brighteners that have been launched? And which woman hasn't sat at the hairdresser, wondering what on earth she's let herself in for? Or whether she should have her forehead Botox'ed or her teeth bleached? That's why we wrote this book for you. To bring you the inside track on what really works, the insider knowledge that gives you everything you need to look and feel gorgeous – in no time at all. (Almost.)

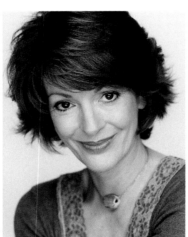

Because in the 21st century, time's the one thing we don't have enough of. What we hear constantly, as health and beauty experts, is that women want maximum results in minimum time. So the emphasis throughout this entirely new book is on just that: the tricks, the tips, the wisdom that help you take a shortcut to looking – and feeling – better. And while cosmetics and good haircuts are a godsend, we hope you'll also learn more about enhancing beauty from the inside out with food, juices, yoga, DIY massage and even how to think yourself gorgeous!

The big question we're asked all the time, though, is: "Which products really work?" Well, we've been privileged to try plenty – and are happy to tell you about our favorites here. (Alongside those of some beauty editor gurus from around the world who've also dipped, dabbed and daubed their way through literally tons of makeup, haircare and skincare.) But our signature – as in our previous bestselling books *The Beauty Bible* and *Feel Fabulous Forever* – has been to carry out Tried & Tested surveys on real women, using products in real-life situations. Not – as with many magazine T&Ts – just one beauty editor sampling moisturizers on her forearm.

So, in *Total Beauty*, we bring you the results of what we believe to be the biggest consumer survey of cosmetics ever carried out, anywhere in the world. Over a period of six months, 1180 women – who we divided into panels of 10 – tested literally thousands of products (generously supplied by the manufacturers) –100 brands, in 32 categories, from 'miracle creams' to hair removers. Which means that each score isn't just one woman's subjective viewpoint: it's an average taken from ten different women's experiences. As research goes, it's exhaustive. We hope it will save you from having to scan shelf after shelf, counter after counter, of endless options – all of them claiming to be *the* product you can't live without.

As well as women feeling increasingly "time-poor", there's been another shift in the eight years since our first book was published. While some women want super-high-tech products that rely on the very latest anti-aging technology, a growing number look for more natural and holistic skincare that fits with a more natural and holistic lifestyle. (And that includes us.) But here, you'd be forgiven for becoming even more confused. What's natural? What's not?

In reality, the only way you can be sure a product is 100 percent natural is to make it yourself, so we've brought you quite a few recipes for do-it-yourself beauty treatments. (Because if you can make a salad dressing, you can make cosmetics). In cosmetics manufacturing, however, many ingredients start out natural and end up being chemically processed into something that's decidedly not. (Take, for instance, the detergent sodium lauryl sulfate, originally extracted from coconut oil but so highly processed that it bears no relation whatsoever to the yummy coconut it's supposedly related to.)

To find out which products on the market really deserve to use the word natural, we went half-blind scanning ingredient labels and asked manufacturers endless questions in order to come up with our "daisy rating" for naturalness. Any product that claimed to be natural (and plenty did) was examined very, very closely – and if it was mostly petrochemicals, silicones, synthetic 'fillers' or detergents, or used chemical sunscreens (which penetrate the skin) rather than sun-blocking minerals (which sit on the surface), it did not get a "daisy"❀.

For some women, this isn't an issue. And that's absolutely your choice. But we think it's good to know what's what. So, throughout the book, you'll find products that we've awarded one or sometimes two "daisy" symbols ❀❀. One daisy means that although the product is not 100 percent natural, it does contain generous – and sometimes extremely high – levels of botanical ingredients, very often only minimally processed and in a more natural base than many you'll find on the shelves. Two daisies, however, mean that a skin/hair/body product succeeds in being totally natural, avoiding the use of synthetic ingredients. And the good news for wannabe-natural beauties is that many of the "daisy-rated" choices scored incredibly well in the Tried & Tested surveys.

We can't promise that you'll never, ever make an expensive beauty mistake again. (We can't even promise that you'll love every single thing our testers raved about.) But we do believe that this book will save you time and money. Because, in the beauty jungle, every woman needs a guide with insider information to help her find her way around. And after all our years in the beauty industry, we truly believe this book is it!

Sarah x   Jo

www.beautybible.com

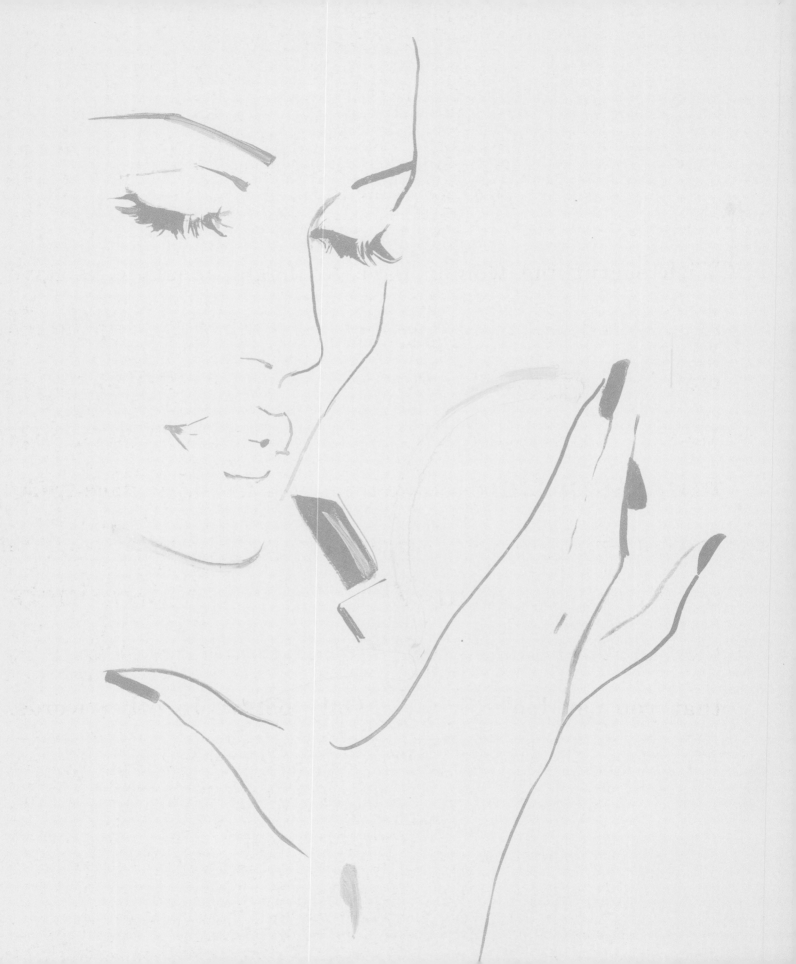

MAKEUP

With everything women have to juggle, most of us have about **five minutes** – tops – to apply makeup in the morning, or to get our faces ready to go from desk to dinner. What we all want is **maximum results in minimum time.** So we bring you fast-track face tricks from beauty pros for makeup-in-a-flash – and steer you towards the ultimate **high-performance products** that are the best that science and nature have to offer. So that you can look like you. Only better. In other words, **Pretty Damned Gorgeous.** Pretty Damned Quick.

YOUR FASTEST-EVER FACE

Who has time to use ten different products every morning or evening? We don't. (Nor does anyone we know.) Two of the world's leading make-up pros – Bobbi Brown and Stila's Jeanine Lobel – give their tips for fast-track faces

As hardworking mothers, nobody understands the pressures of getting ready fast better than Bobbi Brown and Stila founder Jeanine Lobel. They're all for simplification. But, as Bobbi says, "There are certain products that are must-haves in every woman's makeup bag: concealer, foundation in your skin-tone-correct shade, a pretty shade of blush and mascara."

Beyond that, different skin tones and colorings will have different can't-leave-home-without-them makeup items. To help shave time off your routine, Bobbi recommends identifying the products that make the most difference in how you look. Experiment in front of a mirror and try different combinations until you find a minimal combination with maximum impact. "My beauty philosophy is about creating a beauty style that works for you. Trends come and go. Style endures." (So if the world's suddenly gone pink-eye shadow-crazy, you don't have to.)

For blondes: Most blondes find they can't live without mascara, taupe eye shadow (which can double as brow color and eyeliner) and cream blush, according to Bobbi. Lipstick colors that work for blondes are soft pinks, with salmon or pink blush, and bone (creamy-white) shadows.

For brunettes: Most can skip mascara or eyebrow color, but foundation is often a must for evening out skin tone, together with blush and lip gloss. "Good shades are rose, raisin, brown and mahogany," advise Bobbi.

For redheads: Eyeliner is great for emphasizing pale skin and light lashes – and can double as an eyebrow definer. Lip gloss is great on redheads, too. The best shades? "Caramels, rich browns or brown-reds on lips,

apricot or muted pink blush, brown mascara and camel and toast brown eyeshadows."

For grey hair: Just eyebrow pencil, mascara (if your lashes are pale) and a blush and/or lipstick can work wonders. Bobbi's recommendations: "Pink, rose, red, apricot or peach lipsticks; use rose tones, soft brights or soft pastels for cheeks."

Bobbi's 3-minute countdown

3... Start with concealer under the eyes and in the most recessed corners of the eyes, near the nose. It makes you look awake.

2... Put on a tinted moisturizer or, if your skin is smooth and even-toned naturally, sweep a natural blush color or bronzer on your cheeks. If you use foundation, cover any blemish or redness around the nose.

1... Apply brown or black mascara to your lashes, and put a sheer or slightly tinted gloss on the lips.

Bobbi's 5-minute countdown

5... Start with concealer (one shade lighter than your foundation). Apply to the under-eye area and at inner eye corners, and blend into your skin.

4... Apply foundation that perfectly matches your skin tone (see page 14) where needed to even it out, and set with yellow-toned powder (see page 22).

3... Smile, then apply blush to the apples of your cheeks with a brush, blending downward and outward for the most natural effect. Or stroke on a creamy-textured blush – see page 45 for more on these .

2... Brush a light shade of eye shadow over the entire eyelid to open up and brighten the area. Line the eyes, working eyeliner pencil into the lash-line. Brush lashes through with mascara, such as Bobbi Brown Defining Mascara in Black.

1... Go for a slick of lip gloss in a natural shade (like Bobbi's own Petal or Honey).

Jeanine's 3-minute countdown for younger faces

3... Apply concealer to well-moisturized skin wherever you need extra help; use a small brush to disguise blemishes.

2... Apply concealer/cream foundation to eyelids. Use a multi-purpose product on eyes, lips and cheeks as needed. (Stila's All Over Shimmer is perfect for this, in shades 4 – a browny shade – or peachy 5.)

1... Sweep mascara through lashes and, if you like, add clear gloss or tinted lip balm to lips.

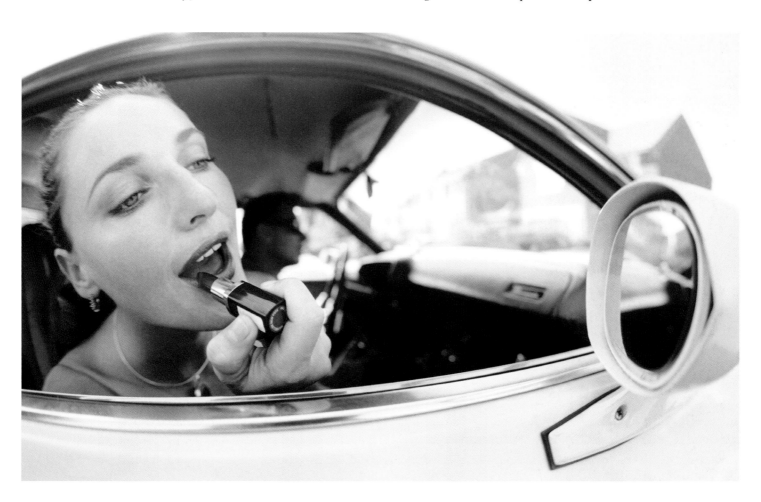

WHAT WE USE

Jo

✳ *Lancôme Teint Idôle Hydra Compact:* delivers amazing density of coverage – enough to cover the broken capillaries to which I'm prone – without ever looking thick or caked. I dab onto a well-moisturized face and blend, adding more where needed to conceal imperfections. I press it into skin in areas where I need maximum coverage. With this particular foundation, I don't need powder – which saves time and mess.

✳ *Lancôme Blush Focus in 04 Caramel Toffee Matte:* a lovely, easy-to-blend, peachy-toned cream blusher. (Pink blushers accentuate my too-red cheeks.)

✳ *A dark aubergine eyeshadow from By Terry:* from a wonderful Parisian makeup boutique, where I once had a personal consultation with makeup guru Terry de Gunzberg herself. She recommended this dark purple-navy shade for lining—rather than shading—my blue eyes.

✳ *Bobbi Brown Mahogany Eye Shadow:* a dark brown that I use as an alternative to Terry's aubergine, for eye lining. As I've aged, I've found that wearing shadow on my lids and/or in the eye socket is aging, making my eyes look heavy. Instead, I blend foundation – see above – on my eyelids, and line the eyes with dark powder shadow, for an effect that looks younger and fresher (I'm told!)

✳ For everyday, I love *Dr. Hauschka Mascara*, which

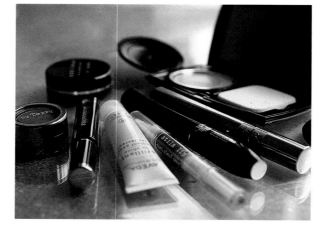

gives a very natural effect – just enough to darken my blonde lashes. It's incredibly easy to remove at night – and I love the fact it's all-natural, and the lovely rose smell. When I need more impact, I choose *Yves Saint Laurent Luxurious Mascara* for a false-lash effect or *Lancôme Amplicils*, in brown/black, both of which are amazingly volumizing – so you never need more than one coat.

✳ *Stila Lip Glaze:* I have several of these ultra-glossy, fruit-scented lip glosses, which deliver sheer, shiny color without that sticky feeling you get with some glosses, and appeal to my "inner girly-girl". They taste and smell of fruit (and I go through so much that I fervently hope they're calorie-free). My fave shades are Raspberry, a sheer pink, and Strawberry, a clear red.

✳ *Aveda Lip Tint SPF 15 in Berry:* adds glide-on sheer color (with a hint of shimmer) to make lips look just-bitten, and is deliciously flavored with refreshing cinnamon leaf, clove and anise oils.

✳ *Aveda Lip Shine:* I like the way that glosses make my lips look fuller, especially this one, which has tiny iridescent particles as well as uplifting and spirit-soothing oils of vanilla and peppermint. Brilliant Lip Shine looks wonderful over lipstick (when I bother to wear it), and in winter I keep some of these in different coat pockets as a weather-beating lip balm.

SARAH

✳ *Bobbi Brown Moisture Rich Foundation in Sand:* this is my staple base which also covers enough to be a concealer for the red areas round my nose and the odd broken capillary—curiously, these have gotten better over the years, an unexpected bonus of aging. It's moisturizing – essential for my very dry skin – and never leaves a cakey finish. I put on as little as possible, dabbing with my ring fingers and always starting in the center of my face – or else I get over-enthusiastic and end up with a mask. A recent discovery is *Lancôme's Adaptive foundation*, which is fab for older skin. I always apply base over *Estée Lauder's Idealist Skin Refinisher*, which is fantastic.

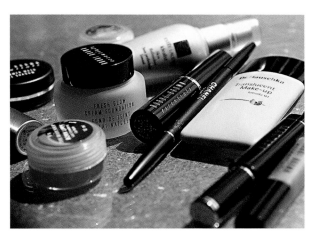

✳ *Dr. Hauschka Translucent Makeup:* this is like a mix of tinted moisturizer and foundation and is perfect for summer or winter days when my skin is looking good (usually when I've had plenty of exercise and sleep). I use the shade called Intrada. (And, of course, it's 100 percent pure and natural.)

✳ *Bobbi Brown Cream Blush Stick in Tawny:* blush makes a colossal difference as I tend to be pale and look like Lady Macbeth's first cousin when I'm tired. This cream formulation is almost foolproof. Powder is too drying for me nowadays.

✳ *Dr. Hauschka Mascara in Brown:* like Jo, I love this gentle mascara and particularly the scent of rose oil. I have long thick lashes – though they're pale at the ends – and they tend to look overly made-up with more than one coat.

✳ *Bobbi Brown Shimmer Wash Eye Shadow in Fawn:* I smear this soft, pale, smoky shade over my upper lids for evenings – but not above, or I look ill. Then I dab a bit of eyeliner on – see below – for a stab at vampy eyes.

✳ *Chanel Precision Eye Definer in Charcoal*: New York hairdresser John Barrett commanded me to make up my eyes "smoky/sexy" for a big party we were going to, and this eyeliner plus some Nars shadow does the trick in a jiffy – even if you're a klutz like me.

✳ *Jurlique Natural Lipstick in Mahogany:* since we eat such a lot of our lipstick I prefer natural products whenever possible. I use Jurlique with a top gloss of *Dr. Hauschka's Dolce Lipstick* in a deep sandy shimmer called simply 09.

✳ *Bobbi Brown Shimmer Lip Gloss in Rose Sugar:* for evenings, I simply can't do without this slightly pearly, infinitely sexy gloss.

✳ *The Body Shop Born Lippy:* these fruit-flavored lip balms – I like Strawberry – not only moisturize and give a bit of shine, they also have an extraordinary effect at parties. (I smeared some on my lips on a freezing New Year's Eve as midnight struck and got kissed – gosh!)

FOUNDATION – BACK TO BASICS

Nobody minds being complimented on a lipstick. But you never want to hear the words "I love your foundation"! Base is meant to camouflage imperfections – yet disappear like magic into the skin, delivering instant flawlessness...

Getting foundation right is a major beauty challenge – which is why bathroom cabinets tend to be cluttered with bottles, jars and tubes of foundation that didn't quite work, but seem too extravagant to throw away. The right base takes just moments to apply – but (sometimes) hours to track down – in order to find the perfect shade. We are huge fans of foundation, believing that base – plus mascara and blush – are the true makeup must-haves, especially as we age and skin tone becomes more uneven. (As Trish McEvoy observes, "If you're looking for one product that makes a difference to older faces, it's foundation.")

SHOPPING FOR FOUNDATION

✳ Take a hand mirror or a compact with you so that you can easily walk to daylight and check the shade.

✳ Remove existing base before trying on foundation. Swipe away from the jawline with cleanser or toner before sampling. If possible, go foundation-shopping bare-faced, so when you've pinpointed a "maybe" shade, you can apply it all over.

✳ Thanks in part to the pervasive influence of Bobbi Brown, the majority of foundations today are based on yellow pigments – which create an infinitely more realistic effect than the pink tones of yesteryear. Too-pink foundation, in the words of Hollywood's Carol Shaw, "looks like calamine lotion".

✳ Don't even think of using foundation to "perk up" your skin by changing its color.

✳ Gun Novak, founder of the FACE Stockholm brand, suggests trying vertical "stripes" of as many as three shades of foundation, from under your cheekbone to jaw-line – applied in a downward stripe with a Q-tip – before heading for a window or door with your mirror. Then you can make up your mind in full, natural light. "The right color will simply disappear into your skin. Try to match it to your neck – which is always lighter – rather than your face. You can always use blush to add warmth." Gun advises shopping for foundation during daylight hours, not after dark: "That's when mistakes are often made."

✳ If for any reason you don't want to try foundation on your face, the next-best place to test base is the inside of your forearm – most definitely not the back of your hand. Test for depth of coverage (but not for color) on the blue vein on the inside of your wrist.

✳ If you have trouble finding the perfect shade, consider investing in a Prescriptives Custom Blending – which saves a lot of searching. A trained consultant mixes up a complexion-matched shade, of which a record is kept for future orders; you're given a bottle of foundation (which can be customized with additional moisture, light-reflecting pigments and more), plus a tiny pot of matching concealer. Custom Blending doesn't come cheap but we think it's worth every penny.

✳ There are literally dozens of foundation "finishes" available today, as well as a thousand shades. What we find most flattering are all the formulations that feature "light-reflecting pigments", which bounce light off the face to create an optical illusion of softness and flawlessness. In our experience, a slightly dewy finish is more flattering than totally matte (especially on more mature skins.)

✳ Estée Lauder – which has excellent foundations – occasionally runs promotional giveaways that let you sample miniature bottles of foundation before investing in a full-sized bottle. Alternatively, it's worth taking a tiny plastic bottle to the counter and asking the beauty consultant to pour in a little liquid foundation in a shade that you both agree *should* suit you. For how to apply foundation perfectly, turn to page 17.

TIP: Be sure you're using the right moisturizer for your skin type; if it's delivering too much moisture – or not enough – your makeup will disappear more quickly and need retouching more often.

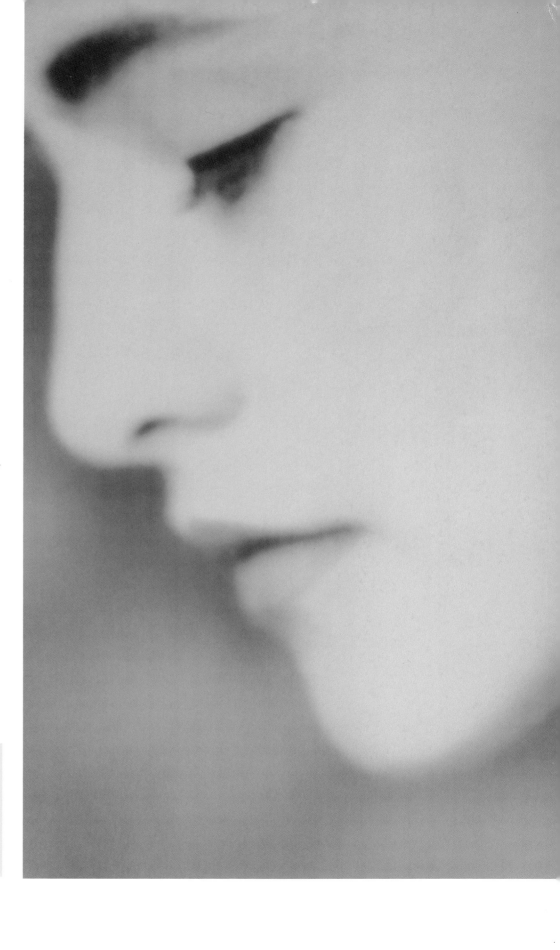

ALL-IN-ONE COMPACT FOUNDATIONS

Tried & Tested

These are a real time-saving option: a few swipes deliver long-lasting cover with no need to powder, as the creamy formulation transforms into powder in seconds. The downside is that they can be drying, so you may need extra moisturizer underneath, but they're great for slipping into a handbag for day-long retouching.

SHISEIDO THE MAKEUP COMPACT FOUNDATION

8.33 points out of 10

Shiseido's range had the input of top make-up artist Tom Pecheux, which may be one reason this refillable compact foundation earned such rave reviews from our panellists. It features a "Prismatic Powder" to bounce light off the face and deliver a flawless finish.

UPSIDE: "I have used lots of foundations but this is the best ever – very natural yet covered everything" • "lasted better than many – 7-8 hours" • "very smart compact – great design – and a lovely, dewy feel" • "I especially liked the fact this compact could be refilled rather than thrown away" • "just the right texture – I don't usually use foundation but found this very pleasant to use: it went on easily, wasn't too 'noticeable' and the compact is a very sensible size – you can actually see your whole face in the mirror".

DOWNSIDE· "I have dry skin on my nose and cheeks and the product 'clung' to this, making them look worse".

GUERLAIN DIVINORA TEINT EXPERT CONFORT

7.95 points out of 10

As you'd expect from Guerlain, this compact has a high 'glam' factor. Some loved the hefty gold compact – some found it was a little too "ritzy"-looking, but most agreed that the formulation itself delivered great results.

UPSIDE: "Glides on easily with damp sponge" • "divine smell – light and sexy" • "very comfortable on the face" • "very easy to build coverage to disguise veins and my red cheeks" • "natural, dewy finish" • "I'd been dying to try an expensive foundation – and this far exceeded expectations" • "good staying power".

DOWNSIDE: "When used dry was patchy, cloying and uneven".

ESTÉE LAUDER SO INGENIOUS MULTI-DIMENSIONAL MAKEUP SPF 8

7.88 points out of 10

Estée Lauder's latest innovation is QuadraColor Technology™, said to help foundation adapt to the way the face moves, for a non-caking finish that makes for easy-to-build coverage.

UPSIDE: "I love this – it made applying foundation effortless and gave a great result" • "evened out skintone without looking like too much makeup" • "I don't usually wear foundation but this was a great product: good coverage, light as powder – and no oily T-zone showed through" • "loved the product – couldn't fault it and will definitely buy again".

DOWNSIDE: "I didn't feel the coverage was as good as with a liquid foundation".

BEST BUDGET BUY
REVLON NEW COMPLEXION COMPACT MAKEUP

7.87 points out of 10

This creamy formula features an SPF 15 and is oil-free. Designed for long-lasting cover, it comes in an impressive choice of 16 shades.

UPSIDE: "A dream to use" • "went on easily, didn't clog pores and left skin looking smooth and moisturized" • "I'm a convert – it didn't irritate or look heavy, and would be great for dull winter complexions that needed a boost" • "coverage even and flattering".

DOWNSIDE: "A little unforgiving on dry skin areas" • "packaging a little cheap-looking".

CLARINS SOFT TOUCH RICH COMPACT FOUNDATION

7.63 points out of 10

Water-based technology gives this product a featherlight formula, which is also designed to offer great skin comfort. Clarins tells us that it contains an "Auto-Focus Pigment Complex" for a 'halo' effect to conceal fine lines and imperfections, while ensuring color stays true.

UPSIDE: "An all-around excellent product – smart design and very easy to use; it doesn't take long to apply and covers blemishes well, without looking heavy" • "great coverage for daytime" • "sheer and natural-looking" • "nicely packaged and easy and pleasant to use, providing a very natural finish".

DOWNSIDE: "Too drying for me – it tended to show up my dry patches" • "this looked and felt lovely initially but after three hours or so, 'caked' on drier areas".

The lowest score in this category was 5.86 points out of 10.

IT'S ALL ABOUT SKIN

You probably need less foundation than you think you do. (In fact, you may not even need foundation at all – just some well-blended concealer, set with powder, as you'll see.) Too much foundation is aging. And old-fashioned. End of story...

The ultimate foundation secret is to find your perfect shade (see pages 14–15), so that it works to conceal flaws and lightly even out skin tone, while letting your own skin show through. But application techniques help, too. So here are the best secrets we've ever learned.

✳ Never apply base/concealer to un-moisturized skin – and try to leave at least 10 minutes between applying moisturizer/primer/eye cream and making up. If you can't do that, the trade-off is that your makeup may not stay put for as long. (Also, we find that makeup just looks so much better if you can take that vital time between moisturizing and putting on base: everything seems to settle down.)

✳ Up close – particularly in magnifying mirrors – everything from open pores or broken capillaries to blackheads and wrinkles looks like a flaw, and is therefore a prime candidate for 'erasing' with concealer or foundation. But caution! Andrea Horwood, spokeswoman for the Australian brand Becca (see Directory, page 246), which boasts – hurray! – an amazing 20 shades of concealer, advises: "Never use a magnifying mirror to apply base or concealer or you'll be tempted to slap it all over. Instead, stand about two feet away from an ordinary mirror and observe from there, dabbing base or concealer where it seems needed from that distance. Then go close to the mirror to blend. Remember: very few people see you up that close." (And if they do, you're probably already in a clinch – and they won't give a damn.)

✳ Some professionals swear by makeup sponges to apply foundation but we're with makeup artist Mary Greenwell

on this one: fingers warm the foundation as you work, and are less fussy. (They can also be cleaned more easily.) One rule: always wash your hands thoroughly before applying makeup, for hygiene's sake.

✳ If you're going to apply foundation with fingers rather than a sponge, Barbara Daly advises putting a small amount on the back of your hand, then picking up

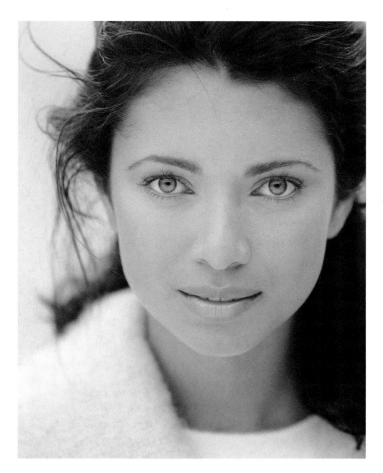

what you need as you go along. "That way you won't overload your skin."

✳ For really quick application, try a synthetic foundation brush – Prescriptives and Make Up For Ever both make them. You dab foundation on with the brush where you need it, then pat it into skin with fingers, delivering amazing results.

✳ You'll almost certainly need two shades of foundation and concealer in your "wardrobe" – one for summer, one for winter. As seasons change, you can custom-blend the two in the palm or on the back of your hand.

broken capillaries. We know countless women who swear by Yves Saint Laurent Touche Eclat Radiant Touch for under-eye circles, which works by "bouncing" light off the face (it won Tried & Tested Concealers category hands-down, see opposite) – but when applied to pimples, it simply draws attention to them.

✳ To disguise pimples, Trish McEvoy recommends using a stiff concealer brush (see page 51) to apply a dab of concealer "on the tip of the pimple – not the sides," she says. "Blend in using your finger, patting the edges till they blur with skin." (You can use a Q-tip for this, if you prefer, but the warmth of fingers enhances blendability.)

Never use a magnifying mirror to apply base or concealer, or you'll be tempted to slap it all over

✳ The debate's still raging among makeup artists about whether concealer should go over or under foundation. We say: the only way to be sure which works best for you is to try it both ways and analyze. Overall, though, we prefer concealer after foundation – otherwise you're wiping away the concealer when you blend the foundation. (Jo gets around this problem by using a foundation that can double as a concealer – Lancôme Teint Idôle Hydra-Compact – and applies it slightly more densely over areas with redness. Bobbi Brown's Foundation Stick is also excellent: the chunky, swivel-up stick can be dabbed directly onto skin, then blended with fingers for super-swift cover.)

✳ When applying concealer, use your middle or ring finger to blend; this makes for a lighter touch (so you don't rub it all off) and a more natural-looking finish.

✳ Be aware: the same concealer may not be perfect for camouflaging both under-eye circles and blemishes or

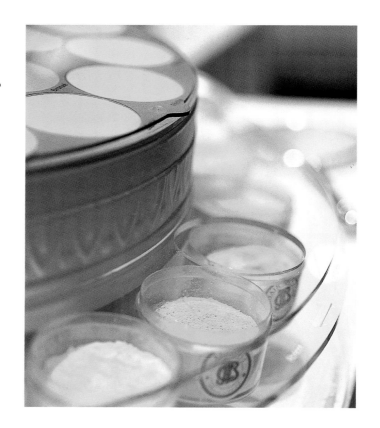

CONCEALERS – *Tried & Tested*

In the last decade, concealers have come a long way from the cakey, chalky, panstick type products that some readers will remember from their young days. They are much more natural and lightweight, without losing effectiveness. We asked our testers to try these on a variety of 'flaws' – broken veins, dark circles, small scars, spots and patches of uneven skin tone.

YVES SAINT LAURENT TOUCHE ÉCLAT RADIANT TOUCH
9.33 points out of 10

A truly outstanding mark for a truly outstanding product that's right up there in the Hall of Beauty Fame: you'll find one of these gold, pump-action magic wands in the kit of virtually every celebrity and makeup artist anywhere in the world today. It can be dabbed along fine lines to make them "disappear" (through light-reflective technology), and our testers were highly impressed with the way it makes dark circles vanish.

UPSIDE: "Brilliant, especially when used on frown-line and nose-to-mouth laugh lines" • "really gives oomph to your complexion" • "most amazing! Covered dark circles under eyes that nothing else has been able to do; truly a miracle" • "like having a blank canvas on which to paint your face – congratulations, YSL!" • "gorgeous gold packaging – very easy to carry round and re-apply on the run".

DOWNSIDE: "I just wish it wasn't so expensive!" • "slightly drying on skin under eyes".

M.A.C. SELECT COVER-P
8.18 points out of 10

This comes in a slim tube, and M.A.C. advise it can be used under foundation, or on its own.

UPSIDE: "Made my skin look fresh and had a velvety texture" • "particularly good for dark circles" • "the small opening in the tube made it easy to control the amount of product –but a little goes a long way" • "great for eyelids, to help keep makeup on" • "I've been looking for a product like this for years!"

DOWNSIDE: "Tended to accumulate in lines" • "made downy cheek hairs more obvious".

LAURA MERCIER SECRET CAMOUFLAGE
8.15 points out of 10

This concealer palette has two shades, for custom-blending and comes in a range of combinations for different skintones. It's a favorite with celebs, makeup artists and, now, our Beauty Bible panellists. Ideally, apply with a brush after blending the perfect color on the back of the hand.

UPSIDE: "LOVED it – the most effective concealer I've ever tried" • "the two colors in the palette made it easy to match skintone and it stayed on well all day" • "toned down rosy cheeks very well" • "hid an angry red spot, without caking – an impressive concealer".

DOWNSIDE: "Had to make sure I applied a rich moisturiser beforehand" • "fiddly to open".

LA PRAIRIE SKIN CAVIAR CONCEALER
8 points out of 10

Probably one of the priciest concealers on the market, this does offer skincare benefits through Caviar Firming Complex (La Prairie's signature Exclusive Cellular Complex), along with lavender, chamomile, and green tea.

UPSIDE: "Skin really radiant, uplifted and glowing – my colleagues comment that I look flawless when I wear this" • "blended in beautifully – I've given it 10+!" • "one of the best I've ever used – if you have something to hide, nothing does it better than this concealer".

DOWNSIDE: "Quite drying and a bit cakey".

❀❀ JANE IREDALE CIRCLE/DELETE CONCEALER
7.62 points out of 10

The highest-scoring 'natural choice' is 100 percent based on mineral pigments, with nourishing jojoba, avocado, and vitamin K to work actively on under-eye circles. Three 'duos' are available, each with two shades for custom-blending; Jane Iredale recommends applying with a small brush (having first mixed the colors on the back of your hand, if required).

UPSIDE: "Blended well and gave a natural finish – love the fact there are two shades which can be blended to create a perfect third shade" • "light enough for use on bare skin" • "I used this the morning after a late, boozy night so it had its work cut out – but definitely made me look better, covering all flaws" • "made a huge, red, angry spot invisible".

DOWNSIDE: "Better on thread veins than under the eyes"• "quite difficult to remove".

BEST BUDGET BUY
BOURJOIS D'UN COUP DE PINCEAU LIGHT-REFLECTING CONCEALER
7 points out of 10

This was the highest-scoring product among the budget ranges that we tested – a brush-style product in a choice of three shades, with added vitamin E for skin-smoothing.

UPSIDE: "Very light and easy to use – went on silkily, disguised shadows" • "I still prefer Touche Eclat but this is a close second!" • "with this concealer and a little powder on top, I was confident without foundation" • "great for disguising fine lines and dark circles" • "definitely concealed dark circles and improved overall look of my eyes".

DOWNSIDE: "Did not cover blemishes" • "slightly greasy and didn't stay put all day".

The lowest score was 5.25 points out of 10.

WHAT FOUNDATION, WHAT AGE?

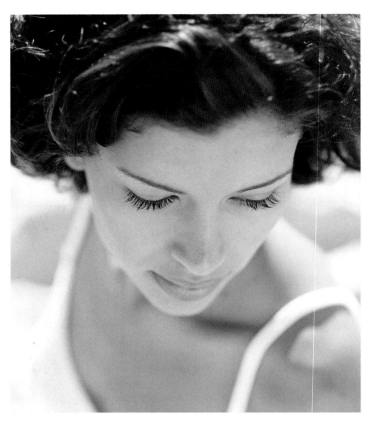

NATURAL FOUNDATION

We admit it: though we choose natural-as-possible skincare, body care and haircare most of the time, we compromise on makeup – which is designed, after all, to sit on the skin, rather than penetrate. But if you're a would-be natural beauty, avoid foundations with mineral oil (paraffinum liquidum) and petrolatum on the ingredient list, as these not only come from a non-sustainable source but can block pores – making complexions prone to pimples. On page 16, find a natural All-In-One foundation that impressed our testers, or check out other bases from Jane Iredale and Dr. Hauschka, whose foundations we consider the best natural options (see Directory, page 246).

Twenty-something: Bask in the glow, says Laura Mercier, leading makeup artist and creator of her own signature makeup line, "because your skin may never look this good – naturally – again. Use foundation only where you need it – to cover imperfections, or to mattify skin. Start in the middle and work outwards only as far as you need to even out the skin tone – but never go near the edges, and avoid all creases."

Thirty-something: You have got the widest choice of foundations: sheer, long-lasting foundations or all-in-one foundation/ powders. But you shouldn't have to go heavier than sheer or medium coverage, with the lightest dusting of powder to set it in areas where you're more prone to shine.

Forty-something: According to Laura Mercier, "Older skins need foundation wherever there are shadows, darkness or broken capillaries. That may include the innermost corner of the eye on the 'nose-bone' (which most women tend to overlook), the inner half-circle under the eye, on broken capillaries on either side of the nose, and just under the corners of the mouth – which can be shadowy in some women." She suggests looking out for formulations with extra moisturizing elements, experimenting with stick foundations – "and whatever you do, avoid 'oil-free' formulations; a little oil in the formulation helps provide a barrier against dehydration."

Fifty-something and above: Says Laura Mercier, "Older women tend to think of foundation and powder like spackle, to fill the cracks. But, in fact, it just draws attention to lines and wrinkles." Laura's approach is almost the same as she'd use for a fresh-faced teenager. "I put a dab of concealer on imperfections – like dark circles, broken capillaries, age spots – blended into the skin, rather than use foundation."

TINTED MOISTURISERS – *Tried & Tested*

For days when skin needs a hint of color but not cover, or for younger skins, tinted moisturizers are the perfect solution: clear, sheer coverage that perks up your complexion and gives the illusion of a healthy glow. (But washes off at bedtime!) They're all available in a range of shades and, as with any foundation, it's important to test on the jawline to ensure the color's right for you. Dry-skinned women may still find they need extra moisturizer underneath. Unfortunately, none of the 'budget' brands our testers tried scored well – so we'd say this is an area where it's worth investing in a premium brand.

STILA SHEER COLOR TINTED MOISTURISER SPF 15

9 points out of 10

It came as no surprise to us when we discovered that this is one of Stila founder Jeanine Lobell's all-time favorite products. Our testers were bowled over by its blendability and even finish. With an SPF 15, it's said to be ideal for normal-to-dry skin (although, Stila insists, "it won't add any unnecessary oil to oily skins.")

UPSIDE: "I don't usually use tinted moisturizer but this was perfect – adding a sheer sheen to skin" • "loved this – I had a cold and was looking very pale and pasty, but this made me appear healthy again" • "lovely, natural look – perfect for day wear" • "just the right consistency – liquid, but not at all runny" • "effective moisturization without being greasy; covers imperfections and lasts for up to 8 hours".

DOWNSIDE: Not one of our ten testers had a negative word to say about this.

DERMALOGICA SHEER TINT MOISTURE SPF 15

8.88 points out of 10

Dermalogica use natural earth minerals of iron oxide rather than synthetic colorings to provide a long-lasting color "wash" in this tinted moisturizer, which is also infused with a potent blend of olive fruit extract – said to offer the highest level of free radical protection for any natural antioxidant.

UPSIDE: "Extremely easy to apply: smooth, with good coverage" • "where has this been all my life? I've never used tinted moisturizer before and now I'm a convert" • "fantastic if you just want to even out skintone" • "very comfortable – and kept T-zone matte, too" • "greater coverage for a tinted moisturizer – better than any I've tried; more like a makeup base but not heavy, yet it covered everything I wanted to disguise" • "absolutely delighted with this product, which is going to become part of my regular skincare ritual".

DOWNSIDE: "Strange, slightly chemical smell" • "dry-skinned women may need to moisturize first" • "made my face feel tight".

YVES SAINT LAURENT TEINT DE JOUR TINTED MATTE MOISTURIZER

8.33 points out of 10

Unlike some tinted moisturizers, this is meant to deliver a matte finish, while maintaining optimum moisture levels for eight hours and shielding skin with antioxidant ingredients.

UPSIDE: "Went on smoothly with no streaking – excellent" • "I didn't feel like I had anything on, but had a healthy, natural glow' • "at long last, a tinted moisturizer which does its job perfectly" • "pleasant, fresh-floral scent; skin still dewy at the end of day" • "liked the matte finish and glam packaging".

DOWNSIDE: "Ran out of the tube – wasting a large amount" • "very highly perfumed – off-putting" • "settled into lines under eyes".

LAURA MERCIER TINTED MOISTURISER

8.22 points out of 10

Available in a selection of six shades, this tinted moisturizer from makeup artist Laura Mercier offers a higher-than-most SPF of 20, for good everyday protection.

UPSIDE: "Skin looked healthy – it provided good coverage to my skin, which is acne-prone with some scarring" • "LOVED this product – it has better coverage than my usual SPF so can replace this and remove the need for foundation" • "very comfortable" • "good coverage – but can I share an application tip? This looked better with a light dusting of powder over the top".

DOWNSIDE: "Forehead and cheeks needed extra moisturizer" • "left skin dry and itchy".

❦ AVEDA MOISTURE PLUS TINT

7 points out of 10

This features a naturally derived SPF – titanium dioxide – and is designed for every skin type, from oily to mature, delivering sheer coverage with a soothing rose scent.

UPSIDE: "Overall good performance: moisturized but wasn't greasy, and went on smoothly" • "smooth, velvety finish" • "lasted well – and could be used near eyes without irritation" • "super texture blended well and stayed on face very well" • "felt cooling when applied" • "gave just as good coverage as my normal foundation".

DOWNSIDE: "Rather inflexible tube which might prove difficult later" • "a special version for dry/mature skins would be good".

The lowest score in this category was 5.04 points out of 10.

UN-SHINE

Many women find that foundation and concealer need setting with powder to keep them from vanishing into thin air, particularly for long evenings. Too much powder, however, looks not matte but dusty – and, worse, accentuates lines and wrinkles. So go lightly...

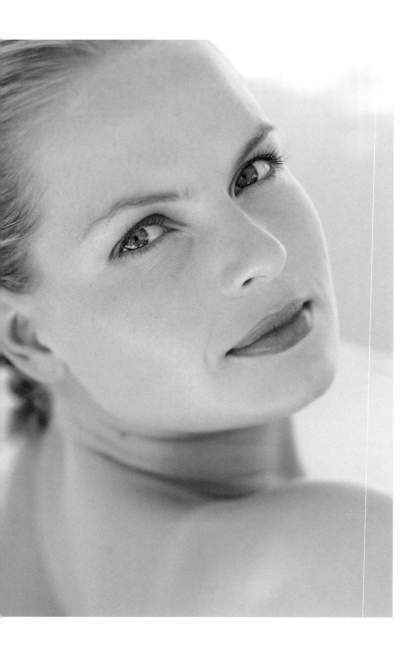

Over the years, we've tried every kind of tool – from velvet puffs to huge, fluffy powder brushes – to apply powder. In the end, we found that this trick – from Mary Greenwell – is the simple secret to powder perfection: "Take a ¾ inch brush (like the one pictured right) – much smaller than most powder brushes – and dip it into translucent powder in a shade close to your skin tone. Tap the brush on the back of your hand to get rid of excess, and work the powder with the brush into the areas that shine most – especially the folds around the nose, which tend to look oily first; it'll keep shine at bay for hours – and you can use pressed powder or oil-blotting tissues for touch-ups later." (See opposite for our Tried & Tested results on these oil-blotting tissues, which are a beauty innovation.)

✳ "If you're prone to shine, consider using a mattifying under-makeup base," says Karen Mason (who's worked on star faces like Patsy Kensit and Debbie Harry, among others). "These contain 'micro-sponges' which soak up oil in the skin and help keep sheen at bay. They're a better option than caking the face with repeated applications of powder, which clogs pores and can lead to breakouts."

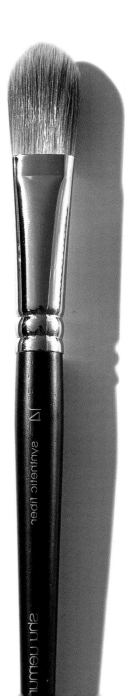

OIL BLOTTING SHEETS – *Tried & Tested*

Adding layer after layer of powder may defy shine – but it cakes makeup. So the beauty world came up with a solution: little sheets of "blotting paper", which can be pressed onto makeup (or oily skin), especially on the T-zone, to mop up shine. Here's what our testers thought of them.

BEST BUDGET BUY
NIVEA VISAGE MATT & FRESH OIL ABSORBING AND REFRESHING SHEETS
8.82 points out of 10

Unlike other entries in this category, these are dual-action – and color-coded. The green side instantly mattifies; the blue side contains cooling, refreshing ingredients so that (as Nivea says) "skin will feel like it's been splashed with water". In reality, while our testers were impressed with the shine-defying results, they particularly raved about this refreshing action. This highest-scoring product is not only the best buy overall, but also the best budget buy.

UPSIDE: "Very effective – leaves skin matte for hours, even after a hard shift at work; nice "chunky" sheets, too – not flimsy like some" • "would be particularly useful in the summer months, with the slight scent of eau-de-cologne" • "brilliant – hygienically packaged, removes shine and refreshes, without taking off makeup; I'll always have a packet of these in my bag from now on" • "excellent to help you return to Zen-like state without splashing cold water on your face and ending up with panda eyes".

DOWNSIDE: "Stung slightly on application" • "nasty chemical smell"

M.A.C. BLOT FILM
8.26 points out of 10

Larger than most, these are made of a special material that has been patented by 3M (who also make Post-It! notes).

UPSIDE: "Absolutely brilliant, unbelievably absorbent, leaving skin dry, free from shine, truly matte" • "decent-sized films that truly do the job – you only need one for the whole face" • "fine once I'd got over laughing at rubbing bits of balloon over my face!" • "very effective – absorbed shine without drying the face".

DOWNSIDE: "Very plastic feel – didn't like pressing it into my face".

CLINIQUE STAY MATTE OIL BLOTTING SHEETS
8.18 points out of 10

These come in a handy pack for slipping into a bag or pocket.

UPSIDE: "Excellent product – really effective" • "really good at absorbing oil; plastic, filmy texture made it very easy to press into the crease around nose" • "delivers everything it promises – eliminating shine, while leaving skin feeling genuinely clean and free from unwanted gunge".

DOWNSIDE: "The relatively small sheets meant I had to use four or five to finish my face" • "plasticky texture of sheets doesn't feel green or eco-friendly".

ANNA SUI BLOTTING PAPERS
7.7 points out of 10

This funky American designer's cosmetics line has gothic purple and black packaging – and a cult following. The papers are lightly scented with rose.

UPSIDE: "Very effective, simple, quick, easy; face looked fresh as a daisy – I even have fewer blackheads!" • "my face definitely didn't get as shiny" • "loved the packaging" • "removes shine instantly" • "I'm a convert to having these cute little papers in my bag".

DOWNSIDE: "Just didn't seem to do anything".

LIZ COLLINGE FINISHING TISSUES
7.23 points out of 10

As well as blotting oil and helping to "finish" makeup by mattifying, makeup artist Liz Collinge – who created this signature range for the British pharmacy chain Boots – likes to use them to catch any specks while combing through eyelashes after applying mascara.

UPSIDE: "Very effective – just absorbs oil, rather than leaving a residue on the skin" • "skin looked fresher and renewed" • "liked the shine removal, without disturbing makeup" • "stylish gun-metal finish plastic tin – slim and secure, for slipping in bag".

DOWNSIDE: "Tended to absorb makeup as well as shine".

The lowest score in this category was 5.5 points out of 10.

An inexpensive alternative to oil-blotting sheets: take a tissue (or even a sheet of loo paper), separate the two layers and place over the oily zone of your face. Press down, but don't swipe; the paper will absorb surface oil and instantly mattify your makeup, anywhere, any time.

A WORLD OF COLOR

Since we wrote our original book – The Beauty Bible – in 1995, we've spent many hours in pharmacies and department stores talking to real women about real beauty issues. And we've lost count of the number of women of color who've stopped us with heartfelt pleas for advice on lines that might suit black, Asian, Middle Eastern and Hispanic complexions…

We're delighted to say that things have improved hugely in the years since that first book. Revlon, Bobbi Brown, Aveda and Origins all offer an extremely wide choice of foundations that include many darker shades. The biggest contribution to improving makeup options for women of color, however, has been made by Iman, the Somali-born supermodel (now Mrs. David Bowie), whose signature line was "born out of years of my own frustration. I would watch professionals like François Nars or Kevyn Aucoin taking an hour to mix six foundation shades just to get the right one for my skin. And I thought: real women can't do that. So where are the products for them?"

Since she conceived her own line, Iman has become involved in every stage of its production – "from mixing up new shades to road-testing products on my dark skin." Says Iman: "I really understand the beauty challenges women of color have – including hyperpigmentation and oiliness." Here, then, are some of the secrets she's learned – for women of color everywhere.

"I really understand the beauty challenges women of color have – including hyperpigmentation and oiliness."

IMAN

✳ "Black skins are surprisingly vulnerable to sun damage," says Iman. "The problem is that you can't see the damage – but it's there. In summer, I'm two shades darker than in winter, and I burn easily. I believe that wearing an SPF 15 daily on the face is a must in summer months."

✳ "Alcohol-based toners destroy the skin, which redoubles its oil-producing efforts to make up for the oil you're removing. You need really gentle cosmetics, because sensitivity is often a problem for women of color, too."

✳ "Many black women have lower lips that are 'split' – the top half being redder, the bottom half darker. For best results with lipstick, even out lip tone first." (You can do this by applying foundation over the lips – which acts as a base to make lipstick more longlasting. Iman has also created a product specially for the task: Lip-Even Corrective Treatment.)

✳ "Don't use base to make your complexion lighter or darker. Test foundation on your jawline, where the neck meets the face. The right color will disappear completely in daylight. I like foundations that have powder built into the formulation, so that you don't get a 'cakey' effect – or powders that are tinted, used over moisturizer, so that you don't even need foundation."

✳ "Dark skins should use a foundation with a yellow base, and it should match your skin tone exactly. If your skin is patchy, always match the foundation to the predominant shade. The foundation must look natural enough to blend in with the neck."

✳ "Use bronzing powder instead of blush for a much more realistic effect."

✳ "Take a cue from your skin tone for your lipstick. If you have light skin, you should wear light berries and neutrals; medium skin looks good in rich earth tones and dark skins should use deep tones."

✳ "Many women fall prey to the allure of brightly colored cosmetics that override their best natural features – and wind up with a face as bright as a box of Crayola crayons. Women, no matter what their skin color, should steer clear of colors that are garish. On eyes, for instance, resist highly frosted shadows and pearls/shimmers, and go for colors that are neutral and closer to your natural skin tone – i.e. taupes and browns."

✳ "I'm a big believer in department store makeovers but the lighting at cosmetics counters lies – so have the makeup artist work on you, wear the look home – and wait for someone to say, 'you look gorgeous'."

Iman's website www.i-iman.com is one of the best cyberbeauty sites of all; aside from tips, hints and the opportunity to ask Iman beauty questions online, you'll find the Makeup Color Coordinator, which steers you towards the best shade choices for your individual coloring.

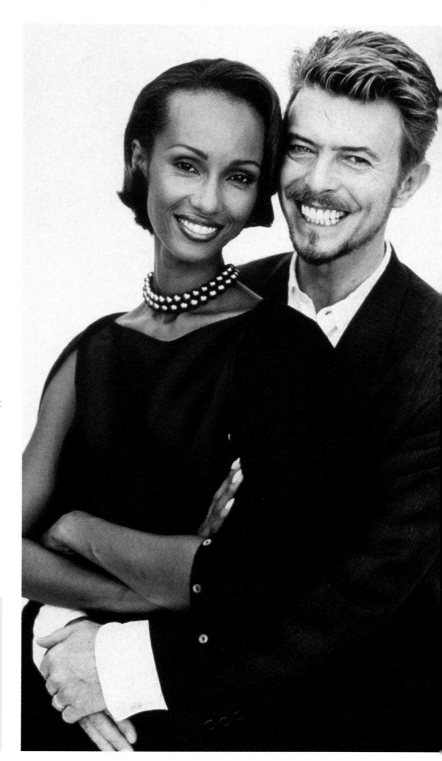

LIPS, LIPS, LIPS

We love lipstick. But we don't like the way it disappears, literally "eaten" off our lips. So here are the secrets of applying lipstick so it stays put, long-lasting lipsticks that live up to their hype – and some good-enough-to-eat natural choices

The secret to long-lasting lipstick (see our Tried & Tested, page 33) isn't just the lipstick itself – it's in the art of application. If you don't already, consider using a liner pencil to extend the length of time your lipstick stays put. Quite simply, use it to outline your lips, using short, feathery strokes rather than long lines – that's when lip-liner tends to wander. If you have big lips and you want to play them down, draw just inside the natural lip-line. If you have small lips and you want to enhance them, you can accentuate the outer edge of the lip-line by drawing along the very outside edge of that line – but don't ever leave a gap between the drawn line and your own lip. You can even try this trick from Trish McEvoy (with a bit of practice): "When you're using the pencil to outline the cupid's bow – just above the middle of the top lip – use the pencil to draw in two soft 'mountain peaks'. The effect is to make lips look plumper." (For more lip-plumping tips, see page 30.)

✳ Once you've outlined your lips, color them in with the liner – just as if you were using a crayon or felt-tip marker in a child's coloring book. This creates the base to which lipstick adheres, and also slightly stains the lips so that when the lipstick/gloss wears off, something's left.

✳ Never use a sharp lip pencil – blunt the ends by drawing backwards and forwards on the back of your hand to soften (and warm) it.

✳ Nobody needs more than one lip pencil – and it should be as close as possible to the natural color of your own lips, so that when your lipstick wears off, your lips aren't encircled by an obvious line. For a softer effect, apply the lip pencil after your lipstick; the liner and lipstick blend, and they'll both last a bit longer. To soften the line, if you need to, you can smudge with a finger.

SHOPPING FOR LIPSTICK

✳ Before trying a lipstick on your lips, Mary Greenwell suggests applying shades to the pads of your fingertips. "That's the body skin that's closest to lip color," she explains. Testing it on your hands lets you gauge the sheerness/matteness and texture – but not how well the shade will flatter your coloring.

✳ We're not paranoid about germs, but we'd never try a lipstick straight from the tester. So, advises FACE Stockholm's Gun Novak,

"Make sure they sterilize the lipstick with alcohol or a germ-killing spray, or even slice off the top before giving it to you to test. And apply lip gloss with a clean Q-tip."

✳ Gillian Dempsey – creator of the celebrity favorite Delux line – gave us another excellent tip for lipstick shopping, illustrated below: "Before you try lipstick on your lips, use it to draw a life-size, upside-down pair of lips on the back of your hand, with the cupid's bow nearest the thumb. Stand two feet back from a mirror and hold your hand up to your face – and you can tell, instantly, whether the color 'lifts' your face or makes it look drab. If it looks flattering, then go ahead and try it on your lips."

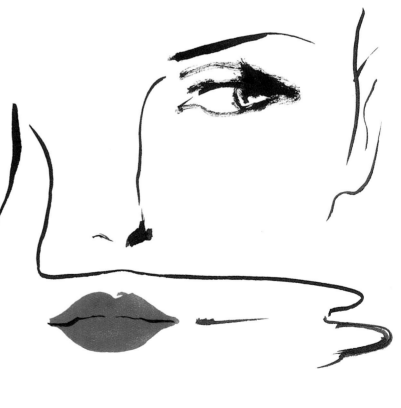

LIP-LINERS – *Tried & Tested*

Makeup artists all rave about lip-liners – to create definition or (applied all over the lips) to act as a long-lasting 'base' for lipstick that doesn't fade when shine or gloss has worn off. We asked our testers to use these lip-liners both for outlining and 'coloring in'. In line with the pros' advice, our testers were given very natural shades to test. (Incidentally, makeup pros advise always using neutral shades. Don't even think of matching your lip-liner to a shade like burgundy or bright red – too, too Cruella.)

❀ ORIGINS LIP PENCIL
9.18 marks out of 10

This scored exceptionally well: a long-wearing formula (so Origins promise), which should also prove water- and feather-resistant; the ingredients are more natural than most.

UPSIDE: "Love this – very smooth and creamy but 'sticky' enough to stay put three or four times as long as a lipstick, when used all over the lips" • "very natural, defined well, no bleeding" • "a very easy-to-use, pleasantly textured pencil that lasted most of the evening" • "I love this and will continue to use it; my lips get very dry but this lip-liner kept them from drying and bleeding" • "brilliant! – only had to apply lipstick twice in an eight-hour day; a must for my makeup bag from now on".

DOWNSIDE: There were no negative comments about this product.

CLINIQUE QUICKLINER
9.11 marks out of 10

This is like a 'propelling pencil' and doesn't need sharpening, which can be an advantage in lip-liner. (Once you've got down to the wooden part of a lip pencil, don't ever, ever use it on lips before sharpening again or you'll risk badly scratching skin).

UPSIDE: "Didn't bleed and lasted ages – yes, yes, yes!" • "good enough to use as a base for lipstick – lasts for ages, even after something to eat" • "used as a base, lipstick stayed on longer; as a lipstick, lasted for several hours – survived two cups of coffee and even a sandwich" • "my favorite lip-liner" • "very creamy but long-lasting and comfortable to wear; small amount does the trick, so economical in the long run".

DOWNSIDE: "Slightly grainy" • "texture a bit lumpy".

ELIZABETH ARDEN LIP PENCIL
7.88 marks out of 10

Designed to complement Arden's range of lip gloss shades, this long-wearing pencil sharpens to the finest-possible point, for precision. Our testers particularly praised the brush at the opposite end, finding it very useful for applying lipstick or 'blurring' the lip-line, if desired.

UPSIDE: "Love the handy brush at the end and the creamy but not-too-soft texture" • "I normally use a propelling, self-sharpening type of pencil these days – but I was really impressed with this product" • "probably the smoothest lip-liner I've ever tried – a pleasure to use" • "I haven't used a lip-liner before and was pleasantly surprised how easy it was to outline lips – and how it prevented my lipstick from bleeding."

DOWNSIDE: "Could be softer and creamier – a little too matte, I found, compared to some pencils I've tried".

BEST BUDGET BUY
MAYBELLINE LIP EXPRESS
7.7 marks out of 10

Maybelline Lip Express is actually a chunky pencil, created by the No. 1 mass market cosmetics line as a two-in-one lipstick and lip-liner. This should certainly avoid the all-too-common problem with lip-liner: an obvious line as lipstick wears off and leaves an outline of liner underneath.

UPSIDE: "Stayed put for a very long time – up to four hours – but I needed to touch it up after a couple of coffees" • "a nice, soft pencil that I will definitely be buying in future" • "excellent, considering its price" • "a very versatile product – lovely color and sheen, long-lasting, easy to use – with no bleeding or feathering".

DOWNSIDE: "No good if you have dry lips" • "realistic – but not as sharp a line as you get with a traditional lip-liner".

The lowest score in this category was 5.12 marks out of 10.

THINK NATURAL

According to Aveda's Horst Rechelbacher, lipstick-wearers chew and lick anything from one-and-a-half to four tubes of lipstick off their lips in a lifetime. (Yes, that's where it goes.) So you may want to think about "greening" your lipstick...

As Horst points, out, that's a lot of petroleum and other chemicals that we're directly ingesting. If you're still concerned, the good news is that today, the natural, more-natural-than-most (and even organic) alternatives deliver better results than ever before – making a more holistic beauty lifestyle a real possibility.

Top of the list in the "truly natural" stakes are Dr. Hauschka, Jurlique and Logona, three of the leading names in "holistic" beauty. Next-best-thing, in our view, are lipsticks made by Jane Iredale, Aveda and Origins, which are free of petroleum-derived chemicals. (We especially love Origins Sheer Sticks, which deliver a swipe of sheer color that's ideal for summer, and are wonderfully easy to use.) Aveda, meanwhile, offers a range of lipsticks colored with *uruku* (say it "oo-roo-koo"), a pigment from the *Bixa orellana* plant which grows in the Brazilian rainforest.

Petrochemicals are widely used in cosmetics – including lipsticks – because they're incredibly cheap ingredients; they make products nicely gloppy – and trap moisture in the skin by creating a "film" on the surface. But in the truly good-enough-to-eat natural lipsticks we've just mentioned, you'll find ingredients from renewable resources, like carnauba wax, beeswax, shea butter, vitamin E and jojoba oil, which can be equally effective. The "downside" of natural lipsticks – if you see it that way – is that with fewer pigments available, the range of lipstick shades is narrower, tending towards a more neutral palette rather than traffic-stopping fuchsias, scarlets and purples. (But we'd say: more wearable as a result.)

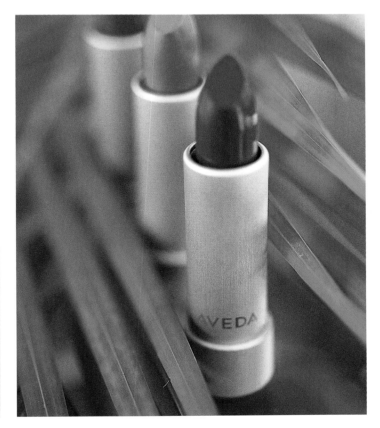

TIP: Bliss Spa's Marcia Kilgore has this tip for de-flaking chapped lips in an emergency. "Exfoliate with Scotch tape," she says. The how-to: moisten lips, then apply a strip of tape across them. Gently remove the tape and the rough surface flakes should come off.

TIP: Condition rough lips with balm, allowing 10 to 20 minutes for it to sink in before applying your lipstick, says makeup artist Maggie Hunt.

PLUMP UP THE VOLUME

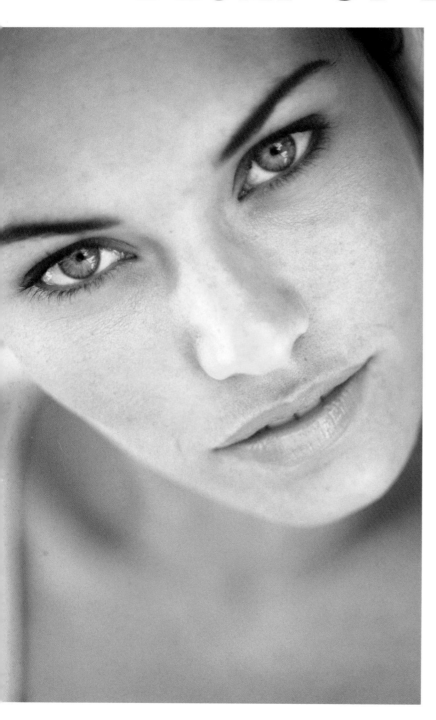

Makeup is all about the art of illusion. Dark colors make areas of the face recede, while lighter colors make features stand out. (Rembrandt definitely knew a thing or two about that.) So if you have a less than Bardot-esque pout, there are tips and products that can literally "fake" fullness.

✳ The first trick for creating a fuller-looking pout is to leave just the center of the bottom lip free of color when you're applying lipstick. Color from the rest of the lips will "travel" to that spot but since it's not as intense, it will create the illusion of plumpness.

✳ Add a dab of shimmer lipstick to the middle of your bottom lip, and smack lips together. A dab of gloss does the same thing. (It's a light trick.)

✳ Fuller Pout Trick No. 3: Dab a bit of lightweight concealer on the center of the lips over matte lipstick, then blend out towards the corners by smacking your lips together lightly.

✳ To make the upper lip appear to stand out more, run a white pencil lightly just above the center of the cupid's bow or add a touch of gold, silver or white shimmer there. (Be careful not to add so much that it looks sweaty!)

There is also a new generation of lipsticks and bases designed to make lips look fuller – and more sensual than Nature made them. Some give impressive results, as you'll see in our Tried & Tested, opposite.

LIP PLUMPERS – *Tried & Tested*

Contrary to marketing hype, these can't really 'plump up' lips – except by delivering a slick of hydrating ingredients – but they do incorporate light-reflective pigments, and often high gloss, to create the beauty illusion of a fuller pout. Some of these come in the form of 'invisible' treatments; others are more like a lipstick or gloss, also delivering color. No natural beauty companies have targeted this niche of the beauty market yet.

LANCÔME PRIMORDIALE REVITALIZING LIP TREATMENT
7.79 points out of 10

The key ingredients in this specific anti-aging lip treatment are pure vitamin E, a red seaweed extract (gatuline) and Flexium (based on nourishing waxes, oils and soft powders, which – so they tell us – "forms an ultra-comfortable and supple mesh which is highly resistant to water and changes in temperature"). On the whole, our testers liked this product more as an age-defying, moisturizing treatment than for its plumping action.

UPSIDE: "My lipstick almost glided on; no feathering or bleeding – and stayed in place longer than normal; fantastic" • "loved this; after five days use, lips were definitely more moisturized" • "definitely made the lip outline stand out more – my daughter, who has a more generous mouth, loved this product and her friends could tell when she was wearing it" • "lips rehydrated – and look younger" • "gave extra definition to the outline of the mouth" • "lips much fuller – very Liz Hurley!".

DOWNSIDE: "Moisturized but did not plump" • "lips looked soft and perhaps slightly fuller but not as dramatic as I had expected".

L'ORÉAL PARIS GLAM SHINE
7.6 points out of 10

This is described (by L'Oréal Paris) as "a sparkling, semi-transparent liquid lipcolor, for a visible lip-plumping effect". It has a fruity fragrance and comes in a wide range of shades including a "Crystal" version, for a somewhat holographic effect on lips.

UPSIDE: "My lips looked shiny, fuller, softer - and very kissable!" • "glamorous and shining, sparkly and special" • "lovely and moist" • "an excellent product, overall".

DOWNSIDE: "A bit too gloopy to feel nice" • "too greasy for me".

CHRISTIAN DIOR DIORIFIC PLASTIC SHINE
7.36 points out of 10

With a lower concentration of waxes than most lipsticks (so Dior tell us) – 6 percent rather than 20 percent – this instead contains a reflective "Shine Booster" to bounce back light, while delivering an ultra-glossy finish. It's also specifically designed to be long-lasting.

UPSIDE: "More instant fullness than most – definitely one for parties" • "a shiny, full pout with impressive staying power" • "roll on Christmas parties!".

DOWNSIDE: "Has its drawbacks – after a night out, there was no confusing which glass was mine" • "too glam for day-wear" • "a lovely, soft gloss which made my lips look smoother – but alas not more voluminous".

MOLTON BROWN WONDER LIPS GLOSS LIP LIFT GLAZE
7.15 points out of 10

A 'sister' product to Molton Brown's existing Wonder Lips Liplift Formula treatment, this mirror-shine gloss – which scored higher than the original – features what they refer to as Maxi-lip™ technology, to boost lip definition, condition and moisturization by up to 40 percent, when used over time.

UPSIDE: "Loved this – I have quite full lips and it made them look even plumper; I have almost used up my sample and will be buying a second one" • "lips looked very full, glossy, smooth and kissable" • "I loved this and my husband thought that my lips looked very kissable!" • "nice gloss, not-too-sticky, comfortable on lips".

DOWNSIDE: "The quantity's too small – this wouldn't last a week on Scarlett Johansson's lips!" • "you had to be careful to smooth color over lips – otherwise you could get a 'clump' of color on top of lip".

The lowest score in this category was 5.03 points out of 10.

TWIST AND POUT

More lipstick secrets!

✳ The sheerer and glossier the formulation, the quicker it is to apply – because you don't have to worry so much about precision. (We can now put on lip gloss in the dark!)

✳ Lip gloss has a tendency to slide off more quickly than any other formulation, but Stila's Jeanine Lobel has this advice: "To give lip gloss more staying power, line lips first with a coordinating lip-liner, then 'fill in' by drawing all over the lip with the liner. Lip gloss will naturally wear more quickly than lipstick, but the liner will make the lips matte and provide a base for the gloss to adhere to, so it won't slip and slide around quite so much."

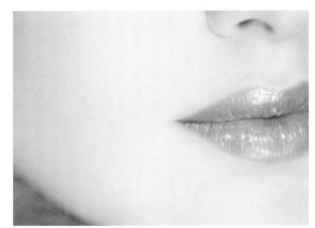

✳ It's up to you whether you apply lipstick straight from the "tube" or with a lip brush – but a brush gives a more polished look and makes lipstick stay put longer by pressing the color into the lips.

✳ To make any lipstick last longer, apply, then slip a tissue between lips and press down on it with your lips. Add a second coat of lipstick. (Alternatively, some makeup artists like to powder lips after the first application – using a velvet puff – and apply a second coat over that.)

✳ There's a red lipstick for everyone, insists Bobbi Brown, but warmer complexions, including olive skin and ones that tan easily, look best in reds that have yellow and orange in them. Cooler tones (fair skin) should stick to blue reds. When in doubt, try red in a sheer texture.

✳ To make sure you avoid getting lipstick on your teeth—a Gloria Swanson effect that nobody wants—purse your lips as though you were about to give a kiss, then put your index finger in your mouth and pull it out. Any excess color will end up on your finger rather than on your teeth.

✳ Don't throw out a fave lipstick just because it's broken off. Swivel it up so that the broken base is exposed. Then, hold the decapitated top with a tissue – so it doesn't slip – and slowly wave a lit match under the chunk of lipstick to warm it. (Be careful not to burn yourself!) When it starts to soften, gently place it back on top of the broken base. Twist the lipstick all the way down and place it—uncovered—in the fridge for five minutes. (Just make sure not to twist the tube up so high next time.)

✳ Got to the end of a lipstick and don't want to waste the last bit? Scrape out the remains with a cotton swab or an orange stick, and mash with Vaseline or lip gloss in a lipstick palette (Bobbi Brown's is perfect).

✳ Some shades make teeth look brighter. Makeup artist Jenny Jordan says: "The best range from watermelon to the fruity, berry colors. Avoid too-bright oranges, or any colors that are muddy or brown-based. They seem to highlight the yellow in teeth." Another point from Jenny: "If skin is really pale, teeth look more yellow. Against a

LONG-LASTING LIPSTICKS – *Tried & Tested*

Is there really a lipstick out there that survives meals, drinks, kissing – but doesn't leave your lips as dehydrated as if you'd just stepped off a 24-hour flight or camel-trekked across the Sahara? That's the challenge we set for our panelists. (There were no natural products that did well enough to be included in this category – presumably because this stay-put technology is based on synthetic ingredients, rather than natural waxes.)

CLARINS LE ROUGE LIPSTICK
8.06 points out of 10

This uses an "innovative polymer resin" in order to form a "sheer, adherent microfilm of color on the lips". (Well, that's what Clarins tell us.) Wheat germ oil, castor oil, shea butter and protective vitamins C and E shield in this lightly fragranced (think vanilla, iris and violet), elegantly-packaged product.

UPSIDE: "Lips felt hydrated and wonderfully smooth – fabulous" • "survived tea and a banana" • "looks and feels fantastic" • "left lips in lovely condition" • "love the classy packaging – very eye-catching" • "plumped lips making them appear very full – and color stays true".

DOWNSIDE: "Did not last all day – none of them do – but a good quality lipstick nevertheless" • "strange taste".

MAX FACTOR LIPFINITY
7.6 points out of 10

More like a 'paint for lips' than lipstick, concedes Max Factor. This is a two-step process: the first delivers intense color (thanks to "permatone", a complex which attaches color to lips with a flexible mesh effect), followed by a moisturizing balm-like top coat which can be re-applied throughout the day.

UPSIDE: "The only lipstick that really does last all day" • "unbelievable; this innovative product really does work" • "had to be removed with baby oil because of its staying power!" • "loved the glossy moisturizing balm" • "the only product I tried that really lasted all day".

DOWNSIDE: "A little flimsy" • "needs to be applied very carefully to avoid a harsh outline".

SHISEIDO STAYING POWER MOISTURIZING LIPSTICK
7.15 points out of 10

Shiseido claims that this features ten times more glycerine than most regular moisturizing lipsticks to keep color glossy and vibrant hour after hour. (The glycerine makes it more comfortable to wear, too.) It also boasts what Shiseido hype as "Advanced Luminous Technology and Color Fidelity" – which, translated for us mere mortals, is meant to ensure that the color stays true as well as stays put.

UPSIDE: "A just-kissed look emerges as this fades – I liked this a lot" • "amazing – not a single trace on my cup after two drinks" • "lustrous, moisture-rich finish" • "excellent staying power without looking too heavy" • "nicest packaging I've ever seen – and so convenient to apply".

DOWNSIDE: "Very lasting, but extremely drying on the lips" • "left lips surprisingly dry, though color stayed true'.

LANCÔME LIP DIMENSION
7.58 points out of 10

The volatile oils in this immediately evaporate – or "set" – to leave what Lancôme describe as a "clinging but supple" film on the lips, which intensifies the color through (again their description) a "magnifying glass effect".

UPSIDE: "Wonderfully glossy, smooth and long-lasting – excellent" • "lasted seven hours – survived a messy bun and some plums; I loved it" • "high-glamor, high-gloss, no need for collagen" • "this had great staying power for a gloss-style product and once set looked really stunning" • "very comfortable to wear".

DOWNSIDE: "Gloss didn't last" • "didn't survive corn on the cob".

ELIZABETH ARDEN EXCEPTIONAL LIPSTICK
7.2 points out of 10

This creamy formulation actually takes the technology for its long wear from the ink industry, combining that staying power with the nourishing effects of moisturizing ceramides (which are a bit of an Arden speciality).

UPSIDE: "Exceptional – long-lasting, fabulous color and moisturizing" • "altogether it lasted two tea breaks and through lunch" • "a beautiful, lasting finish" • "moisturized and looked stunning".

DOWNSIDE: "Very nice cover but lost all gloss very quickly" • "left my lips dry, not supple" • "very drying and made lips appear lined".

The lowest score in this category was 3.28 points out of 10.

SHADOW PLAY

As with most makeup, the simple mantra is that as we age, less is more when it comes to eye makeup. Seventeen-year-olds can get away with glossy, Vaseline-like textures, glitter and rainbow shades – in fact, experimenting is part of the fun of growing up. From thirty on, though, a little carefully chosen makeup is definitely more flattering – and at fifty-plus, eye makeup should be truly minimalist: a dark shadow used as liner, a tad of shadow and mascara, on lids that have been "evened-out" with a light covering of foundation. And here's what else you should know...

EYE KNOW-HOW

✳ The time-saving option, when it comes to choosing shadow colors, is to go for neutral shades – from bone to mahogany. The brighter the color, the harder it is to get it right and to blend seamlessly. As you'll see from a sneak peek inside our makeup bags (on page 12), we are particular fans of Bobbi Brown, whose classic palette features variations-on-neutral that are virtually foolproof.

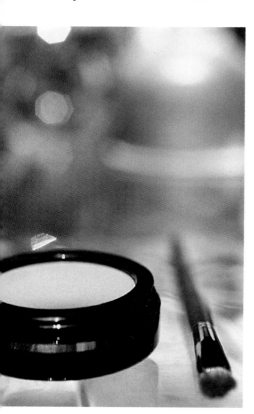

✳ If you want to be a little more daring – say, for evening – choose your eyeshadow to enhance the color of your eyes. This means opting for a shade that contrasts with, rather than matches, the color of your iris – otherwise, says Bobbi Brown, "what you see is the eyeshadow, not the eye. Slate blue and navy look good on brown eyes; browns and taupes are best on blondes." (Think about it: would you display sapphires on a blue cloth?) Green eyes look good in cool colors such as soft mauves and lilacs.

✳ When shopping for shadow, you can test it on the inside of your wrist, where skin tone is similar to eyelids. Preferably, of course, try on lids themselves, (using a cotton swab to apply, for hygiene's sake, then blending with your finger).

Opt for a shade that contrasts with, rather than matches, the color of your iris. Think about it: would you display sapphires on a blue cloth?

✳ Vincent Longo has this tip for making eyeshadow last: "First prime the lids with foundation and lightly dust with translucent face powder to create an even base." (If you use an oil-free formulation, you can skip the powder.) As we age, lids get pink, gray or blue as blood vessels become more visible, so this also helps turn back the clock.

✳ To make close-set eyes seem farther apart, take a concealer one shade lighter than your skin, apply and blend it at the inner corners of the lids. (Don't forget to include those gray shadowy areas on the side of the nose.)

✳ To keep stray "specks" from ruining your eye makeup, always tap the handle of your eyeshadow brush sharply on a hard surface – either the back of your hand, or a tabletop – to remove any excess before applying to skin.

✳ Almost all eye shapes look best when the emphasis is on the outer corner of the eye – imagine a "V", on its side. This creates a wide-eyed, Bambi-like effect. If you apply too much makeup on the inner corner, it makes eyes look closer together.

✳ A dab of white or cream shadow on the center of the browbone – in a dewy or a matte finish – can really open up the eyes. The golden rule: this zone must be perfectly plucked (see page 40), otherwise stubble/brow hairs become super-obvious. (For night, you might try a dab of sheer silver or sheer gold in this area, well blended with the finger; you can even use the tiniest amount of a pale, iridescent lip gloss for the same trick.)

✳ Says Barbara Daly: "cream eyeshadows won't blend well over powders, so don't even attempt to layer cream shadow over powder shadow. For blending cream shadows, the middle finger is ideal – you'll exert the least pressure, thus preventing tugging at delicate lid skin."

✳ The quickest and most effective way to line eyes is with a pencil – but the downside is that these tend to smudge easily. (With the notable exception of Revlon ColorStay, which is specifically designed to be long-lasting.) To "set" eyeliner so that it won't budge, apply an eyeshadow in exactly the same shade over the

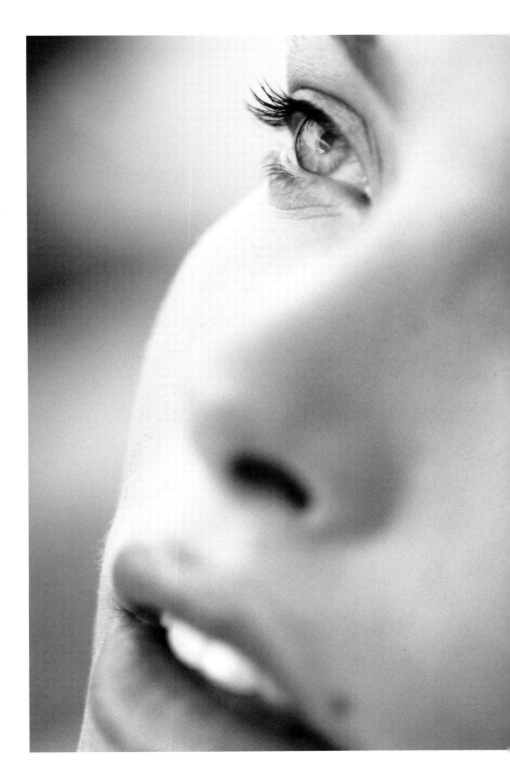

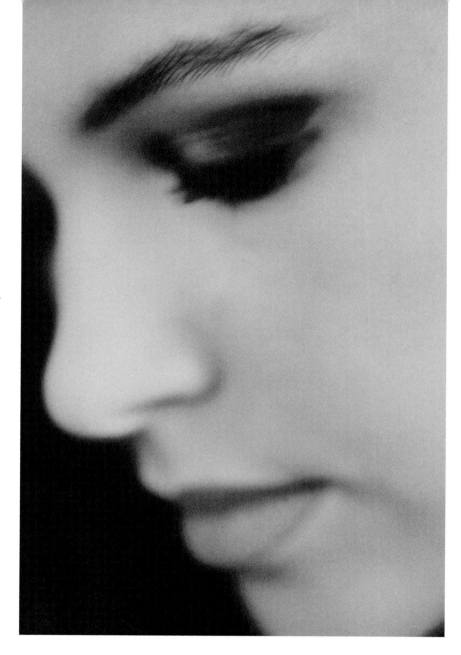

liner, using a fine brush. For even longer-lasting color, dampen the eyeliner brush before dipping in the shadow. (Once eyeshadow gets wet, it's almost impossible to use it as a powder in future; it's only good for lining. So create an imaginary line down the center of your eyeshadow – and always keep one side for dry application, one side for wet.)

✳ Concentrate on getting your eyeliner as close to the lashes as possible – this creates an optical illusion of lash length. And, as the late Kevyn Aucoin said, "There's nothing worse than seeing white space between lashes and liner." He would work the shadow or pencil between the lashes to create a seamless look.

✳ Every so often, liquid eyeliner sweeps back into vogue. In our experience, the occasions when women would be likely to wear it – big dates, glamorous soirées – are nerve-wracking enough to make it even harder than usual to apply liquid liner in a smooth, wiggle-free line. If you still love that Marilyn Monroe look, try this hand-steadying technique: place your mirror flat on a table and lean into it. Rest your elbow on the table and draw close to the lashes, as thickly or thinly as you like, in an outward direction. (An upward "flick" at the outer corner is optional.) Never attempt this for the first time just before an important event; sloppy or misplaced lines stick out a mile and are hard to correct.

✳ Younger eyes look exotic when sultrily kohl-rimmed. (We'll be blunt: older eyes just look silly made up this way.) To achieve this straight-from-the-harem lusciousness, dot a soft but well-sharpened eyeliner pencil as close to the lashes as possible, beginning at the inside and moving outward. Then sweep a pointed brush across the lid, connecting the dots, ending with a slight tip upwards at the edges, for more drama. Blend with a finger if you want a subtler, smokier look. For sexy definition under bottom lashes, dot on pencil then use your finger to "wipe" away the liner, creating a deliberately smudgy effect.

MASCARAS – *Tried & Tested*

Mascara is a highly individual choice – but these versatile options each scored well with our ten-women panels. To prove you really don't need to break the bank for beauty, the top scorers are also Best Budget Buys, and congratulations should go to Max Factor for living up to their longstanding reputation for mascara excellence.

BEST BUDGET BUY
MAX FACTOR 2000 CALORIE MASCARA
8.56 points out of 10

Touch-proof, rub-proof, smudge-proof, snooze-proof – those are the claims Max Factor make for this "dramatic look" mascara, which uses special waxes and polymers to prevent melting through the day, while remaining flexible – so lashes don't become brittle. It's fragrance-free, hypoallergenic and suitable for contact lens wearers.

UPSIDE: "10/10 – good for lasting all day" • "excellent product – value for money and looks fab on" • "dramatic look and glossy, thick long lashes" • "very natural effect" • "two coats for evening looked dazzling yet not over-the-top; thick wand, but easy access to all lashes" • "would recommend to anyone – even those with sensitive eyes".

DOWNSIDE: "Tendency to clump a little" • "wipe wand before applying, as one blink with a clump and you'd be gutted!".

BEST BUDGET BUY
MAX FACTOR MORE LASHES
8.4 points out of 10

Max Factor worked with film makeup artists to solve the problem of clumpy lashes (which are extremely evident in close-ups on a panoramic cinema screen).

UPSIDE: "I liked that my lashes were more defined but still looked natural" • "an excellent long-lasting mascara which caused no irritation to my contact lenses – and no smudging!" • "a well-designed wand lengthened and thickened evenly" • "I'm a convert!".

DOWNSIDE: "By the end of the day this had started to flake".

YVES SAINT LAURENT LUXURIOUS MASCARA
8.27 points out of 10

Despite the full lash effect delivered by this glamorously packaged product, it's said to be suitable for sensitive eyes and contact lens wearers – and none of our testers had a bad reaction.

UPSIDE: "Excellent lengthening properties" • "best mascara I've used: lovely long, lustrous appearance – just like false lashes, after two coats" • "very user-friendly wand for accessing all lashes; who needs eyelash curlers?"

DOWNSIDE: "Difficult to keep the wand clean and I found it a struggle to get off my lashes at the end of the day".

CLARINS PURE VOLUME MASCARA
8.27 points out of 10

This has a creamy texture – based on "vegetal waxes", say Clarins – and delivers (they also say) "thicker, supple, more radiant lashes"!

UPSIDE: "Glossy and lush – made for impressive-looking lashes" • "lashes appeared thick, natural, and healthy" • "lasted well all day" • "made my lashes look massive – going to Dublin for the weekend, and this is coming with me for evening wear; really made my eyes open and look bigger".

DOWNSIDE: "Smudged ever-so-slightly" • "pretty average mascara!".

LANCÔME AMPLICILS PANORAMIC VOLUME MASCARA
8.22 points out of 10

Designed to amplify, curl and separate, this features an exclusive formula of conditioning waxes for maximum thickening, and beeswax for softening to maintain lash suppleness.

UPSIDE: "Plumped up my otherwise weedy eyelashes beyond belief – as good as wearing fakes!" • "thickens and lengthens in one application; I was very impressed – the long-lash look was visible even through my glasses" • "absolutely fantastic – really frames the eyes" • "easy to remove at the end of the day".

DOWNSIDE: "Very clumpy finish, even with only one coat" • "lashes looked spiky".

✿ ORIGINS FRINGE BENEFITS
8.05 points out of 10

Natural ingredients in this product include Damascene rose, chamomile, and carnauba wax.

UPSIDE: "Nice compact brush; bristles make it easy to apply for a natural look" • "stayed on well; made my lashes look longer and quite natural" • "good for those who don't need 'special effects' like thickening or curling" • "brilliant for daywear and very natural-looking".

DOWNSIDE: "Felt sticky and heavy" • "needed plenty of time to dry – or smudge–ville!".

The lowest score in this category was 5.37 points out of 10

LASH FLASH

Applying mascara is one of the fastest ways to look "done". (We know women who name it as their Number One desert-island beauty must-have)

✳ Pros swear by lash combs for separating and preventing clumps—but we find them fussy and time-consuming. Get rid of excess mascara by wiping the wand on a tissue, eliminating blobs before you start.

✳ An alternative to a lash comb is to have a second mascara wand, clean and dry, which you sweep through lashes to separate them while mascara is still wet. No need to buy one: when you finish your next tube of mascara, swish the wand in a capful of eye-makeup remover, then wash with soap and dry. Keep it clean by washing whenever you clean your tools.

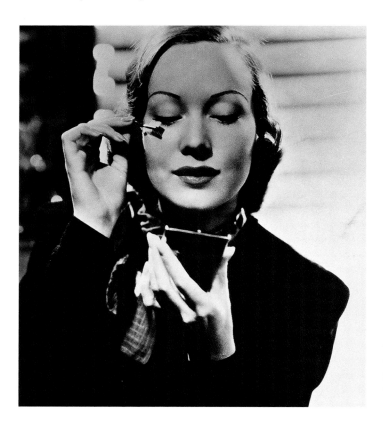

✳ Aimee Adams insists that with modern high-tech mascara formulations, "one coat should be enough to thicken, lengthen, and curl. The more you apply, the more you run the risk of 'spider lashes'." Skipping that second coat saves time. (And prevents that Tammy Faye Bakker look.)

✳ Colored mascaras look great in glossy ads but rarely work in real life, we find. The simple rule is: black works for everyone except blondes, who look best in brown/black by day, reserving black for after-dark.

✳ Lash-lengthening and/or thickening mascaras use tiny filaments to extend and fatten lashes, but many women find that these shed their fibers and encourage smudging as the day wears on. If this is your problem, switch to a lash-curling mascara instead, or ask at the beauty counter for a mascara that's "filament-free".

✳ When applying mascara, wiggle your mascara wand in the base of the lashes. It's the mascara placed near the roots – not the tips – that gives the illusion of length.

SAFETY FIRST

"Hygiene is a real issue when it comes to testing shadows and mascaras in a store," says Bobbi Brown. "Powder shadows can't really transmit germs because they can't survive in dry conditions, but mascaras, cream shadows and liquid liners can be breeding grounds for infections. If you're applying shadows or mascara to the eye zone, always ask the consultant for cotton swabs and a disposable mascara wand. Don't dip and dab or you're asking for trouble".

WATERPROOF MASCARAS – *Tried & Tested*

The challenge: to find a mascara that will survive weepy movies, emotional encounters, rainy days, swimming, and steamy showers. Judging by the results – which weren't exceptional by a long shot – we'd say that waterproof mascara technology still has a way to go, as even the highest scoring products did not work for all the testers. (There were no natural contenders in this category, presumably because lots of synthetic ingredients are required for the 'rain-coating' of lashes.) All of our testers commented that these mascaras are really hard to remove, so the bottom line is that we'd recommend waterproof mascara for times when you know you're going to need it rather than for everyday, when it's best to stick to a high-performance, non-waterproof formula. We have only included a very short list of products here because – in view of our testers' (very detailed) comments – we really didn't feel the others warranted column inches (or your money!).

BEST BUDGET BUY
L'ORÉAL SUPERIOR LONGITUDE WATERPROOF LASH OUT MASCARA
7.88 points out of 10
Features a patented Extensel® formula, to lengthen lashes by 30 percent (so L'Oréal tells us), with a "high-definition" brush featuring more bristles than most, which is designed to improve separation of lashes and "stretch" them at the same time.
UPSIDE: "Outstanding product – I'm still using it; the real test is when you touch up later in the day, and it still looks good" • "curled lashes upwards attractively – and survived the swimming pool at the Datai hotel, Langakawi" • "completely waterproof in pouring rain" • "I was told three times while wearing this that I had amazing eyes – so I think it's brilliant".
DOWNSIDE: "Just don't go swimming in this – it won't stay put" • "I looked a bit like Nosferatu's female double next morning, due to smudging" • "only buy this if you want to look like a racoon after four to five hours".

CHANEL CILS WATERPROOF MASCARA
7.2 points out of 10
With a thick, surprisingly chunky brush, this is designed to coat lashes from root to tip – with no clumping. It contains lash-conditioning pro-vitamin B5 and ceramides.
UPSIDE: "Good wand, and lashes looked lovely and natural; I tried it in the rain, in a steamy bathroom and crying, and then tried to remove it with water and an ordinary cleanser – it wouldn't budge!" • "stayed in place while swimming, but was easy to remove with eye-makeup remover" • "very good, lustrous results" • "delivered longer, glossier lashes".

DOWNSIDE: "Lashes looked dry and 'set'" • "product didn't survive a dental visit – I looked as if I'd just gone a few rounds with Mike Tyson" • "didn't like smell – like a mechanic's overalls, somehow – and brush was cumbersome".

ESTÉE LAUDER ILLUSIONIST WATERPROOF MAXIMUM CURLING MASCARA
6.94 points out of 10
Estée Lauder's popular curling mascara is now available in waterproof form, but received somewhat mixed reviews.
UPSIDE: "I'm not a lover of waterproof mascara but this was one of the best I have tried" • "a fantastic mascara – no clumping on lashes and the brush seemed to be loaded with just the right amount of product each time" • "totally waterproof – in the shower, the gym, cycling on a windy day".
DOWNSIDE: "Wouldn't come off with cleanser or after several attempts with oil-based eye makeup remover".

The lowest score in this category was 4.3 points out of 10.

EYEBROW ESSENTIALS

It's time you got well and truly plucked!

There is probably nothing that makes a face look groomed faster than well-plucked eyebrows. They "open up" the eye, instantly counteracting the droopiness that tends to come with aging. If you're a "plucking virgin", however, we recommend – if possible – going to a professional first-time around, who can assess your perfect brow shape and create a "blueprint". Then, in the future, you simply pluck the hairs that are growing back.

Brows can be tweezed, waxed or removed by "threading", a Middle Eastern technique which – with amazing sleight-of-hand – involves grasping the brow hairs in a loop of thread, then swiftly yanking them out. (We know several smooth-browed beauties who swear this is the ultimate brow-grooming technique, but it's too time-consuming for us, entailing a salon visit each time you need to get your brows "done".)

If it's not possible or affordable to visit a pro to create your brow "blueprint", follow this advice from Eliza Petrescu to help establish the ideal shape for your brows. Manhattan-based Eliza is the ultimate star-plucker, with a perfectly groomed client list that includes Ingrid Casares, Jennifer Grey, Natasha Richardson and Yasmeen Ghauri (who possibly has the most beautiful brows in the world).

1 The space between your eyebrows should be equal to, or a little wider than, the width of your eye. Hold a brow pencil parallel to the side of your nose. The inner edge of each brow should start above the nostril. Do this on both sides of your face. You may want to draw a tiny line at brow-level (with a soft eye pencil, held against the brow pencil) to guide you the first few times.

2 To work out where your brows should end, hold the brow pencil diagonally from your nostril, following the outside edge of your eye. Extend the pencil past the outer corner of your eye, as in the drawing (right). Where it meets the brow line is the correct length.

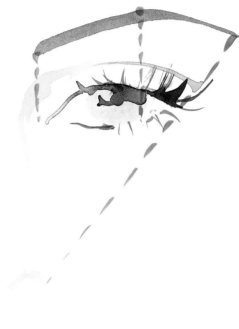

3 To determine your arch, hold the brow pencil parallel to the outside edge of the iris. This is the highest part of the arch. (It's a myth that brows should never be tweezed from above: if the skin below is tweezed super-smooth, then the top should be smooth too – otherwise your brows will look half-finished. But go slowly and carefully.)

TIP: "The ideal time for brow-shaping – or any other painful procedure (such as bikini-waxing) – is the week after your period," says Maribeth Madron, New York-based National Makeup Artist for Laura Mercier. She adds that tweezing when you have PMS is not only more painful, but may result in a zealous, frenzied brow assault. To help resist temptation, she advises storing tweezers in the freezer leading up to your period – so you can't touch them!

And as for technique...

✳ Tweezing should be done after a bath or shower, when skin is supple, using natural light.

✳ First, apply a dab of witch hazel or tea tree oil.

✳ Brush eyebrows upwards and outwards.

✳ Hold the skin with the opposite hand and gently stretch. Place tweezers close to the skin, near the roots of the hair, then pull the hair with a quick motion in the direction of growth. Pluck strays and any hairs that fall under the browline one at a time, all the way across the brow.

✳ Pluck a few hairs from one brow, then stop and pluck a few from the other. Be sure to check that the shape is even on both brows.

✳ Holding tweezers straight and pulling the skin up towards the forehead, pluck any stray hairs from between the brows.

Jenny Jordan – an extremely experienced makeup artist who runs a London brow clinic, and who's worked on Isabella Rossellini and Yasmin Le Bon – has these additional tips:

✳ "I numb brows first with Orajel, a gel which is actually designed for tooth and mouth pain."

✳ "After plucking I apply aloe vera gel, which calms down the redness right away."

✳ "Pluck brows in daylight – facing a window – or using an illuminated mirror; don't try and pluck in artificial light as it's harder to see where the hairs are."

TIP: Eliza Petrescu's Eyebrow Essentials Kit contains everything you need for perfect plucking, including two styles of tweezer (pointed and slant), brow powder and gel, a grooming booklet and an invaluable leaflet. If you're simply searching for a great pair of tweezers, though, we think that Laura Mercier for Tweezerman are the ultimate, ergonomically designed to make them much easier to grip than most.

We have one more tip: don't use a magnifying mirror for eyebrow-plucking – unless you would otherwise have to wear glasses (in which case they're a lifesaver, as Sarah can testify). Although they're good for showing individual hairs, magnifying mirrors don't give the "overview" vital for gauging the correct brow shape, so it's easy to over-pluck (and regret it later).

If you are unhappy with the shape of your brows, don't pluck them for 6-8 weeks. It takes time for brow hair to grow back fully; then you can try again.

SOME BROW DON'TS...

✳ If you're unsure, don't pluck hairs at the outer ends of the brows; simply brush and fix with gel.

✳ Don't be a brow fashion victim. Brow shapes-of-the-moment come and go, but what you should aim for is a classic, elongated shape that will stand the test of time, as Eliza Petrescu describes opposite. Unlike most hair on the body, brow hairs grow back only reluctantly – which is why many women who over-plucked in the 1970s, going for the most minimal of arches (which was then oh-so-fashionable), now have almost no brows to speak of, and are slaves to the brow pencil (see next page).

BROWS – THE FINISHING TOUCH

Brows are like "face architecture" – and for some women, doing their brows, lashes and lips is all they need. Even if you don't usually accentuate your brows, experiment: you may find you need less makeup altogether if you do

✳ Get the shape right, of course, and you're halfway there – your eyes will look groomed, but (unless you're blessed with naturally dark brows), they won't necessarily have enough impact. Many of us need pencil – or better yet, powder – to achieve that.

✳ Eliza Petrescu explains: "Pencil and powder selection should be determined by hair and skin color. Go one shade darker if hair is light; go one shade lighter if hair is dark." (Even if hair is dark brown, she advises, avoid black.)

Of the brow products available, powder gives the most natural look

✳ The only way to test a brow color when makeup shopping is on the brow itself. Either shop bare-browed or remove your color at the counter. (A hand mirror is useful, once again, for judging the color in daylight. If a shade looks natural there, it'll look natural everywhere.)

✳ What you're really looking for are mousy brown tones of pencil or powder – and check to make sure there isn't a hint of red in the pencil/powder, even if you're a redhead. Because brows aren't naturally one color, you might opt for two very slightly differing shades. Brow powders are specially designed for use on this area, and have a slightly waxier texture – but if you can't get the right shade, use powder eyeshadow. (M.A.C. and Bobbi Brown offer brow-friendly shadow colors.)

✳ Before coloring brows, brush them upwards to make sure they're even – and then brush out horizontally. (This is something we skip when we're in a hurry – which is most of the time – but could be a must if yours are unruly.)

✳ Stephen Glass recommends Kanebo's eyebrow pencil in Muted Brown, "a really natural-looking taupe which works on almost all brows". Another rather miraculous product – recommended by Valentine Gotti, aka the "Makeup Doctor" – is Brenda Christian Brow Shaper Pencil, which adjusts to the color of every brow (from blonde to brunette) as if by magic.

✳ We'll be frank: we feel that of the brow products available, powder gives the most natural look, but if you still prefer pencil, start at the inner corner and work outwards using light, feathery strokes. You're trying to color the hairs – although when it comes to "filling in" gaps, you can draw directly onto skin.

✳ When using powder, you need a brush specifically designed for brows—which is stiff and angled. Tap the handle on a hard surface (or the back of your hand) to remove excess, then start at the thickest part of the brow and work outwards using feathery, light strokes. Again, you're trying to get color onto the hairs, not the skin – and be sure that the outer corner ends in a very fine point.

✳ For maximum staying power, Vincent Longo likes to use pencil followed by powder shadow to "fix" the pencil. This is fine for special occasions, but may be too time-consuming on an everyday basis – it certainly is for us.

✳ There is an increasing range of colored "brow mascaras" on the market but in our opinion, they're a nightmare to use in a hurry and don't look natural – brows can appear stiff. In the same way, many experts recommend using brow gel or hairspray to fix brows in place, but, once again – unless your brows are constantly trying to escape – we say skip this, except for the outermost ends if necessary.

✳ If you have the time, sweep brows through with a (clean) mascara wand after you've applied your brow color – either one you've bought, or one you've adapted for the task by first dunking it in eye-makeup remover, then washing it in gentle soap – to give your brows a tended look.

Having brows tattooed with semi-permanent makeup may seem like the ultimate time-saving beauty gesture, but beware: we've seen some horrendous results in which all you notice are the brows, not the woman they belong to. (Remember, too, that brows fade naturally as we age – and what works with your hair color now may well not work when you've gone grey/lighter/darker, in a few years' time.) If you're considering having semi-permanent makeup done, ask to see – in person – several people who've been treated by the person you're considering so that you can gauge the results with your own eyes. Do not be fooled by photos, which sometimes show another therapist's work, or are promotional shots taken by the company that supplies the tattooing equipment. There is also a theoretical risk of contracting HIV or hepatitis C if an unsterilized needle is used. Meanwhile, never have brows or lashes dyed with hair dye; in many countries, it's even illegal.

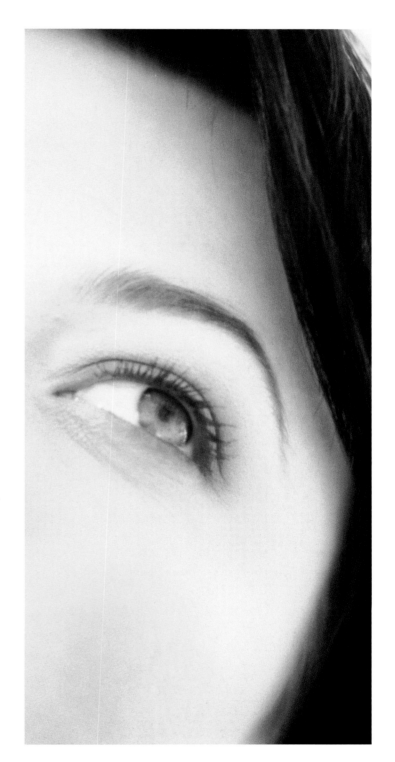

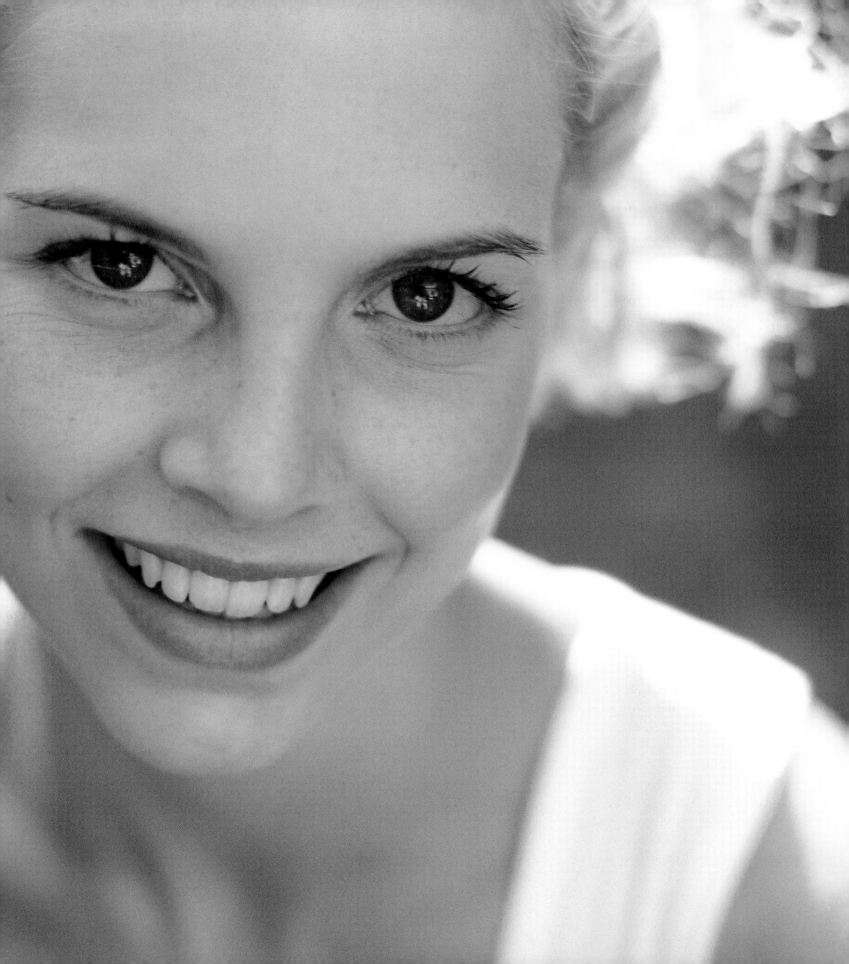

CHEEKY!

*Cheek color gone wrong is enough to make anybody red-faced –
so here's how to get it right!*

Blush – not foundation – is for perking up your face, super-fast. But today, there's a bigger choice than ever of textures as well as shades. Let's start with the right color choice. Before you invest in colors that turn out to be not quite right once they're on, follow this simple rule of thumb from makeup pro Fulvia Farolfi:

Ivory skin tones (which tend to be pale, and therefore need subtle, rather than intense colors) should stick to light beige tones for contouring (see How to Lose Five Pounds in Five Seconds, page 46) and soft pinks for blush.

Pink skin tones also need pale beige for contouring (see overleaf), with a stroke of warm peach to highlight and play down the rosiness of the complexion. (This applies to women with broken capillaries, too, who should opt for more peachy/apricot shades – otherwise the blush picks up that redness and emphasises it.)

Yellow skin tones – perhaps a bit on the sallow side – do best with a honey-colored contour, with a peachy/coral blush.

Black skin tones should choose a fudge-colored blush for contouring, topped off with a brighter, but still dark, shade of auburn – or bronzer (see Iman's advice, page 24).

✳ According to FACE Stockholm's Gun Novak, "The only way you can tell if a blush shade suits you is by applying it to the cheeks, not the back of the hand. So you should really test it on a 'naked' face, or over foundation only, or chances are it'll be a wrong choice and end up in your cupboard. Always test with a cotton pad – or a brush that you've actually seen them sterilize."

✳ To avoid obvious "stripes" of blush, apply it mainly to the apples of the cheeks, rather than all along the cheekbone. Smile, and the center of your cheek will puff out; this is where to apply blush, then blend outwards towards the hairline. According to John Gustafson – a British TV beauty pundit and independent skincare advisor who's trained with all the major-league beauty houses: "If you can just see your blush from about five feet away, the shade is about right." If you overdo blush, don't rub; apply some pressed powder over the top to tone down the color.

✳ If you're feeling tired, you can use blush to give your face an instant "lift": sweep it high on the outer part of the cheeks, near the eyes and up towards the temples.

✳ According to our pros, women with oily skin should use a blush that's a shade lighter than the one they want to end up with. This compensates for the darkening effects of oil on the blush's pigment.

CHOOSING A BLUSHER TEXTURE

Gel blush is good for flawless skins that don't really need base, as it's best applied just over moisturizer; but it doesn't work very well over powder or foundation. Be aware that there's very little "playtime" because if you don't blend it into skin super-fast, you can be left with circles of pigment.

Cheek stains are for the experienced only – they're even harder to blend in, but are incredibly long-lasting. (Good on casual weekends for that just-got-back-from-a-windswept-walk look – again, on already flawless skins.)

Cream blush is our top choice, especially the easy-glide formulations that can be dabbed onto skin – either bare skin (with a bit of concealer if needed), or over foundation – then blended outwards with your middle finger. There's much more "playtime" than with gel blush, although the creamy formulation does slowly "set" to a powdery finish. Barbara Daly has this tip for using cream blush: "Because these blend beautifully, you don't have to worry so much about 'placing' the color. If you have the time, warm it on the back of your hand, then dab it onto the center of the cheek and blend. But because you're heating the skin with the rubbing action, you may look pinker – so wait a minute before you add any more product."

Powder blush should be applied with a very light touch, always with a generously sized, domed blush brush. Sweep the brush across the color, then tap it firmly against a hard surface (to get rid of absolutely all the excess) before applying to your face; never, ever go straight from the compact to your cheeks— that's what creates the "clown" effect.

Bronzing powder is applied in the same way as powder blush, but can be used to create a sun-kissed look elsewhere on the face. Follow the same guidelines as for powder blush – but when it comes to placement, John Gustafson advises: "For a natural effect, apply the bronzer to the places that would catch the sun. Sweep the color up over your nose, the tops of your cheekbones, the brow and the chin."

HOW TO LOSE FIVE POUNDS IN FIVE SECONDS

Makeup can also be used to slim down a less-than-svelte face – provided it's used carefully, and the makeup artists' mantra of "blend, blend, blend" is observed at all times. As makeup artist Jenny Jordan emphasizes: "I can't stress the need for careful blending enough. If you don't do it right, you'll look like you've got smudges of dirt on your face." It's all about optical illusion; using makeup that's a shade or two darker than skin tone can create cheekbones where there aren't any and make double chins and flabby jawlines look more sculpted.

Jenny Jordan's trick is to apply blush in the usual way, and then use the lightest dusting of a light-toned matte bronzing powder – like Bobbi Brown Bronzing Powder – in a sweep, just under the cheekbone. (Suck in your cheeks to locate your natural hollow.)

The bronzer can be used under the chin, too. Alternatively, experiment with a shade of face powder two or three shades darker than you usually wear, applied in those same zones. (For tips on color choices, see Fulvia Farolfi's advice on page 45.)

You can also try using foundation that's two shades darker than your regular choice and apply to those same areas. This is even more subtle, but just as effective – provided you're careful to avoid streaks. Above all, contouring requires practice before you go out in the big, wide world with your new—*subtly*—sculpted features!

SKIN BRIGHTENERS – *Tried & Tested*

Skin brighteners are a whole new beauty category, designed to go over moisturizer and under foundation. They're great for perking up skin that's dull or basically looks as exhausted as you feel. These products tend to contain light-reflecting particles to create the illusion of more luminous skin and are particularly good under evening makeup. Skin-brighteners are especially suited to more mature skins – it's a fact: matte, flat skin looks older – but can be used on their own on younger faces, for a dewy finish that's particularly good at night. Some women find that a skin illuminator plus powder on top is all they need for flawlessness – so they can skip the foundation stage.

The how-to's simple: apply like a moisturizer, all over the face. (They look pretty, too, massaged into the décolletage.) Then apply foundation – or just powder – over the top (or leave as is, if you're a flawlessly complexioned teenager).

CHANEL PRÉCISION MAXIMUM RADIANCE CREAM
8.3 points out of 10
Prettily fresh-scented, this apricot-colored light cream scored extremely well for a product in this category and almost all of the ten testers said that they'd invest in it, in future. Chanel suggest a specific massage technique – outlined in their leaflet – for further enhancing the cream's effect.

UPSIDE: "When I first tested this, my baby was three weeks old and I looked pale and tired – but after using this I looked refreshed and alive – absolutely amazing! The baby is now nine weeks old and I am very tired, but with this cream, I glow! I love it!" • "Skin looked healthier and moisturized, felt very soft and supple – and radiance was increased" • "I had lots of comments about how healthy I look with this" • "the glow from this lasted all day – I even received compliments on my complexion!"
DOWNSIDE: There were no negative comments about this product.

❀ AVEDA TOURMALINE CHARGED RADIANCE FLUID
8.25 points out of 10
A lightweight gel, packed with antioxidants including organic aloe, green tea leaf and vitamin C, this is designed to work longer term to reduce fine lines and wrinkles – but for this category, our testers were asked to assess its power to improve radiance instantly, another of Aveda's claims.

UPSIDE: "Makes skin look like I've been for a brisk walk by the beach – and I love the fragrance, which is typical Aveda: woody, mossy, natural" • "a lovely product to use, particularly during the winter months when skin can look quite grey" • "my skin looked wonderfully glowing and healthy, with or without foundation".
DOWNSIDE: "When I used this twice a day – as recommended – it was rather drying".

GUERLAIN DIVINORA PURE RADIANCE
7.93 points out of 10
Reflective particles of real 24-carat gold are suspended in this clear gel – explaining why it makes skin look radiant (and the price tag!). Guerlain claim that this can work as a moisturizer – it has vitamin E and hyaluronic acid in it – or smoothed on after your regular cream.

UPSIDE: "Blended beautifully for a glowing, even-toned, long-lasting and flattering finish" • "skin definitely looked more radiant" • "definite radiant glow, golden sheen – slightly glitter" • "my face appeared more youthful, with a subtle, shimmery glow; I liked the all-over softness this gave to my face."
DOWNSIDE: "Too shiny to use alone".

ESTÉE LAUDER SPOTLIGHT SKINTONE PERFECTOR
7.72 points out of 10
Lauder call this "the millennium's answer to fresh, luminescent skin". It contains micro-prisms for an instant radiance, with a blend of antioxidants and skin-brightening botanicals that work on a longer-term basis to help fade the appearance of sunspots and blotchiness over a period of 3–4 months.

UPSIDE: "A reflective glaze giving skin a healthy and polished look – lovely!" • "wonderful! It needs care and a light application for daytime, but makes you look very healthy and glowing" • "sexy – a golden glow" • "worn on its own, this revitalized and brightened my face, bringing it to life".
DOWNSIDE: "Too glitzy for day wear".

BEST BUDGET BUY
NIVEA VISAGE SIMPLY GLOWING
6.6 points out of 10
If you're looking for a budget choice, this is your best bet, according to our testers: a light-reflecting cream, which nourishes with apricot oil and "energizes" with vitamin E.

UPSIDE: "No waiting time – I found I could put makeup on immediately" • "very moisturizing, with a wonderful brightening effect" • "liked the light-reflecting particles, which did make my skin glow".
DOWNSIDE: "Too oily for my liking" • "I saw no difference in radiance" • "didn't like apricot smell".

The lowest score for this category was 4.9 points out of 10.

DAY AND NIGHT

We'd love an hour – or two – to get ready to go out at night, and then be whisked off in a glass carriage. The reality is that we're lucky if we can grab five minutes until we have to dash out the door. So here we bring you quick-change secrets that help create a party-perfect look faster than you can say "fairy godmother"...

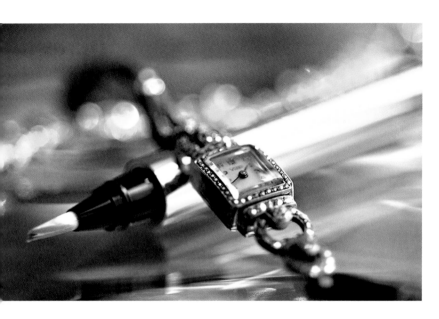

Valentine Gotti is known as the "makeup doctor", jetting between London, Paris, and New York to provide one-on-one consultations to help women discover their perfect shades and techniques – thus helping to streamline not only their makeup kits but their lives as well. She's particularly good at evening makeup, so we asked her to share some insider wisdom.

If you have the luxury of time, you can start from scratch. But since time is precisely what most of us don't have enough of, Valentine suggests we opt for a quickly achievable evening look that freshens and slightly intensifies our day makeup. The secret is to be prepared. "Keep a special day-into-night makeup kit in your desk, at work, or somewhere handy at home – so that you don't lose valuable minutes searching for the right equipment."

Day-into-evening countdown:

✳ "For 'repair' work, you need a good magnifying mirror and cotton swabs to get rid of mascara flakes, etc."

✳ Seek out the best light. "Daylight's best, fluorescent (typical 'ladies' room' lighting) is worst. If you're making up at home, after dark, take the shade off a table lamp and put on your makeup sitting about 2 feet [60cm] away from the lamp, facing the light source."

✳ "Use blue-tinted eyedrops to take away any redness from the day especially if you've been sitting at your computer, which strains eyes."

✳ Reach for your magic wand. Valentine swears by Yves Saint Laurent Touche Eclat Radiant Touch for repairs. "Pump a little Radiant Touch onto the back of your hand, roll a cotton swab in it and use that to pick up any smudges or flakes around the eye area. This works better than eye makeup remover, which takes too much off."

✳ Roll back the years. "Radiant Touch also works instantly to minimize the appearance of lines. Once you've brushed on a tiny amount, pat lightly with your ring finger to blend. Apply down the lines that run from nose to mouth, and between the brows, to subtly highlight the forehead. And apply it to dark circles under the eyes and on the inner corner of the nose, next to the tearducts."

✳ "You don't need to reapply base; simply take a creamy cover stick and apply it to blemishes or broken capillaries."

✳ Add a touch of blush. "Use just a little blusher or bronzer in a very slightly darker shade than you'd usually wear for day. The key is to tap the brush to get rid of excess, and whisk it very lightly over cheeks."

✳ Freshen your face. "If you finish with powder right away, makeup will look cakey. So spritz first with a mist of Evian mineral water spray. Allow it to dry, then add a super-light dusting of loose powder."

✳ Emphasize lips. "Lipstick should definitely be more intense for evening—a dark red or prune. If you're not comfortable with the intense effect of a dark lipstick straight from the tube, turn it into a 'stain': apply, then place a tissue between your lips and press down on it; the sheerer color that remains will last for hours. You can add gloss, if you choose – or just use a dark-toned lip gloss."

✳ Add a touch of shimmer. "Jane Iredale's 24-Karat Gold Dust mineral shimmers (see Directory, page 246) are perfect. Dip your finger to pick up a tiny amount of powder, then add a touch to the eyelids directly above the pupil and blend with your finger till it's sheer. It's also good on the brow, or on the center of the lips over lipstick. I don't really like shimmer anywhere else; it's more flattering to have a triangle of faint shimmer just above the eyes and on the lips."

✳ "If you apply just one coat of mascara in the morning, you should be able to curl your lashes (with an eyelash curler) in the evening, then apply a second coat. The best I've found for doing this without looking 'spidery' is Clinique Long Pretty Lashes Mascara," says Valentine.

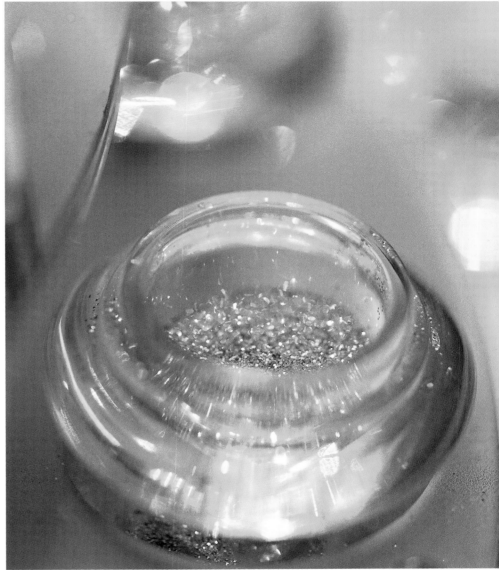

✳ Darken the eye line. "Line your eyes with dark pencil, then brush over the line with an eyeshadow powder in the same shade, and it'll last all night." (See page 34 for advice on choosing eyeshadow colors.)

✳ Spray on your favorite sexy scent. Nothing gets you out of "work" mode and into a "play" mood quicker. Then get out there and have a ball!

MORNING-AFTER MAKEUP

Hangovers make us feel—and look—awful. Alcohol and late nights take their toll on our entire systems – but thankfully, makeup was created for those days when we look less than perfect. (The "hangover look" is also due to tiredness or a cold...)

So you've overdone it. Or you've got the sniffles. Well, staying in bed all day to recover is one option – but it's not very work-friendly. John Gustafson has these tips for morning-after-the-night-before faces...

✳ "Avoid the temptation to pile on makeup. Dry, dehydrated skin will look crusty with masses of extra makeup on. Instead, apply two layers of moisturizer, allowing the first to sink in for ten minutes to give skin a moisture boost, then a fine layer of foundation."

✳ "Avoid a completely matte finish. Loads of powder won't do you any favors when your skin is tired. Restrict powder to the shinier T-zone only – or skip it altogether."

✳ "Use bronzing powder in place of blush, as it won't pick up any redness in the eyes or cheeks."

✳ "Spiky black mascara won't flatter red, puffy eyes. Use a softer navy or grey and stop at one coat, maximum."

✳ "A natural flush of cream blush will give your skin a fresh, dewy look – place it on the apples of your cheeks and blend, blend, blend."

✳ "Use a slightly brighter lipstick than normal to perk up your complexion – but in a sheer, glossy formula so it won't overwhelm your face."

✳ We also recommend an under-makeup "skin brightener" to give skin back its healthy gleam – see page 47 for Tried & Tested results. And if you can remember, before bedtime, drink at least one tall glass of water and slather skin in Guerlain's Issima Midnight Secret. This is pricy – but (in our opinion) worthy of its reputation as "eight hours' sleep in a bottle". (For more fast fixes for faces, see page 110.)

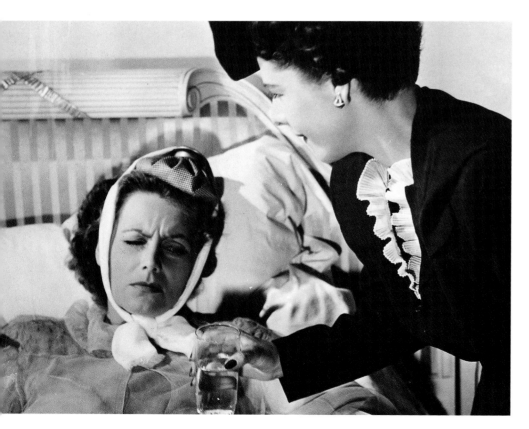

BRUSH ESSENTIALS

Nobody but a professional makeup artist needs an arsenal of different brushes (especially now that so many makeup textures can be applied with fingers) – so here's your ultimate kit...

British-born Tina Earnshaw – who's worked on famous Hollywood faces from Gwyneth Paltrow to Anjelica Huston (and kept Kate Winslet from looking waterlogged in *Titanic*) insists that most non-pros can easily create a perfect, flawless face every time with just five brushes.

1. A blush brush. "The bristles should be slightly domed, so that you don't get any hard edges when you apply blush," she advises. "A blush brush can double as a powder brush, but get rid of any excess of one product before using it for the other."

2. A lip brush. "It's fashionable right now to apply lipstick straight from the tube, for a soft, sexy effect, but if you want it to last on your lips, nothing beats applying it with a brush."

3. A concealer brush. "This should be flat, with a slightly domed top. It's perfect for covering pimples without smearing and for covering up dark circles – especially on the inside of the bridge of the nose, beside the eye. That area's often overlooked, but camouflaging it makes all the difference."

4. An eyeliner brush. "Only go for a very fine liner brush if you like a 1950s-style line; otherwise opt for a 'flatliner' brush, which can be used to press dark shadow into the base of the lashes. That's what emphasizes the eye-line – and creates the illusion of longer lashes."

5. An eyebrow brush. "Ideally, this should be shaped like a mascara wand – or you can clean an old mascara brush with makeup remover and improvise."

We'll add two more optional extras to this list: a ¾ inch [2cm] brush for applying powder (if you wear it) and – if you wear liquid foundation – a synthetic brush, which can be used to paint on foundation where you need it, pre-blending.

Mary Greenwell advises: "Clean brushes with a tiny bit of liquid wool wash in warm water; just dip them and swish the hairs gently with your fingers, but only go as far as the metal; never get the wood wet because then brushes can fall apart. Rinse, then let dry with the bristles hanging over the edge of a table." (Some makeup artists use spritz-on brush cleaners – but these are packed with chemicals, which leave a residue on the hairs. Do you really want that on your skin?)

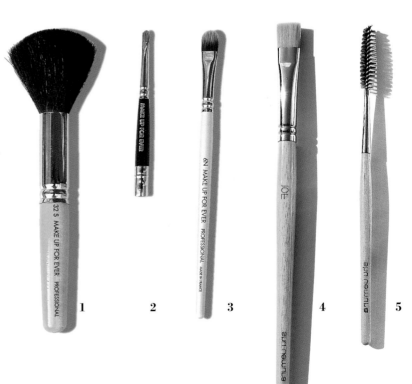

1   2   3   4   5

DO YOU WANT TO BE A NATURAL BEAUTY?

Queen Elizabeth I's lead-based makeup is said to have poisoned her. If you want to be sure that your makeup's safe, four centuries later, read this...

We admit that we compromise a lot when it comes to makeup, often choosing on the basis of performance rather than naturalness. Our makeup bags are far from all-natural. But, there are several very natural lines which we believe are worth checking out, and which we use ourselves for some products.

Dr. Hauschka now makes an entire line of makeup (both Jo and Sarah love the mascara in particular), as does an all-natural German brand called Logona (see Directory, page 246). Jane Iredale's makeup line is based entirely on powdered minerals, and is preservative-free. We're also highly impressed with Living Nature's (albeit small) range of lipsticks, and with Jurlique's (likewise). All of these can be hard to track down in mainstream retail outlets, however, so we recommend that if you want a more natural makeup that's easy to find, Aveda is your best bet.

Makeup is designed to sit on the skin - unlike skincare, which is intended to be absorbed, at least into the top layers. But if you're trying to lead a more natural lifestyle – eating organically, for instance, and seeking out holistic health care – you may have some concerns about your makeup. Makeup often contains preservatives – some of which may trigger irritation. Foundation may include lanolin, from sheep's wool—which may contain organophosphate pesticide residues. Paraben preservatives can set off allergies in some, while a commonly used ingredient in concealers – imidazolidynil urea – may also trigger contact dermatitis.
Many eyeshadows and powder-type products contain aluminium – which some experts believe may be linked to the development of Alzheimer's disease – or talc, which, if breathed in enough, might trigger respiratory problems in vulnerable people. Our advice: hold your breath when you're applying powder, so you don't inhale it.

Some colors which are preceded by the letters "FD & C" are derived from coal tar and may even be carcinogenic. And most makeup is based, at least in part, on ingredients derived from the petrochemical industry: mineral oil, chemically derived pigments and preservatives. (If you're concerned about these issues– and would like to understand more about these and other potential risks associated with beauty products, we highly recommend a book called *Drop Dead Gorgeous*, by Kim Erickson, with a foreword by cancer expert Professor Samuel Epstein – see Bookshelf, page 246).

If you're eager to buy makeup that's "greener" – from an environmental standpoint, or because you're concerned about personal health – you need to put on your specs (or eat your carrots) and start reading the fine print. (Usually on outer cartons.) Here, then, is a list of some of the more natural and sustainable ingredients that you'll find in makeup – and what they do:

Annato – a natural vegetable dye (in the yellow/pink spectrum) which may be used to tint lipstick.

Beeswax – can be used as a lubricant in concealer, lipstick, gloss and mascara.

Carmine – a red pigment from crushed insects (so it's unacceptable to vegans and vegetarians).

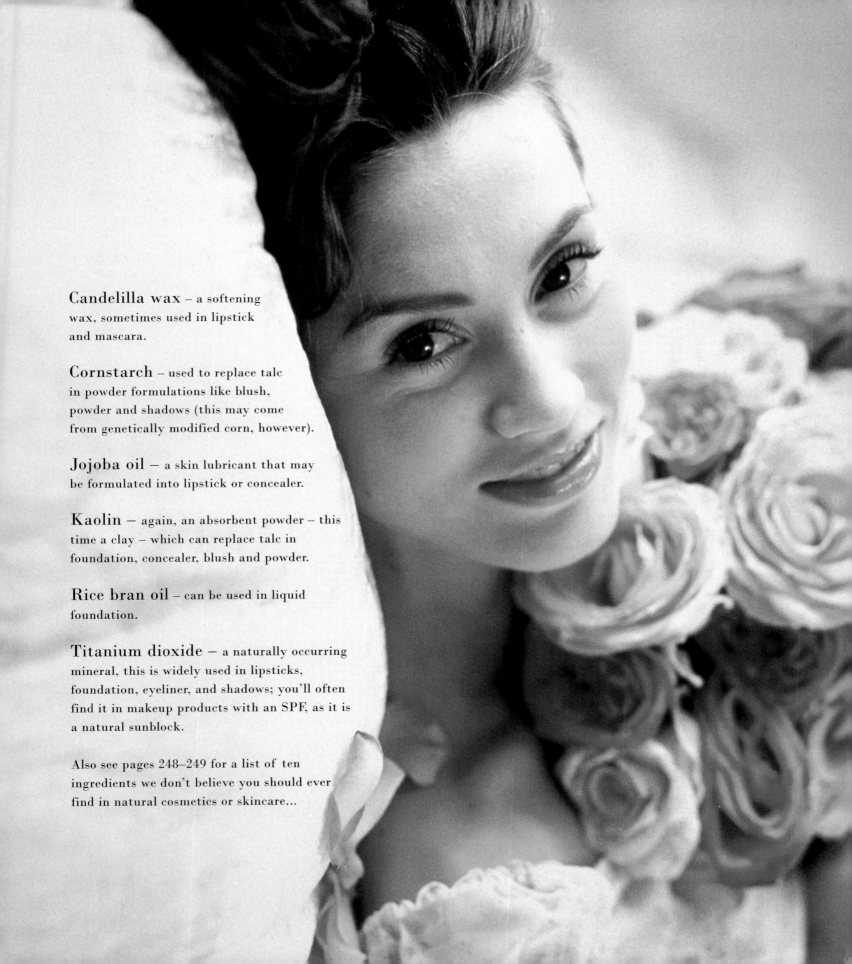

Candelilla wax – a softening wax, sometimes used in lipstick and mascara.

Cornstarch – used to replace talc in powder formulations like blush, powder and shadows (this may come from genetically modified corn, however).

Jojoba oil – a skin lubricant that may be formulated into lipstick or concealer.

Kaolin – again, an absorbent powder – this time a clay – which can replace talc in foundation, concealer, blush and powder.

Rice bran oil – can be used in liquid foundation.

Titanium dioxide – a naturally occurring mineral, this is widely used in lipsticks, foundation, eyeliner, and shadows; you'll often find it in makeup products with an SPF, as it is a natural sunblock.

Also see pages 248–249 for a list of ten ingredients we don't believe you should ever find in natural cosmetics or skincare…

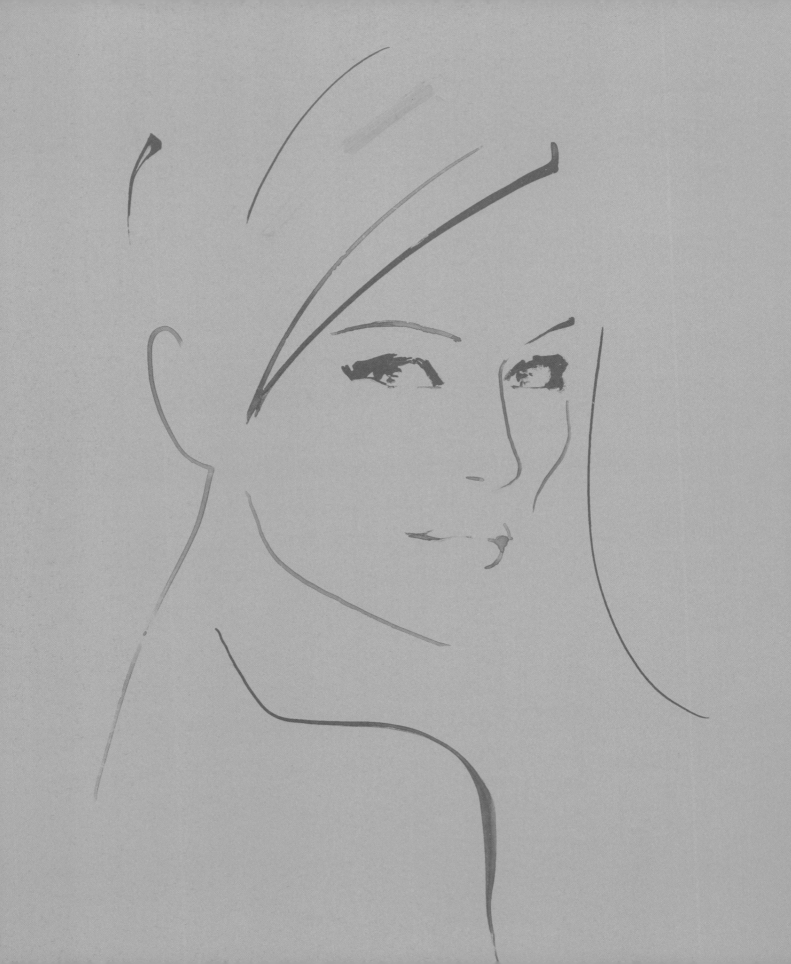

SKIN

Beauty begins with great skin. Skin that glows. That's perfectly in balance. Doesn't misbehave and flare up when you have an important meeting or a hot date. Trust us: it's simpler than you think. (And much simpler than the beauty industry would like you to think...) So: it's time to unclutter that bathroom shelf and get back to (beautiful) basics. Establish an easy as A-B-C regime that you'll love – as will your complexion. Soak up the wisdom of the skincare world's true gurus. And discover the high-tech anti-agers and the natural products that truly work. So that – at every age – you really can love the skin you're in...

GOOD THINGS FOR SKIN

Throughout this book we name products that work wonders for skin. But the good news is that the basics are completely free. So just take a long, slow, deep breath. Because that's where great skin starts.

We breathe all the time. But, because we take breathing for granted, we hardly ever think about this vital process. So stop for a moment – right now, before you go any further. Uncross your arms and legs, let your chest rise gently and your shoulders drop back, then take six deep rhythmic breaths. Inhale through your nose and exhale through your nose or mouth. Do it slowly, taking as much time on the exhale as you do breathing in. Now look in the mirror and see the difference.

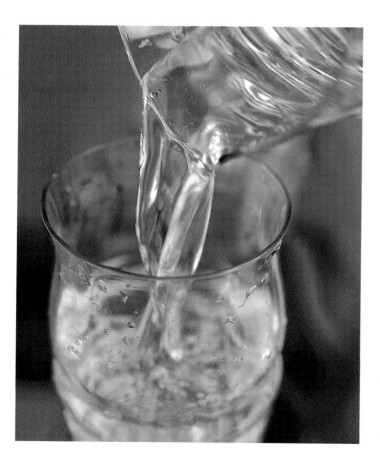

Breathing literally oxygenates your skin so that it looks alive and vibrant. Any activity that makes you breathe more deeply makes your skin glow. Think of those rosy cheeks, when you come in from a brisk walk. So get moving! We're not talking about major athletics here. Just take five minutes to walk, dance, march in place (arms moving as well as legs), run up and down the stairs, or do some yoga (see page 238 for our favorite yoga workout).

Of course, if you have the time to get out in the open, go for a swim or a ride (bike or horse), play a game of tennis or whatever sport you enjoy – just do it. These not only de-stress your mind, they're your skin's (and eyes' and hair's and heart's) best friend. (We head out to the garden to do some weeding or do yoga; Jo swims in the sea and Sarah rides. It never fails.)

Our next freebie skin beautifier is water. Most of us just don't drink enough. That means an unhappy body, inside and out. Headaches, constipation, lethargy and many other chronic problems are largely due to lack of hydration – and these can all show up on our faces, as a sluggish complexion, frown-lines, pimples and just plain "glow" deficiency. After all, two-thirds of our bodies are made up of water. Yet we sit in homes and offices which are as dehydrating as the Sahara Desert and somehow expect to thrive. Think how the water level in a vase of flowers goes down day by day. That's what happens to your skin. Drink at least 2½ pints (one and a half liters) daily – more if you can – between meals (otherwise it flushes away the nutrients in your food). Pure, still water is best but tap water or sparkling mineral water is fine, if that's all there is. (In the East, they prescribe warm water. Try it and see if you like it better.) Whenever you can't think of what to do, or you feel a bit under the

Think how the water level in a vase of flowers goes down day by day. That's what happens to your skin

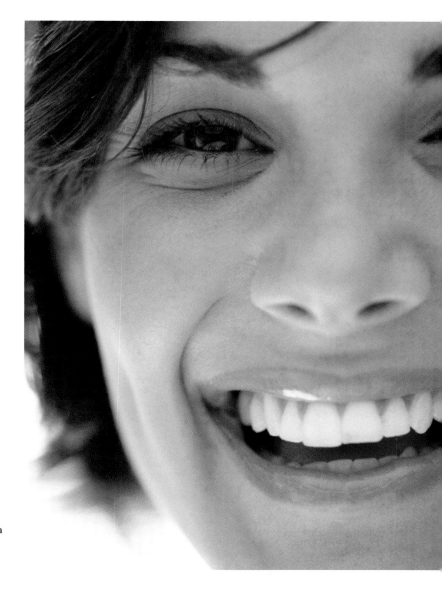

weather, sip a small glass of room-temperature water slowly. Don't chug a big tumbler in a rush – it may make you feel sick.

Use water in the form of steam too. On a bad face day, steaming your face evens out tone and texture, and miraculously softens lines. What's more, it even makes your eye bags go away. If you have time, take a steam bath or sauna (steam rooms have a gentler heat so we prefer them). Or simply boil a kettle of hot water, pour it into a bowl with a couple of drops of your favorite essential oil – rose is bliss for skin – and when the water is very hot but not scorching, drape a good-sized towel over your head to trap the steam, and swelter for five or ten minutes. For good measure, you could treat your hair to a mask at the same time, letting the steam turbo-charge its effects. (Be aware, though, that if you suffer from broken capillaries, heat can make them worse; so keep the water on the warm side of hot and, if you go into a steam room, stay for a few minutes only.)

We also want to teach the world to juice. There's a luminous sparkle that fresh juices bring to your skin which is inimitable. (For more, including recipes, turn to page 235.) Juicing isn't quite free – but you can make two big glasses of vitamin-packed juice, from organic fruit and vegetables, in a modestly-priced juicer, for less than a budget-priced stick of concealer.

Happiness, peace of mind and sleep are essential to skin. Wrinkles really can vanish when your mind and body are rested, and deeper lines soften. (We're not talking about laugh lines – we like those.) These factors are covered in depth in the Well being section at the back of the book (page 212). If you can't sleep, laugh! Call someone you love and share a joke. Or – depending on your circumstance – make love (that might be all you need).

GOOD THINGS FOR YOUR SKIN

- Deep rhythmic breathing
- Water
- Fresh fruit and veggie juices
- Good fats (see page 96)
- Good sleep
- Laughter and joie de vivre

THE CLEAN SWEEP

Fact: the effectiveness of your entire skincare regime hinges on getting this step right. So here's how to wash your face...

We love cleansing. It washes away the day along with the dirt. But it's easy to be overenthusiastic – and using the wrong cleanser can actually be harmful for skin. "If it's too harsh, it strips away the skin's natural barrier along with the dirt and makeup," says Dr. Daniel Maes, vice-president of research and development at Estée Lauder. If you overcleanse skin – with a too-harsh cleanser – it interferes with this vital "barrier function" letting precious moisture out and potential irritants in.

A complexion that feels taut, tight and a little stiff after cleansing is usually an indication of barrier damage. "This makes skin too permeable for too long, allowing ingredients that should sit on the skin's surface – sunscreens, for instance – to get into the skin." Adds Dr. Maes: "We've often found this to be the cause of product sensitivity, in which it's the wrong cleanser triggering a reaction, not the face cream itself."

So: gentle but thorough daily cleansing should be your goal. Although this book is all about shortcuts and saving time, cleansing is one skincare step that you shouldn't skimp on. Personally, we're fans of "pomade-style" cleansers, pioneered by Eve Lom – whose famous fans include Jade Jagger, Sharon Stone and Goldie Hawn – but now much more widely available. (Our favorite is Spiezia Organics, see page 101.) Based on oils that have solidified, they "emulsify" – or melt – at skin temperature. They can't be used with cotton balls, which stick to it – so (opposite) we reveal the perfect cleansing technique.

Do spend at least a couple of minutes on this part of your skincare ritual – otherwise any moisturizer or treatment you apply will just sit on the surface, unable to penetrate the layers of dead skin and remaining grime. Use a warm-to-hot wet washcloth to remove the cleanser. (In fact, we've found that this technique works well no matter what kind of cleanser you choose.)

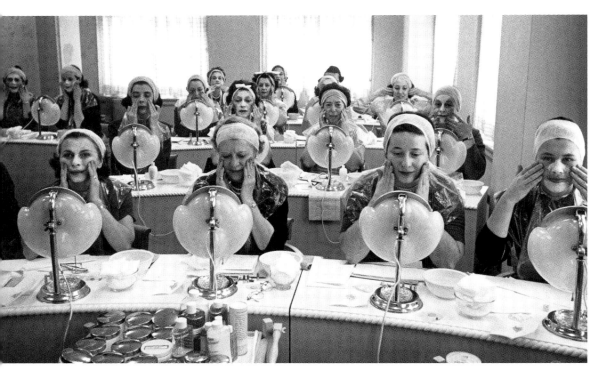

CLEANSING DO'S

✳ Hands should be immaculate before you start; always wash them before cleansing.

✳ Get your hair off your face with a headband or shower cap so you can thoroughly access the hairline and edges of your face.

✳ Smooth your chosen cleanser over your face and neck. Working from the collarbone up, circle the fingertips up and across the neck and face to the hairline. Use the pads of your fingers and some pressure – but remember that the skin under your chin is as delicate as the skin under your eyes. Massage well, all over, which will boost blood flow to the face, bringing nutrients to the complexion. (This technique works wonders for tired faces.)

✳ Cleansing wipes – see our Tried & Tested, on page 62 – are great when you're in a hurry (and 1,000 percent better than falling into bed with your makeup on). But we don't believe they're a long-term substitute for a dedicated cleanser.

✳ The type of cleanser you use should be based on preference, rather than skin type – because you're more likely to use it thoroughly. On page 60, we give the Tried & Tested results for cleansers suitable for all skin types.

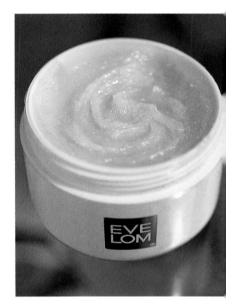

"Cleansing is the most important step in skincare.
If you get that right, then beautiful skin is bound to follow"
EVE LOM

✳ Give the cleanser a minute or two to work on dirt and makeup, and it will all come off more efficiently.

✳ Swish your washcloth in warm-to-hot water and hold the cloth over your face. Pat it down and rub lightly all over your face to remove any remaining grime. Repeat once or twice, until the cloth is no longer grubby. (See page 63 for why this is all the exfoliation you need.)

✳ Washcloths should be used for 24 hours, then machine-washed, preferably with a non-biological, gentle washing powder. (We like Ecover.) Otherwise, bacteria can breed.

✳ Ordinary soap is too harsh for facial skin, upsetting pH balance and leaving it vulnerable. If you're a foam freak, try switching to a gentle foaming cleanser or a special "cleansing bar". But remember that these are basically detergents, which may still be harsh on your skin, so experiment with a richer cleanser using the technique here. You may find it gives you the freshness you crave.

✳ Don't feel you always need to cleanse from scratch in the morning. If you're short on time, simply use your hot washcloth – "or a cotton pad drenched in rosewater," advises makeup artist Sara Raeburn – and wipe it over the face a few times.

SUITS-ALL-SKIN-TYPES CLEANSERS

Tried & Tested

These products are designed to sweep makeup clean away, whether you suffer from dry, normal, oily or sensitive skin – so we tested them across a range of skin types.

BEST BUDGET BUY
❀ LIZ EARLE NATURALLY ACTIVE CLEANSE & POLISH HOT CLOTH CLEANSER

9.5 points out of 10

A truly outstanding result: one woman gave it 11 points out of 10! This pump-action cleanser – from a beauty journalist-turned-skincare-guru – is used with hot water and its own muslin cloths (which also acts as an exfoliator, hence the word "polish"). It's safe to use around the eyes (even our super-sensitive eyes have never reacted to this), and is packed with effective quantities of botanical ingredients including rosemary, chamomile, and eucalyptus, along with cocoa butter and almond milk. It contains no mineral oil or lanolin, unlike many cleansers. Our testers universally loved the fragrance. As it lasts for months and months, we awarded this moderately priced product our Best Budget Buy trophy, too.
UPSIDE: "Skin felt really clean and fresh after use and very soft" • "after a few tries it left skin feeling velvety and radiant; texture just right – felt rich on skin" • "loved – LOVED – this product! Amazing difference on greasy chin, with noticeably smaller pores" • "took off full "Saturday night makeup" easily" • "the muslin cloth was strangely satisfying; good to see all the grime that came off my skin" • "very uplifting fragrance".
DOWNSIDE: None reported.

CHRISTIAN DIOR REFRESHING CLEANSING WATER FOR FACE AND EYES

9.37 points out of 10

This double-duty product is also designed to remove mascara, cutting one step from your cleansing regime. It's clear, like water, but is actually a high-tech formula featuring a hydra-vitamin complex and magnesium, so skin's never left feeling taut.
UPSIDE: "Top points for ease-of-use, requiring no effort to clean thoroughly, leaving my face moisturized and refreshed; a few squirts on a cotton pad go on a long way" • "this is the cleanser I've been waiting for – an amazing, slightly soapy liquid that was wonderful to use and left my skin feeling soft" • "I used every last drop of this and bought some more as soon as it got low" • "loved this – it felt very fresh and silky, and my 18-year-old daughter fell in love with it" • "kind to the eye area".
DOWNSIDE: "It didn't work on waterproof mascara, even though it said it would".

EVE LOM CLEANSER

8.75 points out of 10

A product that's earned its place in the Beauty Hall of Fame – from one of the world's leading facialists. This is a solid cleanser, infused with aromatic oils, which emulsifies on skin. It is wiped away with a muslin cloth and hot water, lightly buffing skin to remove dead cells, and decongesting the face.
UPSIDE: "I was skeptical at first but after massaging my face, as instructed, all the makeup came off effortlessly" • "this is 'the business'; great for skin that needs a zing" • "skin moisturized and INCREDIBLY soft" • "feels like you're giving yourself a real facial, not just cleansing".
DOWNSIDE: "Medicinal smell".

ELIZABETH ARDEN DEEP CLEANSING LOTION

8.5 points out of 10

This, says Arden, "combines the effectiveness of a cream with the lightness of a lotion and leaves the skin feeling smooth and refreshed", removing makeup without stripping skin of moisture. Here's our testers' verdict:
UPSIDE: "At 2 a.m. I wanted something quick and easy to use, and this was it" • "just what I expect a cleanser to do: it smelled lovely, removed all makeup and left skin feeling smooth and comfortable" • "pump-action dispenser ensures no spillage or over-use of product" • "rich cleanser but easy to rinse off".
DOWNSIDE: "Left skin tight – needed to put on moisturizer very quickly".

❀❀ DR. HAUSCHKA CLEANSING MILK

8.4 points out of 10

Dr. Hauschka's biodynamic skincare uses organic ingredients, which are harvested in accordance with moon cycles and other rhythms of nature. This offering features sweet almond oil, clay, and rice germ oil. Again, testers loved the scent.
UPSIDE: "Silky lotion was easily applied and melted off makeup leaving parched, irritated winter skin hydrated, fresh and comfortable" • "cleansed effectively – gently but thoroughly; left skin very moisturized" • "a delicious product which was more like a treatment than a cleanser" • "went into skin easily and left it feeling soft, moisturized and fresh".
DOWNSIDE: Many of the testers would prefer it to be packaged in something other than a glass bottle, for bathroom and travel use.

The lowest score in this category was 5.2 points out of 10

TO TONE OR NOT TO TONE?

We're all looking for beauty shortcuts. Giving up your toner may be a good place to start...

Fact: you probably don't need a toner. Many skincare companies insist that cleanse/tone/moisturize should be the basic, three-step skincare regime, but we disagree. (And so do some of the world's leading facialist "gurus" including Eve Lom, Amanda Lacey and Janet Filderman.) This is especially true if you've got oily, greasy or problem skin. If you cleanse in the way we've recommended in the previous pages, your skin will be perfectly clean – but not squeaky clean; that's a sign that it's been over-cleansed. Many fresheners and toners, however, strip the skin of naturally moisturizing lipids (fats) – leaving it vulnerable. Toners are often alcohol-based – and, as Amanda Lacey explains: "Alcohol is one of skin's worst enemies; it dries out skin – so that moisture escapes even more easily – and upsets oily skin's natural balance so that sebum production goes into overdrive. The more you swipe away oil, the harder skin works to replace it." Eve Lom insists that using toners makes visible pores even more noticeable in the long run.

As an alternative to alcohol-based toners, many brands now produce skin fresheners that are alcohol-free; they may have the word "gentle" on the label (a clue that there's no alcohol in the bottle.) But we'd argue – and so would Amanda Lacey – that if you like the feeling of freshness of a cooling liquid over your face, you're just as well off with good old rosewater. (Amanda recommends Persian rosewater, while Sara Raeburn swears by Baldwin's Triple Rosewater). Orange flower water is another super-gentle option.

Try skipping this step in your skincare routine – and see how your skin (and your bank balance) fares. If you miss the fresh sensation of a toner, try soaking a face cloth in a basin of cold-as-you-can-take-it water, and laying that on your face for a moment or two. Add a couple of drops of your favourite essential oil to the water – we like peppermint – for a real zing.

PORES FOR THOUGHT?

Beauticians often try to tell us that by using a toner during a facial, they're "closing the pores". Baloney. Pores aren't elevator doors which can open and shut. Eve Lom advises: "The best way to minimize open pores is simply to stop using moisturizer on that area and pores will start to appear less obvious. They'll never disappear completely, but they do get better with patience and care."

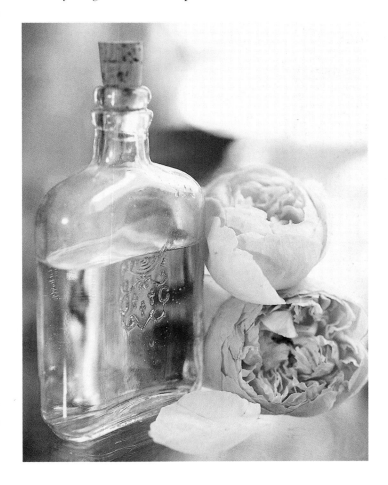

CLEANSING WIPES – *Tried & Tested*

These use-and-discard products have a big convenience factor but personally we'd recommend them as emergency cleansers – kept in your office desk for a quick cleanse before prepping for the evening or for travel – rather than for every day use. However many women do use them instead of normal cleansers for speed and ease: in Spain, we're told, one in two women uses them routinely. We tested lots of these products but overall the points were low. Our ten-women strong panels had mixed reactions, both to the concept and also the side effects. While some liked the convenience, others found they never really felt their skin was clean. The scents were often felt to be overpowering, even chemical. The cloths tended to be on the abrasive side of exfoliating, in some cases bringing out real sensitivity reactions including skin rashes. One of the common problems was eye stinging at the time of using and panda eyes the next morning. The upshot is that we are only listing three products in this category because the next set of points were so low that we couldn't wholeheartedly advise you to buy them.

BEST BUDGET BUY
OLAY DAILY FACIALS LATHERING CLEANSING CLOTHS
7.73 points out of 10
Unlike the other wipes in this category, these have to be wetted with water – which some of the testers found as messy and time-consuming as using a regular cleanser. Other testers, though, liked them. This product is available in three different versions for sensitive, normal-to-dry, or combination/oily skin types.
UPSIDE: "Great for travelling – just stick a couple in your bag, and go"• "they wake up a sleepy face brilliantly" • "lovely, mild soapy smell" • "made skin feel extremely clean and refreshed" • "texture is soft, but it works like a gentle exfoliant".
DOWNSIDE: "Slightly too abrasive on skin" • "very fiddly to use".

BEST BUDGET BUY
BOTANICS QUICK FIX CLEANSING WIPES
7.7 points out of 10
Containing soothing mallow extract to calm skin plus other plant ingredients (as the name suggests), this recent product marries botanicals from sustainable sources with high tech.
UPSIDE: "I would use these again – very efficient, packaging good and nice fragrance" • "my skin felt very clean but quite dry" • "removed eye makeup very well indeed" • "excellent product – large wipe left skin comfortable and clean".
DOWNSIDE: "Used a toner after and got loads more off so it couldn't have removed everything".

M.A.C. WIPES
6.55 points out of 10
Described as "the makeup artist's best friend", these wipe away hard-to-budge smudges and mistakes, lifting dirt and grime, and are more generously sized than most cleansing wipes. Some testers gave 10 out of 10 – but others marked them down considerably, reducing the overall score.
UPSIDE: "They removed makeup easily and didn't make my skin sensitive – brilliant for keeping in a desk drawer and taking away at weekends" • "liked the feeling on skin – didn't leave it greasy or dry" • "didn't upset my irrational skin" • "I could easily rub these over eyes without stinging; skin stayed moisturized but not shiny all day".
DOWNSIDE: "The first few wipes in the pack were very dry, but further down they were moist and more effective" • "awful smell".

The lowest score in this category was 5.5 points out of 10.

SOFTLY, SOFTLY

*Save the scrubbing for kitchen floors. What skin needs is ultra-gentle,
daily exfoliation – not a once-a-week skin blitz*

As far as we're concerned, facial scrubs are another category of beauty products women can scratch from their shopping list. (Scratch probably being the operative word here: many contain sharp particles that can abrade skin when massaged vigorously into the complexion.) Dr. Wilma F. Bergfeld, a leading dermatologist (and past president of the American Academy of Dermatology) makes this point about them: "Dermatologists advise caution in the use of exfoliants; although scrubs indeed slough off dead skin cells, there's a risk of leaving skin dry, red and irritated."

Skin – with all its layers (about 15 on the face) – is designed to protect. Overzealous removal of the top layers is likely to leave it more vulnerable to irritants, as well as to sun damage. Women who use Retin-A – a cream prescribed by some dermatologists to help turn back the clock – are advised to use sunscreen lavishly, as it too works by sloughing away surface layers of skin. Patients

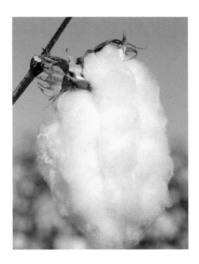

*Dermatologists advise caution
in the use of exfoliants*

who've had facial peels have to follow the same advice. Even over-the-counter products containing AHAs and BHAs – which brighten by removing dull, dead surface skin cells – make it more liable to sun damage.

We believe that simply cleansing skin using a muslin washcloth – a technique popularized by skincare guru Eve Lom, and described on page 59 – gives skin all the exfoliation it needs, lifting away only the very superficial cells which can look flat and dull, and no more. While skin is warm and wet, Eve advises, use the cloth "and concentrate on the areas where dead skin cells build up – around the nose and in the cleft of the chin." The softness of the muslin, she explains, prevents any scratching of fragile facial skin. "And unlike harsh facial scrubs," adds Eve, "it only removes the dead skin cells that are ready to be swept away."

If you can't find muslin washcloths, you could buy a length of muslin from a fabric store and cut it into 12-inch (30cm) squares. Many diaper liners are made of similar fabric, and do the trick beautifully. (Glamorous? Not exactly. But they work – and, as with everything in this book, that's the point.)

COTTON ON TO ORGANIC

Cotton wool is a beauty staple. We always choose organic, which is now widely available. (Natural food stores are a good source, but many supermarkets carry it too.) Cotton is the most heavily sprayed crop on the planet – and inevitably, some of those pesticides and herbicides remain in non-organic cotton wool pads and balls. Buying organic also ensures that you avoid genetically modified (also called genetically engineered) cotton, which is environmentally questionable. Organic cotton wool is just as effective – and really is as pure as it says.

MOISTURE, MOISTURE

Our mothers had it so easy. A dab of Pond's Cold Cream, a smear of Vaseline. But today the shelves groan with moisturizer choices. Here's how to decide what's right for you...

Moisturizers are generally a mix of oil and water with some added ingredients. They should make skin feel gorgeous. Dewy-but-not-greasy. Plump and hydrated, preferably velvety. And, of course, perform their most basic functions – making your skin feel comfortable and helping to create a smooth canvas for foundation, if you wear it. But there can be vast differences in price between a mass brand and a "cult" version (invariably "worn by half of Hollywood", if you believe all the media beauty hype).

The choice is yours. You can get bells-and-whistles moisturizers that tout sun protection (we test these on page 74) and/or their anti-aging benefits (you'll find the best of these in our Tried & Tested Miracle Creams on page 70). And, of course, you can buy high-tech or natural – even organic. But if your goal is to find a good no-frills moisturizer, the key is simply to find one you like using, suits your skin and provides a good base for makeup. And which suits your budget: a moisturizer doesn't have to break the bank to do a good job. So, if you're shopping around, try small sizes (preferably samples), and check out cheaper brands.

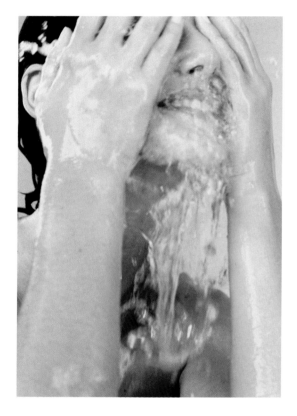

According to the experts, the word "moisturizer" is actually a bit of a misnomer. It's a myth that the moisture in a moisturizer sinks into the skin like liquid into a sponge. Mostly, the water evaporates within seconds of application – that's why moisturizers feel cool when you put them on. A formulation that feels deliciously watery may not actually "moisturize" the skin very well at all. What a moisturizer actually does is sit on the surface of the skin – a bit like a raincoat – and prevent water loss by improving skin's "barrier function".

Hang around in skincare circles and you'll hear the phrase "barrier function" bandied around a lot. When we're young, this barrier tends to behave perfectly – keeping water in and irritants, pollution and even germs out. As we age, the skin thins – partly as a result of sun damage and exposure to pollution and/or smoke, and partly as a natural part of getting older. Water escapes more easily – which is why skin tends to feel drier and tighter (and why we start to need moisturizers). The dry indoor atmosphere in which we live can literally suck the moisture out of skin. If the relative humidity drops from 60 percent to 20 percent, the level of skin hydration plummets by 10 percent, which is a lot

The dry indoor atmosphere in which we live can literally suck the moisture out of skin

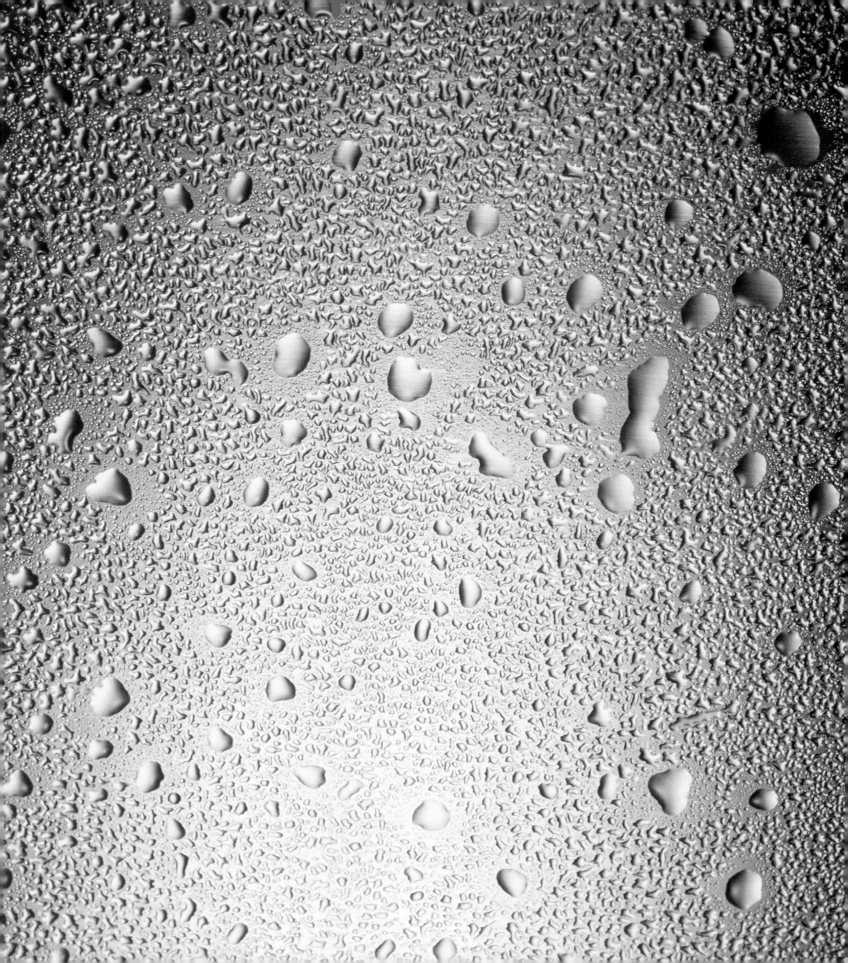

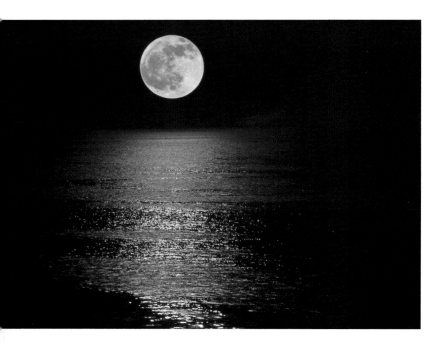

in skin terms. So moisturizers trap the skin's own, natural moisture by putting a fine film on the surface. They generally do this with a combination of oils and skin-compatible "lipids". Lipids are the fats that fill in the spaces between the skin-cell layers (think of the way that mortar holds bricks together), preventing moisture loss.

As an insurance policy against skin damage in summer, your moisturizer should feature an SPF 15. (For more on whether you need that protection year-round, see page 72.) As a better-safe-than-sorry tactic, we definitely advise buying a moisturizer that includes antioxidant vitamins in the mix – such as vitamins A, C and E, as well as pine bark extract and/or polyphenols (from grapes or olive, for instance). They are now available at every price level.

Does every skin need a moisturizer? No, not absolutely every one. For more on your skin type and its needs, see pages 84–8.

DO YOU NEED A SEPARATE NIGHT CREAM?

The cosmetics industry says: "yes". John Gustafson – the TV beauty pundit and independent skincare advisor – insists "No – as long as the one that you're using does everything you want it to. If you're happy with your day cream, sure, use it at night. Let's face it, most of us want a short-cut." (Though you might want to read what we say on page 72 about overloading skin with SPFs before wearing yours at night as well.) Eve Lom, however, in common with facial exercise expert Eva Fraser, counsels clients to go naked, face-wise, at night – no cream, no lotion, no serum—so that skin can "rebalance" all on its own. But the initial sensation of tautness takes some getting used to – we, personally, can't hack it.

WATER WORKS: Most home and office environments are very drying to skin, literally sucking the moisture out of our complexions. If you keep the humidity level higher at home and in the office, your skin will love you for it. Plants can help – especially if you mist them regularly, and keep them well-watered. So can balancing a dish of water on – or near – a radiator. (Jo keeps a humidity-tester on her desk – a freebie from a mineral water company – and takes action if the humidity dips.)

TIP: We've often read that applying a moisturizer to damp skin "traps" the moisture. This just isn't true. What actually happens is that your moisturizer gets diluted so the hydrating ingredients are applied less generously than the manufacturer intended. Always blot skin dry with a fluffy towel before applying any type of cream.

TIP: Never apply moisturizer in a downwards direction – it drags skin; use upwards, sweeping movements that fight the effect of gravity on your face.

MIRACLE CREAMS

*Today, creams and lotions really can turn back the clock.
It's time to start believing in miracles...*

We stopped being cynical about miracle creams a couple of books ago, having sent our testers "anti-aging" lotions, potions and serums to try on half their faces. We started to get letters back from some testers – after just a few weeks – asking if they could start using the creams on both sides, as they felt their faces were starting to look "uneven"! (We've had the same response this time.)

So while medical doctors often pour scorn on anti-aging creams – "women waste thousands in war against wrinkles" was a recent headline – we say: women aren't that stupid. (And certainly only make repeat purchases if they feel a cream has delivered what it promises.) While prevention is always better than cure – a diligent skincare ritual, staying out of the sun, exercising and eating well – we truly believe that some of these creams do have an age-defying effect. This was confirmed, yet again, by the Tried & Testeds carried out for this book – which you can read on page 70.

These products do, however, have tradeoffs. Any cream that has an "action" – for instance, chemically exfoliating the very top layers of skin so that it looks brighter – may trigger a "reaction". (This is why some women experience sensitivity to "miracle" creams, and can't continue using them.) We'd advise always getting a sample to try, whenever possible, just to establish that you like the smell and how the product feels on your skin, and that you don't suffer any reactions to it. If you have sensitive skin, try a patch test on the inner arm, near the elbow. If the

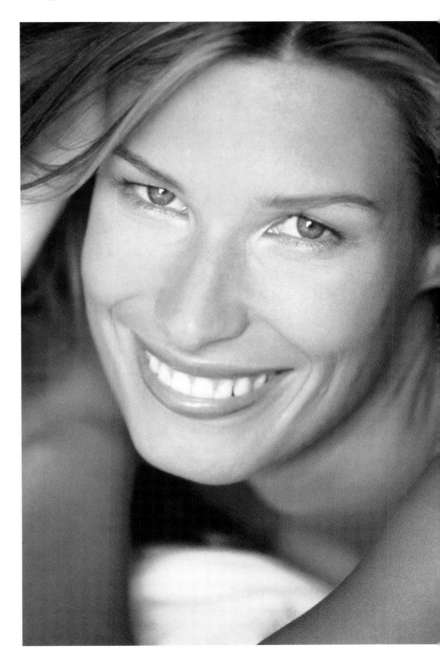

*Medical doctors may sometimes pour
scorn on anti-aging creams but
we say: women aren't that stupid*

beauty counter won't give you a sample, roll up your sleeve and give yourself a patch test – right there and then. Leave the cream in place for 24 hours (no bathing or showering) then look for any signs of redness, itching, swelling or soreness. It's not a foolproof system but it may be helpful, especially if you're prone to reactions. (Remember, just because a product is natural doesn't mean it won't cause problems. Rosehip seed oil, for instance, is rich in vitamin A – and is a potent anti-ager. But when Jo applies this to her skin, she develops sore, flaky red patches, just as she does with more chemically based vitamin A creams. Sarah's eyes swell up whenever they encounter the herb eyebright.)

We're not going to blind you with science about miracle creams. (If you want the optional science lesson, see opposite.) We're just going to help you take a shortcut to choices that real women, with real lives, have found to really work.

CAN YOU MIX AND MATCH YOUR SKINCARE?

Absolutely. Don't believe a salesperson who insists that, for optimal benefits, you should slavishly use an entire product line. In most cases, products do not have "synergistic" benefits which would enhance their individual actions when they are used together. Feel free to mix and match brands, but beware of "overloading" skin with anti-aging products. Never use both an AHA and a vitamin A-based product at the same time; less is definitely more here. When in doubt consult your dermatologist. Or ask at a skincare counter. But be aware that it is basically their job to try and encourage you to buy the most expensive regime, rather than point you in the direction of the simplest.

TIP: Preferably, go skincare shopping with no makeup on so that you can apply a cream to your face and see if you like it. If that's not possible and you can't get your hands on a sample, always buy the smallest size of a product first-time-around. And if you do have any kind of adverse reaction to a product – any kind of rash or stinging – you should be entitled to a refund, so take it back. If the sales person gives you a hard time, ask to speak to a supervisor, then contact the manufacturer, as well as the store manager, and write to them both detailing what happened.)

THE ACID TEST

We'd like to give a word of caution about AHAs – alpha-hydroxy or "fruit acids" – which were all the rage in miracle creams a few years ago, although they are less widely used now. (Incidentally, "fruit acid" is usually a misnomer. While the suggestion is that these ingredients come straight from a bowl of apples or a piece of sugar cane, those used in most cosmetics are mostly synthetic versions of botanicals.) We have both experienced rather extreme reactions to these, when used over a period of time – in Jo's case, they triggered a recurring sensitivity after just one or two applications of products containing different fruit acids, resulting in "facial flakiness". (They do, after all, work by exfoliation.) If you have sensitive skin, we'd advise avoiding fruit acid-based creams – even if the manufacturers make claims for the product's "gentle" action or use phrases like "buffering" to describe how they've been formulated into a product. AHAs work by removing the top layers of skin, to reveal fresher, newer layers beneath. (As do vitamin A-based creams.) But those 15 or so layers of our skin were put there for a reason – protection. Whenever you use an exfoliating cream—wear an SPF 15 by day.

GLOSSARY

Here are some of the ingredients you're likely to find in more high-tech (and particularly anti-aging) products – and what they claim to do. We've also included some terms you might find on packaging, to help you decipher "cosmetic-speak".

AHAs a.k.a. alpha-hydroxy/ fruit acids: Although it's possible to use natural fruit acids, many of those found in skincare are likely to be synthesized to replicate the effect of acids from milk, grapes, apples, olives, and more, which can brighten the skin. They work by dissolving the intercellular glue that bonds dead, flaking cells to the skin's surface, uncovering the smooth skin beneath.

Antioxidants: Today, much skincare includes vitamins – usually A, C, E, and sometimes F – to help fight damage from free radicals, which act like cellular terrorists, attacking collagen, cell membranes, and the skin's lipid layer (where its moisture supplies are stored). Antioxidants work by "mopping up" free radicals in the skin, triggered by exposure to sun, pollution, and cigarette smoke.

Beta-hydroxy acids: These acids are close relations to AHAs and work in much the same way, speeding up cell turnover. The best-known is salicylic acid (from willow bark). The same cautions should apply.

Collagen/elastin: Vital elements within the skin, necessary for skin elasticity and smoothness; over time, production of these slows down. However, you can't boost your skin's supplies of collagen and elastin from the outside.

Enzymes: Enzymes are naturally present in the skin, but when incorporated into skincare, they gently and thoroughly rid the surface layer of dead, dry cells. Enzymes (often derived from papaya) digest dead skin cells without harming living cells or irritating the skin.

Humectants: Ingredients that attract moisture from the air to the surface of the skin, including glycerine, sorbitol, squalene and urea.

Hypoallergenic: Some companies make the claim that their product is "hypoallergenic", meaning that many of the known irritants have been screened-out. But that's no guarantee a product is trouble-free, since some women may be sensitive to ingredients that most of us are tolerant to. In addition, extra chemicals may be added to hypoallergenic products to mask the fragrance.

Liposomes: High-tech skincare "bullets" which can be launched – filled with their anti-aging cargo – into the epidermis, so delivering their moisturizing ingredients deeper than would otherwise be possible. (But remember: they're cosmetics, and so can't actually create lasting physiological changes in the skin itself.)

Nanospheres: A fancy term for small, rounded particles. They're a "second generation" liposome, developed from the same technology.

Non-comedogenic: This means the cosmetics have been specially formulated so as not to clog the pores, and so reduce the risk of producing blackheads and other blemishes.

Oxygen: The idea is that oxygen delivered to the skin's surface in a cream will improve cellular activity and turnover. However, the only foolproof way to deliver oxygen to your skin is to take a brisk walk, or engage in some other physical activity.

Panthenol/pro-vitamin B5: Derived from vitamin B, this can have a cosmetic (and temporary) "skin-plumping" effect; it's highly conditioning as an ingredient in hair products, too. Gentle and non-irritating.

pH: Most moisturizers are formulated to have a neutral pH – neither too acidic or alkaline for skin. Citric acid and sodium phosphate are among the ingredients used to balance pH.

Retinoids: Vitamin A Palmitate, in particular, is a widely used "skin-firming" ingredient. It's a relative of Retin-A – a prescription-only skin drug which is believed to reactivate sluggish collagen production.

SPF: Sun Protection Factor – an indication of how much additional time a sunscreen product will allow the user to remain in the sun without burning. (However, the actual "safe" time may be shorter than you'd think – see page 142 for more details.)

MIRACLE CREAMS – *Tried & Tested*

There's a war on wrinkles – and it's being waged by all the big names in the beauty business, with billions of dollars at stake. The amount of money channelled into diminishing our laugh lines, frown lines and age spots – not to mention sags and bags – is mind-boggling. And so is the hype: you'll have seen the promises in ads in glossy magazines and TV. Hope in a jar? Or false promise?

We tested the claims by giving our ten-woman panels the ultimate challenge: we asked them to apply each product, over a period of months, to one side of their face and compare the results with their usual product to assess the contrast (if any). They were then asked to fill in detailed questionnaires. The benefits were, in some cases, extraordinary – as you can see here – with reports of lines reduced, fresher, brighter, more radiant skin, plumpness, firmer tone, and more.

Having carried out this incredibly exhaustive analysis of literally dozens of creams, serums, and lotions, we've come to two conclusions. Firstly, yes, some do work wonders – turning back the clock just as they say in the ads. And secondly, you don't have to pay a fortune for a cream that works "miracles" – the word our testers used repeatedly – because some of the top-scoring products in this category won't break the bank. Our 'natural choice' (look for the daisy), didn't score quite as highly as some of the high-tech creams, but still did extremely well in this super-challenging category and is also moderately priced.

The good news, then, is that whatever you want to spend on a miracle cream – and whether you want high-science or the power of botanical skin-savers – there's a cream out there that really can make a difference to your skin. However, as you'll see from the Downside comments, your mileage may vary. So always try and get samples before you splash out and buy.

ESTÉE LAUDER RE-NUTRIV ULTIMATE LIFTING
8.4 points out of 10

With its ritzy packaging and sky-high price tag, this is truly in the realm of skin luxuries. Active turn-back-the-clock ingredients include antioxidant green tea and resveratrol, white birch extracts, creatine (an amino acid). Most of our testers agreed that the only downside to this highly-effective cream is the price.

UPSIDE: "This cream is definitely a miracle cream – it changed my skin from dry to glowing and although I didn't have deep lines, my fine lines have almost gone" • "definite improvements in skintone and texture – a gorgeous cream to use" • "reduction in lines on neck, bright radiant glow to skin; my open pores are also diminished. Lovely to use" • "made my skin velvety-soft and even without makeup, my complexion didn't look as sluggish".

DOWNSIDE: "Could see no difference compared to my usual anti-aging product" • "I preferred to use this at night as if I used it in the morning, I had to wait half an hour before applying makeup – it's slow to absorb".

ELEMIS PRO-COLLAGEN MARINE CREAM
8.4 points out of 10

This is the first serious anti-aging cream from the respected international 'spa' brand, incorporating gingko biloba (to boost circulation), seaweed extracts (the 'marine' element), absolutes of rose and mimosa, in a nourishing base incorporating carrot seed extract, jojoba oil and shea butter.

UPSIDE: "This really is a miracle cream – a little goes a long way so although it's expensive, it should last a long time" • "people (men) at work seem to be giving me a second look and I feel much more confident after using it – I've seen a dramatic improvement" • "I was very sceptical that any product claiming to reduce lines/wrinkles would work – but I've been proved wrong, I'm hooked!" • "this will be on my Christmas list as a special treat" • "please send me a bucket-full of this cream!".

DOWNSIDE: "I have oily skin and this seemed to make it more pronounced" • "richness of cream is too heavy for an oilier skin".

BEST BUDGET BUY
ALMAY KINETIN AGE DECELERATING DAILY MOISTURE CREAM SPF 15 (UVA/UVB)
8.28 points out of 10

This rich, nourishing formula features an exclusive ingredient called (you guessed it) kinetin, which used to be available by prescription only: it's a highly stable antioxidant from green, leafy plants. This cream is 100 percent fragrance-free and allergy-tested (Almay is famous for that), and also features an SPF 15. With one exception, our testers were wowed. It was easily the most affordable of the creams that did well – less than one-tenth of the price of some of the winners, in fact – so definitely earns our 'Best Budget Buy' in this category.

UPSIDE: "I'm addicted – fabulous! Gives that "I just had a facial feeling" – soft and smooth to the touch, perfectly moisturized" • "this cream has made a significant difference – lines minimized, especially round the eyes and mouth" • "after eight weeks' use, this melted years off my face" • "overjoyed with the results – skin's smoother, looks younger, glows, elasticity's been restored; my boyfriend and mom have both noticed a difference in my skin" • "perfect under makeup" • "skin brighter, fresher, slightly younger; fine lines improved, some improvement on forehead furrow".

DOWNSIDE: "I experienced excessive oil and a breakout".

PHILOSOPHY WHEN HOPE IS NOT ENOUGH SERUM
8.2 points out of 10

This 'sister' product to the original Hope In A Jar – see below – scored even higher marks with the group of ten women who tried it. A light fluid gel, it can be worn under moisturizer on drier skin, and has amino acid peptide technology with a large dollop of skin-brightening vitamin C.

UPSIDE: "Lives up to its promise – quite noticeable reduction in bigger grooves and wrinkles, as well as a moderate improvement in crepiness" • "brilliant stuff – my skin looks like I've had a facelift, and several people have said that I'm looking well" • "made my skin look like I live on a healthy diet of fruit and water – and I couldn't stop touching its baby-softness" • "it took about two weeks to see the difference but it was worth the wait – didn't even feel the need to wear makeup, some days" • "love the pipet-style dispenser – very scientific, yet the smell is herbal, floral, very 'holistic' and natural" • "also claims to retard hair growth

which amazingly appeared true – upper hair regrowth on my top lip slowed down".

DOWNSIDE: None of our testers had a negative word to say about this.

PHILOSOPHY HOPE IN A JAR
8.14 points out of 10

This cream, with its tongue-in-cheek name. is a favorite with celebrities and makeup artists – and comes in versions for normal to dry skin, (which we tested), and also combination.

UPSIDE: "Fantastic – beautiful texture, and my skin is younger, brighter, firmer and more radiant" • "I have sensitive skin and this is the first product I've had no reaction to – silky, luxurious, a real treat to use" • "skin brighter, almost glowing, with an improvement in fine lines – I loved this" • "fine lines have reduced over 12 weeks – I'm finding it difficult not to use it on the left side; it will have some catching up to do!" • "lasts forever, with the most wonderful velvety texture – skin's 100 percent brighter" • "people are commenting I look younger than my age; my husband can see a difference, too".

DOWNSIDE: "Packaging impossible – I had to resort to scissors!" • "not so much a miracle cream, more a nice moisturizer".

CARITA LA CRÈME PARFAITE
7.95 points out of 10

A delicate, pink cream designed to be used morning and evening, this luxurious product has a very hefty price tag. Carita claim the reason their creams feel so light, soft and easily-absorbed – which our testers certainly all commented on – is that they're spun ten times faster than other creams!

UPSIDE: "I always thought anti-aging creams were fraudulent but have been delighted by the results – much safer than Botox!" • "definitely made skin appear brighter and smoother" • "great as an intensive neck cream" • "a little goes a long way – smoothes on easily and effectively" • "fixed my permanently

dehydrated skin – no more fine lines or scaly bits" • "loved the texture and perfume which didn't irritate my sensitive skin, unlike many creams".

DOWNSIDE: "Smell is a turn-off – too synthetic" • "good moisturizer, but not effective on me as an anti-aging cream".

✿ ORIGINS MAKE A DIFFERENCE
7.85 points out of 10

This was the highest-scoring out of the more natural ranges we tested. Although not 100 percent natural, Origins – a more natural division of the Estée Lauder empire – does pledge to avoid petrochemical ingredients, and use generous quantities of botanicals in their formulations. A lightweight cream-gel, its active ingredients include algae, a corn-derived sugar and Rose of Jericho, known for its ability to withstand almost total dehydration.

UPSIDE: "This really is a miracle cream – by far the best moisturizer I've used, delivering excellent results; work colleagues have commented how well I look" • "my sister said I looked "plumped-up" and my skin definitely looked healthy and smooth" • "I've really enjoyed using this – the smell and texture are gorgeous and it's worth sticking with as the results just keep getting better" • "I look less tired" • "skin is brighter – I just look more healthy" • "I really loved this delicious product and will buy more when it runs out" • "particularly liked using this in the morning as the aromatic smell perked me up – top marks all-round, and I will definitely buy it again".

DOWNSIDE: "Difficult to use under makeup – I tried several times" • "had no effect".

The lowest score in this category was 4.2 points out of 10.

THE TRUTH ABOUT SPF 15

Skincare companies and dermatologists have drummed it into us: "Coat yourself with SPF 15, even in winter, even on a cloudy day, even in cities like Seattle and Stockholm." But you just might be overloading your skin if you follow that advice

Certainly, when it comes to anti-aging, who'd question that prevention is better than cure? But for anyone with sensitive skin, there may be a good reason for slathering on that SPF 15 only in summer months or sunny places.

Put simply, chemical sunscreens can irritate some people. And there's a growing concern among some health professionals about the overall load of chemicals our systems have to cope with – many of which are absorbed through the skin. Certainly, reports of sensitization are rising. As Dr. Daniel Maes at Estée Lauder (one of the companies which actually pioneered daily sun protection

In places where you'd go for a sunny vacation – anywhere from California to Australia, from Italy to the Caribbean (and any ski resort, where sunlight will be reflected off snow) – then yes, an SPF 15 is definitely the absolute minimum daily requirement. For simplicity, you should choose one of the many daily moisturizers that are formulated with this "magic number". It's still best to keep your face out of the sun whenever you can, at all times, though. Think: shade, hats, beach umbrellas. And remember: you'll need to reapply sun protection during the day.

Experience and history have simply told us that people who spend lots of time in the sun end up with wrinkly, damaged skin, say experts

in moisturizers) observes, "There is an increasing amount of data that shows that the regular application of sunscreen on the skin can lead to a reaction."

The problem, he says, is that most chemical sunscreens work by penetrating the skin – and some complexions rebel against that, with redness, stinging, tingling or eczema-like eruptions. (Armed with this information, Estée Lauder now "buffers" its sunscreen ingredients with a special polymer so that they can't penetrate the skin, making sensitivity far less likely. But Lauder – often one step ahead – is in the minority on this.)

But every day, during winter months, in other areas of the world? Experts are unconvinced (and so are we). On overcast, rainy or gloomy days, or times in spring/autumn/winter when all your skin's going to see of daylight is nipping out for a sandwich at lunchtime, or walking from the train station to the office, then SPF 15 is overkill.

One of the arguments against using an SPF 15, explains Mike Brown, a UK-based Boots Scientific Suncare Advisor, is that "SPF 15 ratings only measure protection against UVB rays – the burning rays – but in winter, in northern countries, there's a negligible amount of UVB around. There is, however, a small amount of UVA (aging) light – although even there, winter exposure only adds up to about 10 per cent of annual UVA exposure." Having said that, he adds, "Nobody yet knows what a 'safe' level of UVA exposure is. Experience and history have simply told us that people who spend lots of time in the sun end up with wrinkly, damaged skin."

So tap into your common sense here, says Professor Nicholas Lowe, M.D., Consultant Dermatologist, Cranley Clinic, London and Santa Monica, California, and Clinical Professor at UCLA. "If you're going skiing or spending a lot of time outdoors, if you're playing golf, or walking on a bright winter's day when there's frost on the ground – then yes, an SPF 15 is a bright idea."

If you suffer from melasma – aka "mask of pregnancy", a hormone-linked condition in which patches of skin can darken when exposed to sunlight (which can also be a problem for some Pill-takers) – an SPF 15 "will also prevent worsening, and may even help to lighten skin again," adds Professor Lowe.

We suggest applying a generous dollop of common sense rather than an extra layer of chemicals. Why not try listening to your instincts? Watching the weather forecast? And – when it's raining cats and dogs, or just downright gloomy – giving your skin a sunscreen break?

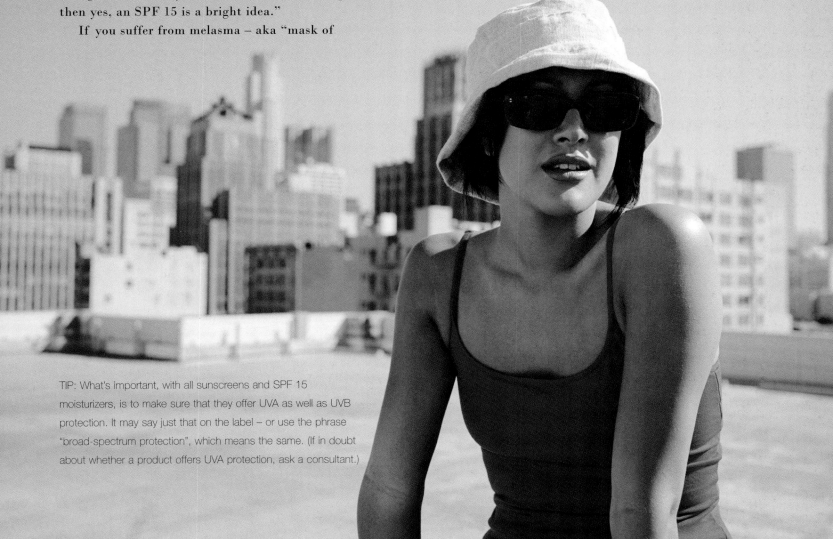

TIP: What's important, with all sunscreens and SPF 15 moisturizers, is to make sure that they offer UVA as well as UVB protection. It may say just that on the label – or use the phrase "broad-spectrum protection", which means the same. (If in doubt about whether a product offers UVA protection, ask a consultant.)

SPF 15 MOISTURIZERS – *Tried & Tested*

As we've explained (see page 72), these offer UV protection in a moisturizer – so that you don't need to layer sunscreen over it. However, scanning the ingredients lists for the products our testers rated, all contain synthetic sunscreens – so we felt that, so far, there's no true 'natural' option in this category. If you're into naturals, your best bet still seems to be layering – putting a titanium- or zinc oxide-based sunscreen over your regular moisturizer. Or you could try mixing an SPF 30 sunblock, half-and-half, with your usual day cream.

L'OCCITANE SHEA BUTTER ULTRA MOISTURIZING DAY CARE SPF 15
8.6 points out of 10

Shea butter, which comes from the crushed ground kernels of shea tree nuts, is used traditionally by the women of Burkina Faso in Central Africa to keep their skins as soft as a baby's. With added vitamin A and sunflower oil, this product proved popular for dry skins.

UPSIDE: "Lovely cream which massaged into skin and felt very nourishing but was then totally absorbed to give good base for makeup" • "I really like this product – skin felt hydrated, had good firm texture and makeup went on well" • "would most definitely buy product – excellent for days out during cold winter months as well as summer" • "felt lovely to apply and afterwards left my skin very soft".

DOWNSIDE: "So thick you have to be careful not to put too much on – a little definitely goes a long way" • "skin looked shiny and I came out in little spots – would be great for very dry skins".

CLARINS HYDRATION-PLUS MOISTURE LOTION SPF 15
8.56 points out of 10

This leading science-meets-nature French brand has now crammed an SPF 15 into one of its bestselling moisturizers – and, according to Clarins' own research, "it not only has an immediate hydrating action but actually increases the skin's long-term ability to retain moisture". Our testers were all very impressed; in fact, none had a bad word to say about it.

UPSIDE: "A classic product and a brilliant moisturizer" • "featherweight – you don't feel it's there" • "excellent; makes you feel a million dollars! And I like the pump dispenser" • "at last – a non-oily SPF lotion for my face" • "a pleasure to use" • "makeup went on really well, within minutes" • "a really good moisturizer, without being greasy or heavy".

DOWNSIDE: None.

OLAY TOTAL EFFECTS TIME RESIST MOISTURIZER SPF 15
8.37 points out of 10

This anti-aging moisturizer features Total Effects' unique ingredient VitaNiacin, which is made up of the skin-enhancing vitamins niacinamide, panthenol and vitamin E. It offers "broad-spectrum" protection, shielding skin against aging UVA rays as well as against burning UVB.

UPSIDE: "Does what it says – reducing fine lines and wrinkles, and improving skin tone; gives skin a healthy glow, too" • "excellent sun protection – even on a week's holiday in Cyprus" • "this product was very effective on my mature skin, nice to use too, and made me feel confident" • "delivered a smoother, slightly firmer appearance after two weeks" • "fresh, summer-flowers fragrance".

DOWNSIDE: "Makeup went on slightly patchily" • "a bit tacky for a while".

BEST BUDGET BUY
L'ORÉAL PLENITUDE ACTIV.FUTUR MULTI–PROTECTION HEALTHY GLOW FLUID
8.06 points out of 10

A synergy of grape polyphenols and pure vitamin E (both antioxidants) offers protection in this lightweight, non-greasy, delicately fragranced moisturizing cream from L'Oréal's advanced scientific labs, which also work on developments for the pricier Lancôme lines.

UPSIDE: "Very comfortable – and makeup went on very well afterwards" • "gave my face a very matte appearance – which is good for immediate makeup application" • "felt expensive and nourishing" • "easy-to-use pump bottle and non-messy; lightweight to travel with" • "my skin actually seemed to glow through my foundation" • "loved this one – makeup glided on and hid lines better".

DOWNSIDE: "I needed to use a lot of this product".

The lowest score in this category was 5.1 points out of 10.

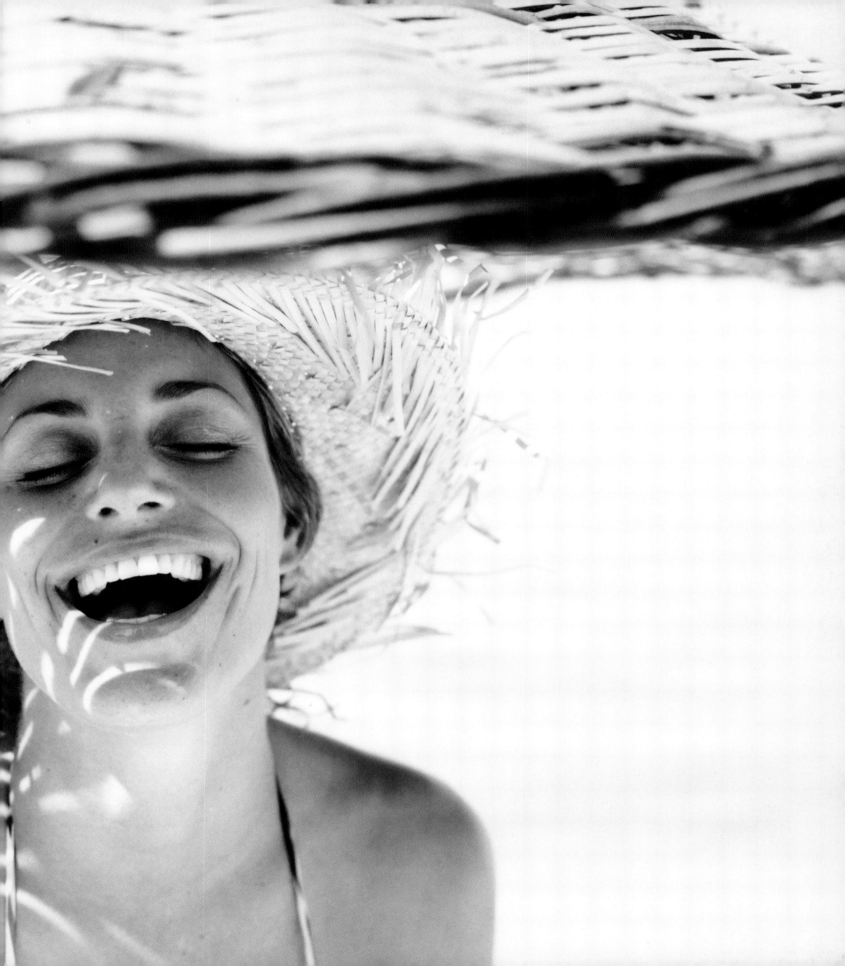

THE NECK'S BEST THING

Photos can be cruel. Those unposed moments when we're captured with a canapé midway to our mouth and not two but three – or more – chins, topping a scraggy neck. Hasn't happened to you yet? Count yourself lucky – and discover how to make your neck zone smoother and more swan-like...

Necks are a serious beauty challenge. With fewer oil glands than elsewhere on the body, they get dry and crepey sooner than our faces. (Often, in fact, giving our age away faster than our passports!)

At the same time, because we move our heads constantly, the collagen and elastin fibers get loosened – leading to sagging. One of the major reasons that women complain of tired and baggy necks, though, is downright neglect. Skincare often stops at the jawline, whereas in some cultures – France, for instance – the décolletage area is treated with as much TLC as a woman's face. And it shows!

But creams, we have discovered, can offer the possibility of truly dramatic improvement (if not quite turning you into Audrey Hepburn overnight). The neck treatments our testers assessed for this book were some of the highest-scoring products of all (see page 78). So while we're all for decluttering the bathroom shelf, this is one product that many women could benefit from adding to their beauty regime. Meanwhile, here's more wisdom on how to keep your neck as unlined and elegant as possible. (While keeping those extra chins at bay.)

✳ Cleanse your neck as thoroughly at night as you do your face, and wipe with a hot, wet washcloth in the morning.

✳ Give necks the "double-whammy" treatment. Every time you apply a moisturizer or sunscreen to your face, include your neck and bosom. And every time you slather on a body moisturizer, sweep it upwards to the jawline. That way, neck skin will never go thirsty.

✳ Always use upward strokes when applying neck creams – it really does make a difference.

✳ Protect the neck area whenever you're in strong sunlight (and throughout the summer months) with an SPF 15 moisturizer. There is no greater age giveaway than mock croc skin and no greater flatterer than a luscious décolleté.

✳ Beware of wearing fragrance in the sun; psoralens (ingredients usually found in citrusy fragrances) can cause permanent staining. In summer, spritz your clothing instead. (Having first established that your fragrance won't stain fabric.)

✳ To help avoid a double chin, keep your reading matter at eye level – which means not reading in bed, unless you lie back and hold the book above you. Do not prop it on your chest and peer down at it.

✳ Take up yoga. We know seventy-something yoga devotees with sharp jawlines and smooth, unlined necks, who chalk it up to the stretching. Also, when you're sitting at your desk or in front of TV, allow your neck to fall gently backwards, then bring it slowly upright. Use your cupped hands to support your head if your neck is stiff. If you hear cracking sounds, don't worry, but if it's painful stop immediately and consult a chiropractor.

✳ If all else fails, resort to turtlenecks. (Note: the most flattering results and neatest neckline come from reversing the "tube", so that the neck material is tucked inside rather than folded outside.)

✳ If you have a short and/or thick neck, create an illusion of length by wearing open necklines with wide collars, and V-necks which reveal as much of your cleavage as you feel comfortable with. Also see our Hair section (pages 174–6) for tips on minimizing thick necks.

TIP: Bharti Vyas (whose stellar clientele includes Cher and Cherie Blair) advises: "Eat one raw carrot after every meal – good for the skin, and chewing gives facial muscles a workout, keeping saggy jowls at bay."

NECK CREAMS – *Tried & Tested*

While neck creams deliver instant nourishing benefits, smoothing and firming the appearance temporarily, long-term results require dedicated daily (or twice-daily) use. So our testers were assigned just one neck cream to try on neck and décolletage over a period of at least two months before reporting back. For such a notoriously difficult area to treat, we were truly amazed – and delighted – by the winners' high scores. The bottom line: some neck creams really do work miracles.

CLARINS EXTRA-FIRMING NECK CREAM
9.19 points out of 10

Active ingredients in this cream include ginseng, mallow extract and honey (which is moisturizing), as well as antioxidant vitamin E and rice extracts. For optimal results, Clarins recommends exfoliating the neck once a week to remove dead cells. (We say: use your muslin cloth – see page 63 – rather than a scrub, which is way too harsh for this vulnerable area.)

UPSIDE: "Increasing improvement, especially in the crepey skin at the middle/front of the neck; lovely, spring-like flower smell, too" • "under my chin is firmer and less saggy" • "neck looks much younger and smoother – my neck seemed really grateful!" • "loose skin tighter and far less lined" • "noticed a fading of brown spots caused by the sun and the Pill" • "the area under my jawline and chin is firmer and more defined" • "will buy it and recommend to friends without hesitation" • "delicious – and a little goes a long way" • "lines on my neck had totally disappeared by the end of the two months' trial period".

DOWNSIDE: absolutely none.

CHANEL ULTRA CORRECTION ANTI-WRINKLE RESTRUCTURING LOTION SPF 10
9 points out of 10

Chanel prescribes a ritual massage to enhance the benefits of this cream, which our testers followed diligently. Some of them were so impressed with the results on their neck they couldn't resist using this on their faces, too. It contains glutamic acid (which helps to strengthen skin's self-defense mechanism), licorice (to regulate hyperpigmentation), emollient canola oil, and shea butter, and a vitamin E derivative – and offers UVA/UVB protection with an SPF 10.

UPSIDE: "My neck has lost its greyness and is not so crêpey-looking" • "skin looked very smooth and 'clean', and bad lines on my lower neck – from sun damage – are less visible" • "wonderful – used it on my face, too, and fine lines are not so pronounced" • "rich texture, smelled like heaven; making the effort to massage the neck makes me aware how much better the skin seemed; in fact, the best cream I've ever used" • "my dermatologist said my skin was very moist and smoother than usual – three weeks after finishing this, I realise how good it was so have splurged out on another jar" • "skin looks plump and well-fed – appears to be 'lifted' ".

DOWNSIDE: "Neck area still felt a bit rough to the touch".

LANCASTER SURACTIF NECK AND DÉCOLLETÉ TREATMENT
8.8 points out of 10

This rich but, say the makers, "non-oily" product delivers retinol (vitamin A) and other "enriching" ingredients including borage to boost cell renewal and leave skin feeling soft, supple and moisturized. It also features a UV filter to help shield against future damage.

UPSIDE: "Melted into skin with a divine, 'couture-like' fragrance – and gave excellent results" • "miraculous improvement – my very fair skin looked white, rather than grey, and was much brighter and dewier" • "chest shows the most improvement in crepiness and the softening of some scarring" • "goodbye ugly duckling neck – I now have the neck of a swan!".

DOWNSIDE: "Used this on my face and got a few pimples – which I don't normally get". (Well, it wasn't designed for the face but for the thinner skin of the neck.)

BEST BUDGET BUY
❀ LIZ EARLE NATURALLY ACTIVE SKIN REPAIR MOISTURIZER
7.85 points out of 10

This scoops both the 'Natural Winner' title and the 'Best Budget Buy', and is actually a facial nourisher that works well when used morning and evening on the chest and upper neck. Botanicals – which are featured in very generous levels (unlike many so-called 'natural' creams) – include echinacea, borage oil, avocado oil, beta-carotene, hop extract, and wheatgerm, which is naturally very high in vitamin E. Our testers clearly loved this cream, which is available in versions for Dry/Sensitive and Normal/Combination skins.

UPSIDE: "My neck area – which has a tendency to be crepey – is smooth and soft, with a significant difference" • "smells divine – nice creamy texture, which left skin smoother and soft" • "luscious, pampering cream literally melts into skin" • "I'm just raving about this – it does more than it says on the jar" • "cleavage – achieved with Wonderbra in Xmas party frock – wasn't as crepey" • "neck looked less like plucked chicken skin and the cream gave skin a lovely sheen and healthy glow".

DOWNSIDE: "Packaging could be more attractive".

❀❀ JURLIQUE NECK SERUM
7.55 points out of 10

This swiftly-absorbed, lightweight gel features high quantities of organic ingredients – and Jurlique (one of our favorite natural companies) assures us that the soy on which it's based is not genetically engineered. Active ingredients include frankincense and myrrh, ginkgo flavonoids, vitamin C and oils of jojoba, rosehip, avocado and evening primrose. (Incidentally, it is not cheap.)

UPSIDE: "My neck looks slightly younger, smoother, more hydrated and clearer" • "definitely less crepiness after just two weeks" • "sinks in fast, with a lovely fresh and natural smell – and lines are less visible" • "without a doubt, skin on neck and décolletage felt noticeably smoother" • "I'm amazed how much smoother my skin feels, with a definite improvement in fine lines".

DOWNSIDE: "Hated the smell".

The lowest score in this category was 6.28 points out of 10.

FABULOUS FACIAL OILS

Facial oils are pure plant goodness – and they work for every skin type. (Yes, even oily skins.) They act on mood as well as complexion, restoring flagging spirits while nourishing, replenishing, balancing, reviving. (And more...)

Many women shy away from using facial oils because they believe they'll leave their skin looking like an oil slick: greasy, shiny, messy. In reality, facial oils are absorbed very quickly, allowing their active ingredients to get to work, delivering intensive skincare benefits. In truth, they're better for nighttime skincare than under daytime makeup – so why not try facial oils to maximize your "beauty sleep", instead of your usual night cream? (Even

once or twice a week, if not every single night, can make a difference.)

We asked award-winning aromatherapist Danièle Ryman – a protégée of aromatherapy's pioneer, Marguerite Maury, and now acknowledged by *The Times* of London as "the Queen of Aromatherapy" – to prescribe suitable oils for different skin types, as well as an aromatherapy facial massage technique which not only

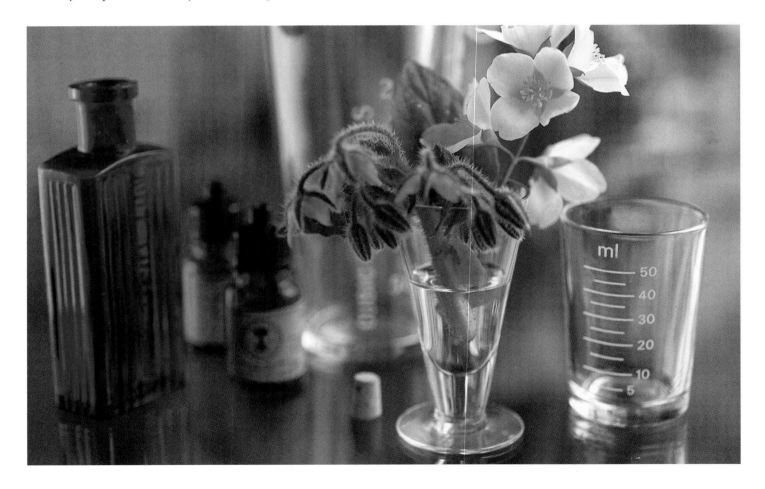

turbo-charges their benefits, but helps put back the glow, fast! Danièle recommends making fairly small quantities of the oil (as in these recipes) and using them while fresh. Ideally, store the oils in blue or amber glass bottles, and definitely keep them in a cool place out of direct sunlight.

Normal Skin

"People with normal skin are lucky as they tend to have few problems," says Danièle. *"But it still needs to be well cared for to keep it supple and balanced."*

1⅗ fl. oz. soy oil (the type used for cooking is fine, but we prefer organic as a lot of other soy oil on the market has been genetically engineered)
⅛ fl. oz. almond oil
2 capsules wheat germ oil (this prevents rancidity – find at health food stores)
8 drops lavender essential oil
4 drops orange essential oil
2 drops geranium essential oil

Pierce and squeeze the capsules to extract the oil; blend with all the ingredients in a 1¾ fl. oz. bottle and use daily or nightly.

Weekly Facial Sauna

Danièle recommends using mineral water for this weekly treatment. Add one drop of one of the essential oils from the facial oil recipe for your skin type to a bowl of hot water; then lean over it and place a thick towel over your head. Stay in that position for a few minutes, then rinse your face with fresh mineral water to which you've added a teaspoon of cider vinegar per cupful of water. (For combination/oily skins, add one drop of geranium essential oil and a pinch of rosemary leaves.)

Combination Skin

"Most of the time you can treat this as if it was normal," explains Danièle, *"but if the sebaceous glands in the T-zone – the nose, forehead and chin – flare up (which they may do in periods of stress or before a period), it's advisable to treat the area with a facial oil prescribed for an oily skin."*

2½ fl. oz. soy oil (see comments, left)
¾ fl. oz. almond oil
1 capsule of wheat germ oil
1 capsule of evening primrose oil
6 drops geranium essential oil
4 drops palmarosa essential oil
1 drop tea tree essential oil

Shake well and leave in a dark place at room temperature for a few days to give the oils time to reach their full potential.

Aging Skin

This recipe's perfect for skin that's lost its bounce, its glow, or is showing any signs of Aging. (It's also good for drinkers, smokers or those who don't get enough exercise.)

1¾ fl. oz. almond oil
⅛ fl. oz. castor oil (available at any pharmacy)
1 tablespoon extra virgin olive oil
1 capsule wheat germ oil
10 drops sandalwood essential oil
8 drops rosewood essential oil
2 drops rose essential oil
2 drops black pepper essential oil

Mix the ingredients together and apply to the skin, preferably using the massage technique on page 83.

Broken Capillaries

"Blood shows through broken capillaries because they are weak and therefore transparent," explains Danièle. "This oil helps to strengthen them."

1 fl. oz. almond oil
½ fl. oz. extra virgin olive oil
3 capsules wheat germ oil
1 capsule evening primrose oil
6 drops sandalwood essential oil
3 drops grapefruit essential oil
2 drops lemon essential oil
2 drops chamomile essential oil

Apply all over the face and neck, morning and night; massage very gently, with no pressure or tugging. (Facial steaming is not recommended for this skin type, as it tends to worsen broken veins.)

Puffy Faces

"This is great when skin's looking puffy – especially under the eyes," says Danièle, "which can happen in people prone to water retention, or sometimes just after an illness."

1 fl. oz. soy oil (see above)
⅓ fl. oz. almond oil
2 capsules wheat germ oil
1 capsule evening primrose oil
8 drops chamomile essential oil
4 drops cypress essential oil
2 drops rose essential oil

Massage into face applying deep pressure around the sinus area and the mouth for a few minutes. Then dip a small towel in a basin of hot water and apply the warm, wet towel to the face a few times. This will help the oil to penetrate and get rid of some of the puffiness.

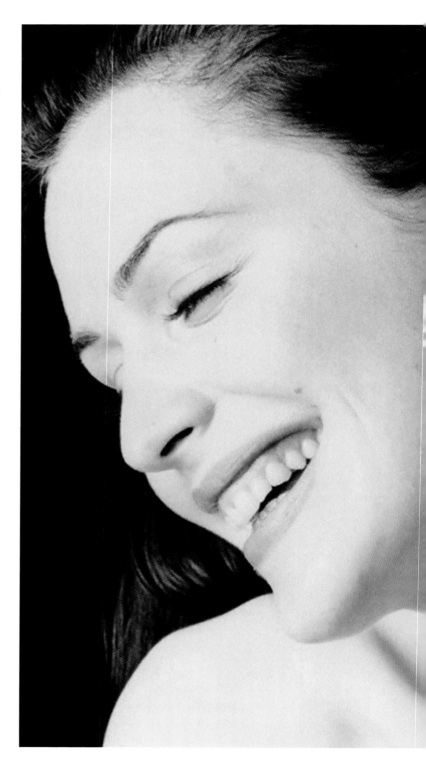

ENERGIZING FACIAL MASSAGE

This technique will optimize the benefits of facial oils, helping to de-puff through lymphatic drainage. "If you do this on a nightly basis, it relaxes the face – relaxes you overall, in fact – and circulates blood to nourish the complexion," says Danièle. (So it's also great for an instant glow before a party.)

1 First of all, secure your hair well back from your face with a headband, so that you can treat the whole face. Apply the oil to your fingertips, and then follow the movements described. Add more oil as required. The oils should sink in within a few minutes, you can then remove the headband without getting your hair oily. (Danièle recommends that, if possible, you also massage the oil into the hairline – but you can skip that if you're not planning on washing your hair or going to your hairdresser in the near future.)

2 Using the pads of your first and middle fingers, and starting between the brows, massage out towards the temples in long, smooth movements. Stop for a moment just at the top of the middle of the brows and press firmly. Stop again at the outer edge of the brow and press firmly. Move up the forehead and repeat the movements, covering the whole forehead.

3 Slide your fingers down your nose and press gently on the sinus pressure points.

4 Put your fingers under your cheekbones and move towards the ears. Move fingers along the bone and press firmly at three points along the cheekbone, between the point where you started and just below the temples.

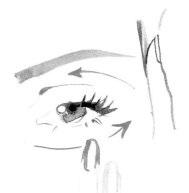

5 Holding the skin around the eyes slightly taut with the fingers of one hand, use the ring finger of the other hand to massage lightly around the orbital bone of the eye, tracing three circles in each direction.

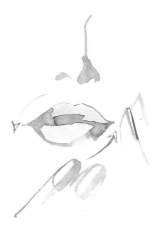

6 Holding your mouth slightly taut, massage lightly in a circular direction around the lips using the first two fingers (as shown on the left), and then reverse. Swap hands, "mirroring" these movements.

7 Using your first two fingers, press the pressure points just under the nostrils.

8 Massage the entire neck, going up behind the ears; press the pressure point just behind and below the ear.

9 Slide your hands up your neck and press into the base of your skull.

10 Use your hands to massage the opposite shoulders, with deep strokes.

SKIN TYPE SOLUTIONS

Different skin types need different care. Here is some wisdom for "problem" skins – sensitive, dry, combination and oily

SENSITIVE SKIN

There's a sensitive skin epidemic. We've got it. You've probably got it. In fact, as many as 63 percent of us claim to have experienced sensitive skin at some point. Even worse, according to some skin experts – like Dr. Daniel Maes, Estée Lauder's vice-president of research and development – it may accelerate the aging process. Says Dr. Maes, "Skin reactions and premature aging go hand in hand." But the good news is that, by following some simple steps, sensitive skin can be calmed, controlled, and even prevented altogether.

✳ Keep it simple. This is (literally) pure logic: the more products you use on your skin, the more likely you are to encounter an ingredient that triggers a reaction. And once your skin's flared up the first time in reaction to an ingredient, it becomes sensitized. So that same "remembered response" happens the next time (and every time) your skin is exposed to it in future.

✳ Do a patch test before buying a new product. If your skin's super-sensitive, this is the only way to know whether it can cope with a new product. Apply a small amount from the "tester unit" in a store to an inconspicuous, soft-skinned spot – such as in the crook of your elbow or behind your ears. (Elbows are easier: if you do it behind your ear, you have to rely on someone else's judgment about whether there's a reaction.) Wait for at least 48, preferably 72 hours to check if there's a reaction: redness or pinkness, flakiness, a raised area or even just a difference in skin texture. If a cream passes the test, try it on a corner of your face – by your temple, for instance – which you can cover with your hair if it flares up.

✳ Introduce new products into your skincare regime one at a time, so you can monitor reactions. Become a label-hound. Scan ingredient lists and see if you can pinpoint "common denominator" ingredients that seem to set off a reaction.

✳ Don't be fooled into believing that "allergy-tested" means "trouble-free". This just means that the most common allergens have been screened out – but it's no guarantee that someone, somewhere, won't have a reaction. Likewise, "fragrance-free" or "unscented" often means there's been an extra dollop of chemicals added to mask the original smell.

The more products you use on your skin, the more likely you are to encounter an ingredient that triggers a reaction

✳ Check your nail polish. Sounds crazy? Formaldehyde and toluene – which are both known irritants – are commonly used in nail polish (and many other products); they can trigger sensitivity because we so often touch our faces, eyelids and necks with our hands. Look for nail polishes that claim to be "toluene-" and "formaldehyde-free", and are now increasingly widely available.

✳ Keep your skin well-watered – literally. Dry skin is often sensitive because its "barrier function" is impaired by tiny cracks in the surface, from the dryness, enabling irritants to sneak in more easily. Replenish your inner reservoir by drinking water – at least eight glasses a day – and create a more humid, complexion-friendly environment at home and in the office with bowls of water (see page 66).

✳ "Summer can trigger many problems for sensitive skins," says Dr. Pat Brosnan, President of the Society for Research into Allergy. "People often have reactions to garden sprays, sunscreens and even to the sun itself. Going on vacation, meanwhile, exposes you to different water, foods, chemicals and temperatures – so you need to boost your immune system by taking a multivitamin supplement to help combat possible flare-ups. And always be sure to rinse skin thoroughly in fresh water after swimming to remove chlorine, which may cause an allergic reaction."

✳ Be aware that chemical sunscreens are very common sensitivity-triggers; look instead for sun products (and facial moisturizers) with mineral sunblock ingredients (i.e. zinc oxide and titanium dioxide), but do a patch test with these, too.

✳ Touchy skin is often a sign of inner angst. (You may notice you're more prone to flare-ups when life's going less than smoothly.) Try stress-busting techniques, get regular massages (or try our D-I-Y massage technique on page 226), and consider meditation. Chill out – and your skin may too.

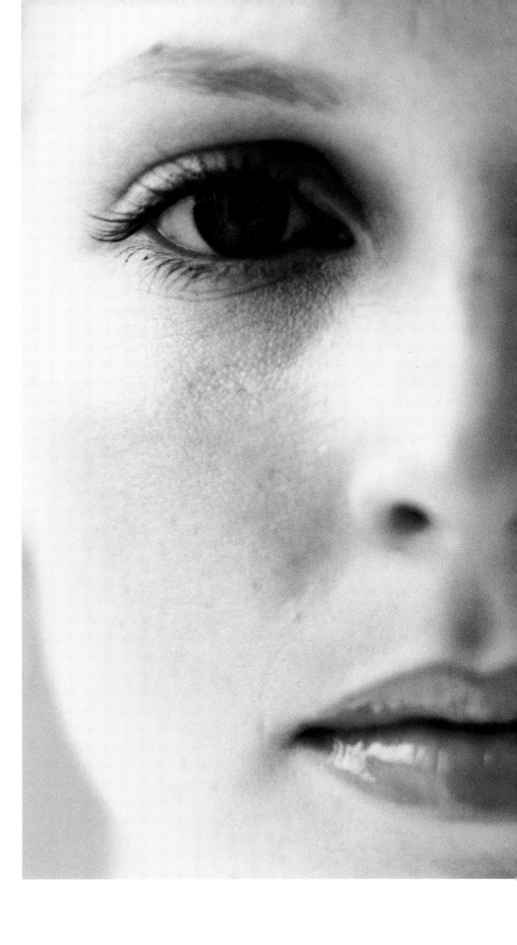

DRY SKIN

It's a myth that dry skin causes wrinkles. (We both have dry skin which is pretty unlined, so we know!) What happens is that dry skin can look papery and, as a result, older. It's uncomfortable, too – so here are some dry skin strategies. (Ironically, in some cases, they're not really that different from the tactics for oily skin – because it's all about bringing the complexion into balance.)

✳   After you've cleansed, pat your face dry and apply moisturizer immediately. If you have particularly dry areas, "double-moisturize" in these zones: apply moisturizer, let it sink in, then apply a second layer. But be aware that what looks like dry skin – especially around the nose – may actually just be a surface build-up of dead skin cells. If you lightly buff these on a daily basis with a muslin washcloth (see page 63), they should disappear.

✳   Again, avoid harsh toners; if you like a feeling of freshness, switch to rosewater or orange flower water.

✳   Make sure you're getting enough EFAs – Essential Fatty Acids – which can help "moisturize" skin from within (see page 97).

✳   Boost the humidity levels of your home and office (see page 66 for how-to's).

✳   Make sure skin is being hydrated from within. According to leading nutritionist Vicky Edgson – co-author of *The Food Doctor* – "I can tell which of my

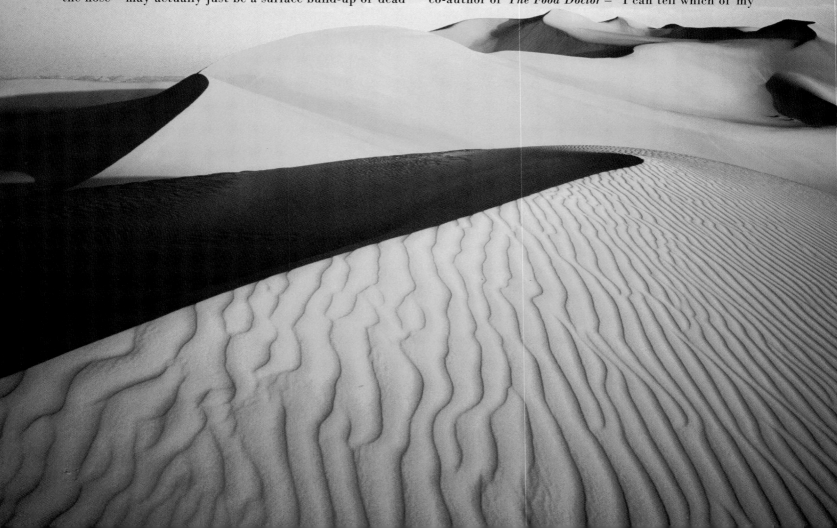

patients have been drinking enough water the minute they walk through the door – because their skin's translucent and clear." The target? "At least 4½ pints (2.5 liters), filtered or bottled, drunk steadily throughout the day." (Vicki's tip: always keep a glass – or bottle – of water on your desk.) The occasional glass of fruit juice can count as part of that total – "but remember that fruit juice interferes with blood sugar levels, so it's better not to substitute. Herbal teas can be included in that 4½ pint total – but not caffeinated beverages. In fact, for every caffeinated drink, you need to drink double that in water."

OILY SKIN

The temptation with oily and problem/acne-prone skin is to strip away oil almost as fast as it's produced. But what happens then is that oil production whirrs into overdrive, producing even more to replace what you've stripped away. We've spent hours, while promoting our books in beauty stores, steering oily-skinned women (and men) away from harsh toners and antibacterial cleansing washes and towards very gentle products instead. Many later told us that their skins have been "miraculously" rebalanced by following this advice.

✳ Try switching to a solid, pomade-style cleanser – like Eve Lom's, Amanda Lacey's Cleansing Pomade or Spiezia Organics Cleansing Cream – and removing it with a hot muslin washcloth (for technique, see page 59). Give skin at least one month (and at least one menstrual cycle) to "settle down".

✳ Give up using harsh alcohol toners – and switch to rosewater, orange flower water or witch hazel instead.

Stress can be a big trigger factor with oily and problem skins

✳ Problem teenage skin doesn't need a moisturizer – which may actually clog pores and lead to acne. According to dermatologist Dr. Sue Mayou, "Getting my younger acne patients to stop applying moisturizer sometimes goes a long way towards improving their skin." More mature-but-still-oily skins should be moisturized with an oil-free, "non-comedogenic" (i.e. non-pore-blocking) lotion – but only on cheeks, forehead and neck. Avoid any products containing mineral oil, as these plug pores – leading to breakouts.

✳ In the sun, and on hot days, you will of course need to apply sun protection. Look for a gel-based facial SPF 15 product – preferably one which is labeled "non-

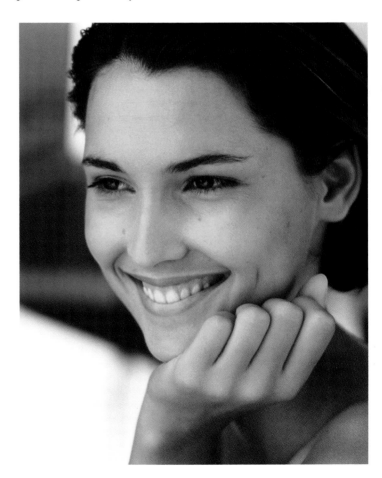

comedogenic" (see page 87) – which will dry to a matte finish, without overloading skin with oil. "Don't go higher than SPF 20," advises Amanda Lacey, "or you'll just overload the skin with chemicals." According to Christine Varret, founder of the French skincare line Epure (which specializes in products for problem complexions), "The sun's drying effect may seem to help oily skins, but UV radiation causes the outer layer to become thicker and block pores. Failure to use protection can trigger outbreaks of blackheads and pimples." To avoid sunscreen build-up, dermatologist Dr. Karen Burke advises swiping skin with witch hazel to remove any residue, then reapplying sunscreen. "Don't layer," is her advice.

✳ If you suffer from breakouts, check if your acne appears in the same area most of the time; if so, it could be triggered by habitual use of a phone, helmet, or glasses that aren't spotlessly clean.

✳ Stress can be a big factor in oily and problem skins. When you're stressed, you produce adrenaline, which has an impact on other hormones – including encouraging the production of sticky, pore-clogging sebum. So find ways of calming down. (For suggestions, see pages 218.)

✳ According to herbalist Kathryn Watson, "problem skins can be improved by taking echinacea, which enhances the immune system. Lavender or tea tree oils can also be applied neat to the skin – if you have a breakout." Look for Bioforce's Echinacea tincture, and take the drops in water, according to the instructions. We are devotees.

COMBINATION SKIN

Many women have combination skin – oily round the T-zone, dry elsewhere. In this case, you can mix-and-match the advice on the previous pages, as required. But if you truly have two extremes, John Gustafson suggests that there is most likely an imbalance in your skincare routine. "Most people tend to be normal in the center and drier on the cheek, or oily in the center and more normal on the cheek, but total extremes are usually caused by over-cleansing/under-moisturizing."

"If you do have those extremes, use products designed for normal skin for 30 days – one body cycle – and then review what condition it's in. Having two products for different zones is overkill; your money will be better spent on a regime for normal skin. But avoid moisturizing the T-zone – and apply a little extra moisturizer to the cheeks." John also recommends looking for products labeled "complexion- or skin-balancing".

THE TRUTH ABOUT THE BIG SQUEEZE

According to Eve Lom, all zits are not created equal. "Squeezing on a daily basis can damage and scar skin. But if you get an occasional pimple, it's OK to squeeze." Her technique? "You have to prepare skin, first by cleansing, then warming it. Ensure hands are spotlessly clean, too. Take a piece of cotton wool and soak it in hot water, then hold over the blemish for about six seconds, repeating five or six times, before squeezing with the tips of your fingers, not your nails – which could break skin. Never try to squeeze a red lump; unless there's a white 'head' on it, you'll just spread the infection and make matters worse. And wipe with tea tree oil, afterwards."

ZIT ZAPPERS – *Tried & Tested*

Pimples aren't just reserved for teenagers. But can any product stop zits and other breakouts in their tracks or zap those that have already come up? That's the tough challenge we set a group of panellists who told us they had problem skins.

DERMOLOGICA MEDICATED CLEARING GEL

8.95 points out of 10

This medicated cooling gel, applied at night, gained high marks in a difficult category. It claims to help clear skin and prevent blemishes by sloughing off dead skin cells with salicylic acid, then reducing the sebum (oil) that clogs follicles, with Alginated Zinc Triplex, which is also antibacterial and anti-inflammatory. All our testers said they would buy it.

UPSIDE: "Easy to use, quickly absorbed, clean fresh smell, didn't sting – I used at night and the pimple was less red and sore on day 1, drying out and fading on day 2, almost gone on day 3" • "pimples seemed noticeably less angry looking after just one night" • "calmed pimples and prevented more over my whole face".

DOWNSIDE: "only disadvantage is that you can't use a night cream (unless you just have a couple of pimples)".

DERMOLOGICA SPECIAL CLEARING BOOSTER

8.2 points out of 10

One of a range of special booster skin preps, this waterbased gel also contains Alginated Zinc Triplex (see above) plus watercress, burdock and ivy to help purify the skin. Designed to be applied to individual blemishes, it leaves a film which, our testers found, was effective at clearing skin.

UPSIDE: "I've tried loads of pimple treatments and was sure this one wouldn't deliver but I'm a big fan now" • "red pimple and whiteheaded pimple both healed much quicker than usual" • "a godsend for my rather bad skin".

DOWNSIDE: "you have to put it directly on the spot and not the surrounding skin or that becomes really dry".

CLINIQUE ANTI–BLEMISH SOLUTIONS CLEAR BLEMISH GEL

7.79 points out of 10

One of Clinique's top-selling products, a neat rollerball featuring salicylic acid (to unblock pores) and non-irritant kola-nut solution, plus astringent witch hazel and alcohol.

UPSIDE: "Can be used on top of makeup and started working right away – a whitehead disappeared" • "my skin seemed much improved" • "liked the rollerball; will definitely keep this near for when I feel a zit coming" • "effective on several red, angry lumps".

DOWNSIDE: "Ouch!" • "slight stinging sensation and drying of skin" • "seemed to make blemish more visible".

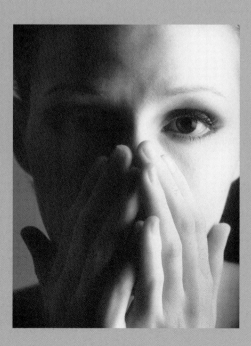

❀❀ AESOP CHAMOMILE CONCENTRATE ANTI-BLEMISH MASQUE

7.55 points out of 10

This fast-acting mask is 100 percent natural. It contains iron oxide and montmorillite (a kind of clay), and is packed with antibacterial botanicals (including tea tree, rosemary, sage and lemon peel oil). It can either be left on skin under concealer or used as a rinse-off, overnight treatment.

UPSIDE: "I used this on huge, bumpy, red pimples and after three days, the whole area looked less angry" • "smelled citrusy and fresh, and calmly and quietly got rid of zits in two days" • "skin felt really silky; it's easy to use – like a mentholy mud face pack".

UPSIDE: "Hated the smell – like stale calamine lotion".

BEST BUDGET BUY
BODY SHOP TEA TREE BLEMISH STICK

7.44 points out of 10

This light, translucent gel – packed with naturally antiseptic and antibacterial tea tree – comes with a sponge applicator, and has added sea algae to help prevent overdrying of the skin. Extremely affordable.

UPSIDE: "Reduced redness in an aggravated blemish" • "after the zit had dried up, there was no red mark" • "pimple had healed entirely in three days; I'll buy this again" • "easy to carry around" • "kept the area clean and fresh".

DOWNSIDE: "I was worried about reinfecting the blemish, so I cleaned the wand after each application" • "dried out my skin".

The lowest score in this category was 4.25 points out of 10

TREATS FOR TIRED AND PUFFY EYES

Tried & Tested

We asked our testers to report on the instant re-sparkling, de-bagging, line-smoothing, dark-circle-diminishing effect of these products – but many opted to take a longer-term approach as well. (Because if it was effective, why not keep up the good work?) Somewhat to our surprise, hardly any testers reported any sensitivity to the following products.

SHISEIDO THE SKINCARE EYE SOOTHER

8.25 points out of 10

This gel gets its de-puffing, bag-erasing power from vitamin E and the leaves of the houttunyia plant, with crushed pearl pigments to "bounce" light off the skin under the eyes. To turbo-charge its efects, Shiseido recommend that it's patted into the eye area using the fingertips, boosting microcirculation.

UPSIDE: "I liked the idea of being able to apply over makeup – it really refreshed the eye area and would be good for flying" • "so soothing – you only need a small amount as it's very effective at cooling the skin" • "reduced dark circles after 2 hours" • "I'd recommend this as an essential item for every woman!" • "eyes were loads brighter and more awake-looking – after a late night they felt almost normal again".

DOWNSIDE: "The gel was quite runny and smudged my make-up when applied on top".

PRESCRIPTIVES SUPER LINE PREVENTOR + INTENSIVE EYE TREATMENT

7.8 points out of 10

According to Prescriptives, this cream-gel is clinically proven to reduce the appearance of lines and wrinkles by up to 48 percent, used over time. It also contains magnolia extract to de-puff and eliminate dark circles.

UPSIDE: "I have problems with puffy eyes because of thyroid and sinus problems, and this is the best product I've tried, up till now" • "brilliant at reducing puffiness; my sister also tried it after a late night out and really noticed a difference" • "eyes were noticeably refreshed next morning with a huge reduction in puffiness" • "eyes feel more taut and look a lot clearer and brighter, so I'm using a lot less concealer, as well".

DOWNSIDE: "Strange chemical smell" • "made my eyes smart and water – perhaps because it's easy to use too much product".

❀❀ DR. HAUSCHKA EYE SOLACE

7.76 points out of 10

Another "natural wonder" from Dr. Hauschka, this features eyebright, fennel extract, chamomile and rose essential oil in a cooling lotion which our testers unanimously found super-refreshing.

UPSIDE: "Relaxed my eyes and took away the strained feeling at the end of the day" • "very cooling and refreshing – excellent when you've had a long day and eyes are red and tired – leaving them much clearer" • "would be excellent before or after a big night out" • "not a quick fix, but great for pampering on a lazy day as it took 10 minutes to soothe, cool and reduce redness" • "eyes felt 'alive' again".

DOWNSIDE: "A slice of cucumber would work just as well".

ESPA SOOTHING EYE LOTION

7.62 points out of 10

The active ingredients in this cooling blue liquid – in a dropper bottle, to be dispensed onto a cotton pad – include cucumber extract and cornflower.

UPSIDE: "Can't use it while you're doing something else as you have to keep eyes closed, but brilliant results – a real brightener" • "even better kept in the fridge" • "a lovely, soothing lotion that chased away fatigue; the whites of my eyes seemed whiter" • "smells gorgeous".

DOWNSIDE: "Bit of a hassle if you're in a rush – a damp tea bag would do just as well" • "not practical for use in the morning before work".

BEST BUDGET BUY
L'ORÉAL PARIS DERMO– EXPERTISE HYDRAFRESH EYES

7.25 points out of 10

A hydrating gel-crème, this is enriched with vitamins and minerals and is specifically designed to instantly combat the appearance of dark circles, helping skin (rather than eyes themselves) regain brightness. The instructions include a special application technique of puffing and pinching (which was not popular with some testers) to optimize results.

UPSIDE: "Immediate improvement – very refreshing" • "within a few minutes, puffiness had gone and eye bags were much diminished, leaving eyes brighter and more awake" • "very refreshing; worked well with sensitive eyes – and I'm a contact lens-wearer" • "eyes look more 'open' and eyelids feel a bit lighter" • "took puffiness right down".

DOWNSIDE: "Stung a bit when I lay down".

The lowest score in this category was 4.8 points out of 10.

GET YOUR EYES RIGHT

Regardless of what comes out of your mouth, eyes speak the truth. They smile. They glare. They make love. They show stress. They cry. So don't you owe them a little TLC?

Eyes may be the mirror of the soul, but they take a real beating, constantly being bombarded with dust, smoke, UV light and irritants of all sorts. Then we slap on makeup – only to scrape it off again with heavy creams. And we still expect eyes to look limpid and beautiful even when we're skimping on the sleep required to rest them.

The skin under the eyes is much thinner and contains fewer oil glands than on the rest of your face – and so can be drier and more prone to wrinkles, puffiness and dark circles. We're often asked if it's necessary to use a separate eye cream for this area. According to Ayurvedic beauty guru Bharti Vyas, the answer is no. "Your regular moisturizer should do the trick," she advises, "but don't apply to the eye area itself; simply dab onto the 'orbital bone' around the eye zone, and it will travel to where it's needed; the fine lines around the eyes act like channels to deliver the product where it's needed."

Definitely don't fall into the trap of slathering eyes with a super-rich cream to replace lost moisture and restore suppleness; that's too much for the eye area to cope with and can lead to puffiness or sensitivity. If you have problems with eye sensitivity, we suggest an eye gel rather than a cream. Some companies also produce eye oils; never apply these directly to the skin; instead, apply a couple of drops to the tips of your fingers, rub them together, then tap onto the orbital bone, as above.

When it comes to eye care, however, caring for the skin in the eye zone is only part of the story. Protection from light pollution is the most instant advice we can give. "Wear sunglasses or an eyeshade everyday," suggests naturopath Roderick Lane. If you are buying sunglasses, remember to buy large wraparound ones (small ones may look chic but they don't give adequate protection) which are 100 percent UVA and UVB resistant. (The label

should tell you.) A wide-brimmed hat – or even a baseball cap (right way round only) – will do nicely if you prefer, although these don't have the double benefit of shielding eyes from flying particles.

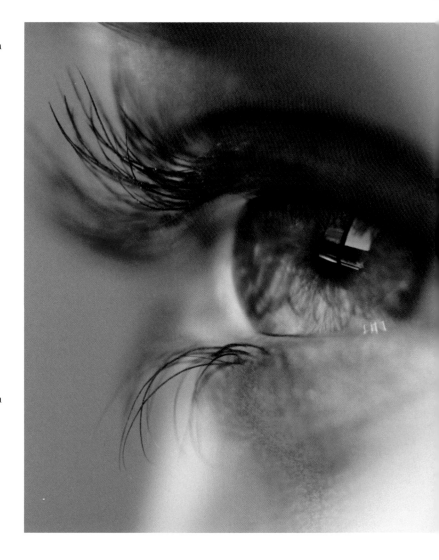

The most obvious eye problem is sore, tired eyes – which often means red and scratchy eyes too. For instant relief, stroke a drop or two of Dr. Bach's Rescue Remedy flower essence on the lids, applied with your finger; try dotting the cream version around the eye too. Soothe them with a compress (see opposite) and – yes, we know this may sound strange – have something to eat. Eyes use up a lot of sugar and oxygen, so fluctuating blood sugar levels will cause fluctuating vision. Go for something relatively substantial as a snack and remember to eat every three hours: grazing on five small meals a day is great for low blood sugar.

Dry eyes and dancing print often indicate a lack of Essential Fatty Acids so invest in a good supplement such as Linseed 1000 and eat plenty of oily fish. If your eyes are often sore after a day at the monitor, or you get headaches, do get them tested. The right prescription glasses can help ease all kinds of eye problems enormously.

GET RID OF YOUR EXCESS EYE BAGGAGE

The bloodhound look is not a great one, but most of us suffer with eye bags at one time or another. There's the temporary kind, which deposit themselves under your eyes after a late night out, or—most unfairly—appear because of a sensitivity reaction to a product, smoky rooms, or an allergy such as asthma or hayfever. (That's often accompanied by weeping eyes.) Anything which affects your sinuses will have the same effect.

Curiously, too much sleep can also puff up the eye area. The problem can be largely due to heredity, too, as can dark circles. Sleeping well and getting plenty of fresh air (provided you're not a hayfever sufferer out in a high pollen count) plus exercise will often do the trick.

For longstanding and intractable eyebags, the only permanent solution is cosmetic surgery – but there are many quick fixes. See opposite for our favorites...

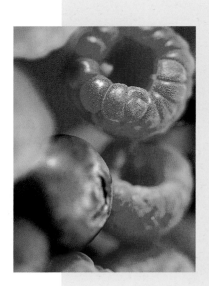

SOS – SAVE OUR SIGHT

As we get older, we run the risk of losing our sight because of cataracts (opacity/fogging of the lens resulting in blurred vision) or Age-related Macular Degeneration (AMD). Cataracts can be successfully operated on but there is currently no treatment for AMD, which can destroy older people's quality of life. There is considerable evidence that we can help prevent these conditions by eating plenty of fruit and vegetables rich in antioxidants. Vitamins C and E appear to be the most effective for preventing cataracts, and two carotenoids, called lutein and zeaxanthin, for preventing AMD. The best way to get these in food is simply to eat the widest array of the most colorful fruits and vegetables you can find, including spinach, corn, sea kale, peppers, broccoli, peas, cabbage, lettuce, squash, oranges, mangoes, peaches, peas, and papaya. There are specific nutritional supplements designed for the eyes. Jo has her own recipe for eye health: she buys dried red berries – a mixture of blueberries, bilberries, cranberries, and sour cherries – and soaks them in enough water to cover, bringing to a boil and allowing to cool. This antioxidant-rich berry mixture is delicious spooned on muesli or yogurt.

IF YOUR EYES ARE SENSITIVE/ALLERGIC

✳ Play detective to try and track down products which may be irritating you. Sometimes it's quite obvious that a new mascara or eye-makeup remover is the culprit. If you use eye drops regularly (and it's definitely not a good idea to depend on these for eye-brightening), take a break and then try a different product.

✳ Always wash your hands before applying or removing makeup and use disposable applicators whenever possible. If you use washable applicator sponges, wash them daily and leave them somewhere warm to dry out completely; brushes should be washed weekly.

✳ Heavy creams are often not suited to the eye area, so use very sparingly, and consider investing in a special eye cream. Use ring fingers to tap on creams; don't drag or pull.

✳ If you use cotton wool, make sure that it is soft and free of tiny rough or hard particles which can damage the eyes. We prefer organic cotton wool (see page 63).

✳ If you work at a visual display unit (VDU), remember that the static attracts a lot of dust which can aggravate tired eyes: invest in an anti-glare screen, which can be fitted over the VDU, and an ionizer for your desk.

✳ Ice it: simply stroke an ice cube around your eye area for a few moments (you can wrap it in a cotton hankie or napkin, or a piece of cling wrap, if you find it too cold on its own); Linda Evangelista gave us this trick – and it works like magic, even when you're getting out of bed for considerably less than $10,000 a day. You can also try keeping teaspoons in the freezer and doing the same. (Silver works better than stainless steel).

✳ Exercise: to drain the puffiness away, do any exercise that involves gravity – so that means walking, jogging or dancing; bouncing on a mini-trampoline is excellent. The yoga routine on pages 138-43 will also help hugely by keeping your whole system "flowing".

✳ Tap tap: with your ring fingers, tap all around the eyes to disperse fluid (see Susan Harmsworth's 2 minute De-Stresser on page 112).

✳ Compress for sore and tired eyes: you need a few minutes to relax with this so it's not an office fix. Brew 2 teabags of German chamomile (*Chamomilla recutita*), cool,

gently squeeze out excess liquid and place over eyes. Relax for five minutes or as long as possible. Alternatively, infuse ½ oz. (15g) of the dried herb with 8⅓ fl. oz. (250ml) of boiling water. Cool, then wrap in a clean piece of cotton or linen to form an eye mask. Squeeze gently then lay over eyes. Be careful not to get irritating bits of herbs in the eyes.

✳ Grated or sliced raw potato is also effective: lay it on some gauze to form an eye mask.

✳ Steam: if you can get to a sauna or steam bath, the puffies will disappear as if by magic.

Eye-makeup Removers
Tried & Tested

If the beauty world could have more than one Holy Grail, then we'd definitely include eye-makeup removers on the list. It's something women ask us about constantly, complaining that removers trigger adverse reactions such as stinging, redness or puffiness. What we would say is that while some women know they have very sensitive eyes/skin – and so are very careful – our experience is that a reaction to both synthetic and natural ingredients can occur out of the blue. Contact lens wearers may have even more problems with sensitivity. So: no magic answers here, but these are the products that did well across the board in our ten-woman panels which tested more than two dozen products in all.

Many of the removers that scored well are what's called "dual-phase": that means you have to shake the bottle to mix the oil and water ingredients. The advantage of this formulation is that it enables the manufacturers to leave out emulsifiers – eliminating some potential sensitivity triggers. (Which is why our sensitive peepers generally don't suffer reactions to dual-phase removers.) Beware, though: the fact that most eye-makeup removers state they're ophthalmologically and/or dermatologically-tested doesn't mean they can't give you a sensitivity reaction.

There is an art to eye makeup removal, however: saturate a cotton pad, then squeeze; press onto eyelid to dissolve makeup and then gently wipe away, from inner to outer corner. Never rub. Use a fresh pad for each eye (and for lips, see below). If you need to get into the 'lash-line' to remove mascara, dip a cotton swab in remover and gently roll it along the lashes. Eye-makeup removers can also be used to remove lipstick – even long-lasting lipsticks – but be sure to choose a fragrance-free version, or they can taste horrible.

Prescriptives Quick Remover for Eye Makeup
9.16 points out of 10

Not a single one of our testers reported any adverse reaction to this liquid formula, which is oil- and fragrance-free and has soothing cucumber extracts.

UPSIDE: "Felt as if it had just been in the fridge (though it hadn't): very refreshing" • "wonderful – didn't need to rub my eyes, which felt clean and fresh and ready for everything" • "skin felt smooth and conditioned after quickly removing all traces of eye makeup" • "great product – especially for people with sensitive eyes, like me".

DOWNSIDE: Our testers had no negative comments to make about this.

Chanel Précision Eye Makeup Remover
8.9 points out of 10

Like many of the removers that scored well in this category, this is a shake-vigorously-before-use product, which comes in that oh-so-covetable Chanel packaging. (Jo is particularly pleased that this product scored well as it's the remover she keeps coming back to, time after time, having tried countless others on her sensitive eyes.)

UPSIDE: "Excellent product: cleaned off eye makeup with no soreness and left skin moist; I am usually sensitive to eye makeup removers but this did not make my eyes water" • "felt luxurious and worked well – and did not affect my contact lenses, which is a bonus" • "removed makeup very easily – even two coats of mascara" • "excellent: left the eye zone very moisturized after use – as if I'd used an eye cream; a real delight" • "fragrance-free – just as described".

DOWNSIDE: "Light but greasy – I needed to wash my face after use".

Sisley Gentle Makeup Remover for Eyes and Lips
8.7 points out of 10

Sisley is a pricey brand, fast becoming a cult favorite, which contains some active botanical ingredients. Our testers particularly loved the straight-from-nature orange blossom scent.

UPSIDE: "A dream to use – no rubbing needed and all the gunk just floated away; wonderful, magical stuff" • "beautiful smell and refreshing on the eyes" • "removed all traces of eye makeup very well, with slightly more effort on waterproof mascara" • "very economical – you don't have to use much".

DOWNSIDE: "Hard to get liquid out of the bottle" • "left skin feeling a bit dry".

Givenchy Secur'eyes Delicate Eye Cleanser
8.56 points out of 10

A water-based formulation, this is designed not to leave any trace of oiliness on the eyes -

although it does have a "soothing, moisturizing agent", say Givenchy. It is specifically marketed as being suitable for contact lens-wearers and anyone else with sensitive eyes.

UPSIDE: "Removed all traces of eye makeup and I did not have panda eyes next morning" • "absolutely thrilled with this product – no stinging at all; eyes felt gentle, stinging and clean" • "every trace of mascara, liner etc. came off effortlessly" • "a special mention for clever design: you turn the top and it smoothly opens, without the bother of un-screwing" • "lovely to use as a cold compress on eyes, too".

DOWNSIDE: "No different to a normal, more budget-priced eye makeup remover" • "left skin slightly dry".

CLARINS EYE MAKEUP REMOVER
8.4 points out of 10

This is a "dual-phase" product: shake it up and the oil-and-water elements mix (but separate again after a few minutes). It contains a cocktail of plant extracts, including cornflower to soften and soothe, rosewater to calm and tone, plus soy protein as a lash-conditioner.

UPSIDE: "No effort required for waterproof mascara, which was gone in a flash; excellent for sensitive skin" • "made eye makeup melt away with the minimum of effort, leaving skin feeling refreshed and clean" • "comfortable and fresh sensation after application" • "gentle, light floral scent".

DOWNSIDE: "Seemed to get through bottle very quickly – in less than a month" • "slight stinging sensation – but it passed quickly" • "made eyes sore".

LANCÔME BI-FACIL DOUBLE-ACTION EYE MAKEUP REMOVER
8.35 points out of 10

A two-toned, dual-phase blue lotion, which (as one tester put it) "looks very cool on the bathroom shelf".

UPSIDE: "Moisturized, with no greasy residue – so I could apply makeup again, if needed" • "leaves skin feeling fresh, clean and soft – and is very gentle; excellent" • "very effective on waterproof mascara".

DOWNSIDE: "Left eyes a bit blurry" • "made my eyes feel very sore and took 90 minutes to recover; I was still affected, next morning".

DERMALOGICA SOOTHING EYE MAKEUP REMOVER
8.3 points out of 10

Alcohol – and oil-free, Dermalogica's remover is suitable for contact lens-wearers, and features lash-strengthening protein silk amino acids.

UPSIDE: "I did enjoy this product – I don't usually use a specific eye makeup remover, but this was simple and easy to use" • "makeup came off easily and quickly" • "moisturizes lids which I tend to miss when applying cream" • "lovely, soothing, refreshing texture with no greasy residue at all" • "no stinging at all, even when I got a drop in my eye"

DOWNSIDE: "Not strong enough for waterproof mascara" • "stung sometimes".

DECLÉOR EYE MAKEUP REMOVER
8.2 points out of 10

Although this contains natural ingredients like rose and Roman chamomile, we scanned the ingredients list and felt we really couldn't give it a "natural" daisy – but our testers liked it.

UPSIDE: "Very soft, water-like and flowery" • "removed mascara easily" • "great for contact lens-wearers, like me" • "very refreshing".

DOWNSIDE: "Not as effective as other brands that I've used" • "possibly too gentle?".

❀❀ JURLIQUE OPC MAKEUP REMOVER
6.83 points out of 10

The highest-scoring of the natural products we tested is actually an all-over makeup remover

milk, but our testers tried it specifically for one of its purposes: eye-makeup removal. One of the biochemist founders of this Australian all-natural skincare brand used to work with Dr. Hauschka, and these products contain herbs grown on Jurlique's own farm. In this product, you will find rosewood and lavender, plus antioxidant green tea, red wine grape seeds, vitamin E and turmeric.

UPSIDE: "No rubbing required even for waterproof mascara; fantastic smell" • "skin felt moisturized and plump after use, soft and rehydrated" • "loved the lavender/herbal scent" • "rich, creamy texture – the smell was fantastic and the skin around my eyes felt very smooth afterwards".

DOWNSIDE: "Would prefer a plastic bottle to glass" • "stung eyes and didn't completely remove makeup".

BEST BUDGET BUY

L'ORÉAL PARIS DERMO-EXPERTISE REFRESHING EYE MAKEUP REMOVER
6.6 points out of 10

This accessibly priced oil-free remover also works on lips.

UPSIDE: "I've used this before and still find it one of the best all-rounders" • "removed all mascara – not even a trace was left; easy-to-use flip-top bottle" • "quite simply, it does its job" • "so easy-to-use and hassle-free – I like anything that makes life easier".

DOWNSIDE: "Left my eyes irritated" • "too gentle for removing lots of mascara, unless you're prepared to use lots of effort".

The lowest score in this category was 5 marks out of 10.

FEED YOUR SKIN

There's always some irritating person who crams in junk food day and night, indulges in every skin vice – and still has skin like a ripe peach. But they're the exceptions – and if you nourish your skin inside and out, it will definitely bloom.

We love treats. (Just try keeping us away from organic chocolate and ice cream.) And there's certainly nothing wrong with them. But we suggest that, in your quest for velvety, dewy, age-defying skin, you try and focus on nature's own skin foods. This strategy is simple and it will help the whole of you, inside and out. We believe in buying organic food whenever possible. It often tastes better – and ultimately, we're convinced evidence will emerge that it's more nutritious because it is grown in soil with higher quantities of vitamins and minerals. Also, because organically produced food doesn't contain lots of

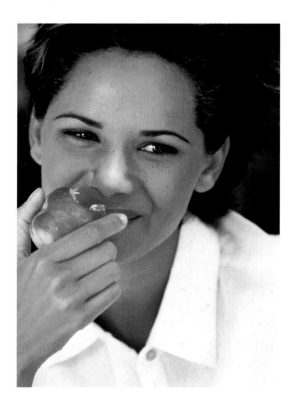

chemicals which our bodies then have to get rid of, using up valuable energy.

We certainly find, eating organically, that we hardly ever suffer from colds, 'flu or the other nagging complaints that have some of our friends running to the doctor so often. And now there's even some evidence that eating organically can help us all stay slimmer – or even shed pounds. The thinking? Our bodies can't deal with the chemicals – pesticides, herbicides and additives – which are found in so much food today. These chemicals disrupt our natural slimming systems and it can be almost impossible to shift extra weight. (If you want to read more about that, we suggest Dr. Paula Baillie-Hamilton's book *The Body Restoration Plan*, see Bookshelf, page 246.) Eating organically doesn't have to be expensive. Cut down on meat consumption (if you're not a vegetarian), cut down on processed foods, up your intake of grains and legumes and veggies, and you'll find that eating organically isn't any more expensive than eating conventionally produced food.

Here, then, is the blueprint for eating for great skin. (But do also drink for great skin: plenty of still, pure water – see page 56 – between meals, otherwise it may hinder the nutrients in your food from being absorbed.)

Fresh fruit and vegetables: Grapes, fresh pineapple, apples, and kiwi fruit are fabulous for your skin, according to Kathryn Marsden, nutrition whiz and author of *Superskin*. Also cabbage, carrots, beets, parsley, and avocados. Have some raw every day. (See Great Juices, page 235.) Don't peel fruit and veggies with edible skins: the nutrients are often concentrated in or just below the surface.

Fresh fish: Aim for oily fish – mackerel, sardines, herrings, tuna, salmon, trout. They contain the Essential Fatty Acids Omega 3 and 6, which plump out your skin and keep it healthy.

Whole grains: Grains are the seeds and fruits of cereal grasses, packed with energy waiting to germinate into a plant. Whole grains are best; they haven't been processed and so haven't had the nutrient-rich coatings (or husks) removed. Look for whole wheat, rye, oats, millet, barley, brown rice, plus the ancient grains – spelt, kamut, faro, and quinoa – which have more protein and less gluten than their modern counterparts.

Nuts and seeds: Have a good variety of these weekly. Always buy unshelled if possible. Keep them in a cool dark place.

Yogurt: Plain natural yogurt with live cultures is a skin boon, and a wonderful help to the gut because it contributes beneficial bacteria.

SKIN SUPPLEMENT

As you'll have gathered, we like tried and tested products. So when we first heard about Imedeen nearly ten years ago, we were frankly dubious. How could a food supplement thicken your skin? But the formula, based on a patented Biomarine complex, did the job for us. After four months (a tad longer than the time on the pack), Sarah's almost transparent skin became noticeably thicker. Many women claim it helps tone as well. And when Jo stops taking it – because she runs out – her skin definitely becomes more papery and less "plumped" quite soon. Imedeen, which now comes in two versions, the original Imedeen Classic and Imedeen Time Perfection (with added antioxidants), is marketed as a dedicated skin

supplement but we also believe in big doses of Essential Fatty Acids, in the form of flaxseed or hemp oil, or our favorite Udo's Oil (a balance of Omega 3 and 6, which we plop on our breakfast muesli).

EMERGENCY MEASURES

When we are very tired and our skin seems to be having a nervous breakdown, we find this nutritional skin support regime very effective as a booster to get us (and our complexions) back on track ASAP. It was devised by leading naturopath Roderick Lane, of London's Eden Clinic. It goes without saying that you should continue eating as healthily as possible (preferably in line with our great-skin guidelines, explained here). Even perfect complexions and Duracell-bunny energy levels will benefit from this boost once or twice yearly. It's also excellent before and after any surgery to help wounds heal faster. Lane recommends BioCare supplements (so do we) but there are plenty of other good brands, such as Solgar or Quest, or Viridian, which is primarily organic.

Roderick Lane's Skin Boost
Take the following supplements daily for 28 days, with breakfast unless otherwise directed.

Vitamin A: 15,000 IU (international units)
Vitamin B complex: 1 capsule
Vitamin C with added bioflavonoids: 1000mg tablet
Vitamin E: 400 IU a day
Linseed 1000: 2 capsules
Trace Mineral Complex: 1 capsule (take with your largest meal)

A NATURAL QUESTION...

Do you want to be a truly "natural" beauty? Or do you want the latest and greatest skin-saving breakthroughs that beauty science can throw at you (and your complexion)? It's up to you...

In the past decade, beauty has gone in two dramatically different directions: the super-high-tech products – packed with "liposomes" and "nanospheres" and other straight-from-the-lab-sounding ingredients – and the more natural skin treatments. These harness the power of botanical skin-saving elements like rose, lavender, and frankincense, some of which have been used for beautification as far back as ancient Egyptian times.

The feedback we get certainly reflects that women are more and more interested in truly natural products. This isn't only for personal reasons: in the production of cosmetics (as with most other industries), synthetic chemicals are often released into the environment, creating a persistent threat to wildlife and a destructive impact on the ecosystem. No wonder, then, that the natural beauty market's booming.

Personally, we veer towards using natural beauty products, because we have taken steps to create a natural lifestyle for ourselves in many other ways. (Which means choosing organic food, no synthetic cleaning products or

If you can make a salad dressing, you can make your own cosmetics and, in that way, you can be sure of everything you're putting on your face

toxic paints, and consulting natural health practitioners, among other lifestyle steps.)

Whenever practical, we tend to choose products from renewable resources, rather than those packed with petroleum derivatives, which deplete the earth's natural

riches. What's more, when it comes to our beauty regimes, we have found that many with long lists of preservatives or emulsifiers make our skins flare up – with redness, soreness, flaking, itching – so we try to opt for products with less complicated ingredient lists. (For more about the increasingly widespread problem of sensitive skin, see page 84.)

We often make our own beauty products, even perfumes – and show how you can do that too, throughout the chapters of this book. Quite simply, if you can make a salad dressing, you can make your own cosmetics. Which in reality is the only way you can be 100 percent sure of everything you're putting on your face, body or hair. We love the idea of cosmetics that are (literally) good enough to eat!

We're concerned about what we put on our skin because some of it, inevitably, ends up in the bloodstream. (As much as 60 percent, Rob McCaleb, President of the Herb Research Foundation, once told us.) Not long ago, doctors used to claim that skin was a one-way street: it let toxins and sweat escape – but acted as a "raincoat", keeping everything else out. Now, that thinking has been reversed, and skin is acknowledged as being a highly efficient way of getting chemicals into the bloodstream – more efficient than taking them by mouth, in fact, because the skin route bypasses the digestive process. (Think of HRT and nicotine patches, and HRT gel.)

Inevitably, some of the ingredients you apply on your skin will end up being absorbed. Sebastian Parsons, Managing Director of the cult organic skincare company Dr. Hauschka, has said that the average woman absorbs over 30lb of moisturizing ingredients into her bloodstream over 60 years – and that's not including the other what's

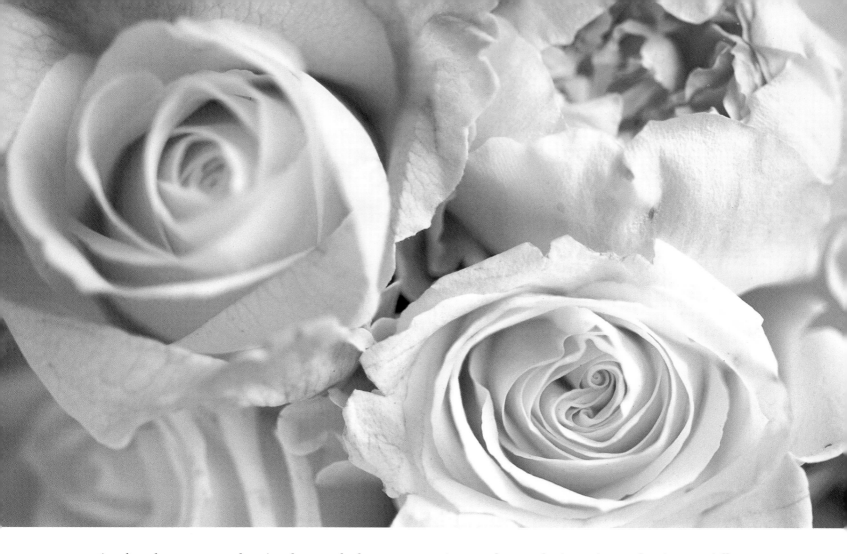

cosmetics that she uses every day. As of yet, nobody knows what the longterm effect of putting that cocktail of chemicals on our skin will be.

THE RIGHT TO CHOOSE

The challenge for would-be "natural beauties" is identifying what's what. If it were as clear as choosing skincare labeled "natural" or "high-tech" (and, of course, marketed the same way in the glossy ads), life would be easy. You'd simply have to ask yourself: do you want to invest in the latest that skin science can come up with – or do you prefer the idea of fewer synthetic chemicals and more active botanical ingredients?

Unfortunately, there is absolutely no legal definition of what's natural and what's not. Many product lines put a back-to-nature, feel-as-if-you're-frolicking-through-a-spring-meadow marketing spin on what is essentially an almost exclusively synthetic product, without much more than a sprig of lavender wafted at it. As "organic" increasingly means "trustworthy and desirable" to shoppers, many companies are even claiming their products to be "organic" – when in reality only a tiny percentage of ingredients are from plants grown without chemicals. It gets more complicated still – sorry – because many natural ingredients go through quite a toxic process in order to become suitable for use in cosmetics. One shortcut is to look for skincare labeled "certified organic," which means the products comply with the USA's stringent standards.

We certainly can't make up your mind for you about what kind of cosmetics to choose: (truly) natural, or those based on (sometimes literally) rocket science. That's a lifestyle decision. Your lifestyle. But, as with every section of this book, we have exhaustively "tried-and-tested" what's out there to help you take a shortcut to the natural (and more natural) products that our ten-woman panels (600 volunteers in all) declared to be truly impressive. In that way, we hope to help you identify which are the more natural choices – through our "daisy" ✿ rating. We scrutinized the ingredient lists of all the products submitted for this book which claimed to be "natural" – and awarded them one or two daisies if we felt they really were more natural and less synthetic than most. (For more about the daisy rating, see our Introduction on page 6.)

But, of course, all of life's a gamble. And, often, a compromise. You may feel – as do many of our friends – that you simply want everything that advanced skincare technology can deliver to your skin, and the more high-tech and space-age, the better. Certainly, when it comes to makeup, it's true that many natural products don't yet perform nearly as well as their high-tech rivals. So peer into our makeup bags and (with the exception of lipstick and mascara) you won't find everything as pure as nature intended. That's where we compromize shamelessly... But

when it comes to skincare, we're increasingly going back to nature.

(P.S. On page 52, you'll find a list of natural, botanical ingredients which tells you what they do. We've also come up with a list of ingredients which we feel have no place in skincare or haircare that claims to be "natural", on pages 248-249.)

All of life is a gamble. You may feel you want natural skincare – or everything that science can deliver to your skin

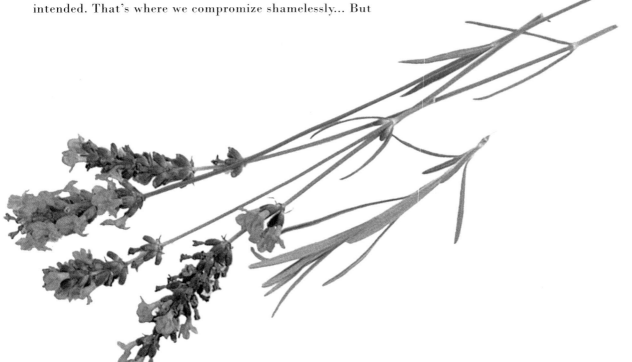

WHAT WE USE

JO

✳ I have what I describe as "beauty editor's skin": after overloading it with new product after new product, there's virtually nothing it tolerates without flaring up in an angry, red reaction – triggered, in the first instance, by a one-shot use of fruit acids almost a decade ago. So now my skincare regime is incredibly simple – and incredibly natural.

✳ For cleansing, I swear by *Spiezia Organic Cleansing Cream* – a certified-organic, oil-based pomade which is miraculous for melting makeup and leaving skin beautifully smooth, and which I remove with a hot washcloth (see page 58).

✳ In the morning, I use a hot washcloth again to cleanse, swishing it in a basin with seven drops of *Jurlique Aromatic Hydrating Concentrate* in Lavender. Since I've been using *Lavera Laveré Hydro-Sensation Anti-Aging Energy Cream* morning and night, which is lightweight but rich – and also happens to be organic – I've never had so many compliments about my skin; it's dewy, glowing and fresh-looking. I also mix up my own facial oils from time to time (see page 80 for how you can do that, too) – or use *Sundari Nighttime Nourishing Oil* if my skin's been dried by travel or central heating/air conditioning.

✳ I like *Green People Eye Gel* as it's instantly cooling and doesn't make my eyes sting (unlike many), alternating with *Sundari Chamomile Eye Oil.* As an occasional skin-booster (especially if my skin's dingy or flaky for any reason), I reach for *Liz Earle Naturally Active Brightening Treatment*: a camphor-rich mask which really gives skin back its "oomph". And, yes, that's it: for a beauty editor, a pretty uncluttered bathroom shelf.

SARAH

✳ I always always (well, almost always) cleanse and moisturize before bed. In the summer, I like *Cleanse & Polish* from the *Liz Earle Naturally Active Skincare* line. My biggest new discovery is the *BKamins* range from Canada, especially formulated for older skins and based on a unique bio-maple extract which really does work miracles. The *Maple Treatment Night Cream* is sensational.

✳ When my skin is feeling tender in the winter, *Spiezia Organics Cleansing Cream* (more like a wax) or *ESPA Cleansing Balm* are wonderful. In general I don't use toners, but if I'm covered with grime after riding, I like to swipe my face with a cotton pad (organic because I don't want pesticide-ridden or genetically-engineered cotton on my face) soaked in rose water. I've learnt to love the organic range of skincare by German company *Laveré*, particularly the moisturizer.

✳ For puffy days, I swear by ice cubes and *Liz Earle Brightening Treatment*, a three-minute mask which is simply a miracle. (Don't leave it on too long, though; its tightening effect can go too far!) I have fantastically sensitive eyes but they love *Jurlique Eye Gel* to calm the puffies and moisturize. *Jurlique Herbal Recovery Gel* is an anti-aging favorite, while *Estée Lauder DayWear Plus Multi-Protection Anti-Oxidant Creme SPF 15* is still my favorite day cream, with their *Idealist Skin Refinisher*, which seems to make my foundation last far longer into the night than I can.

✳ And an absolute must-have: for lines on forehead and lips and tough, rough places anywhere, *Superbalm*, again from the *Liz Earle Naturally Active* line, which is – well, super.

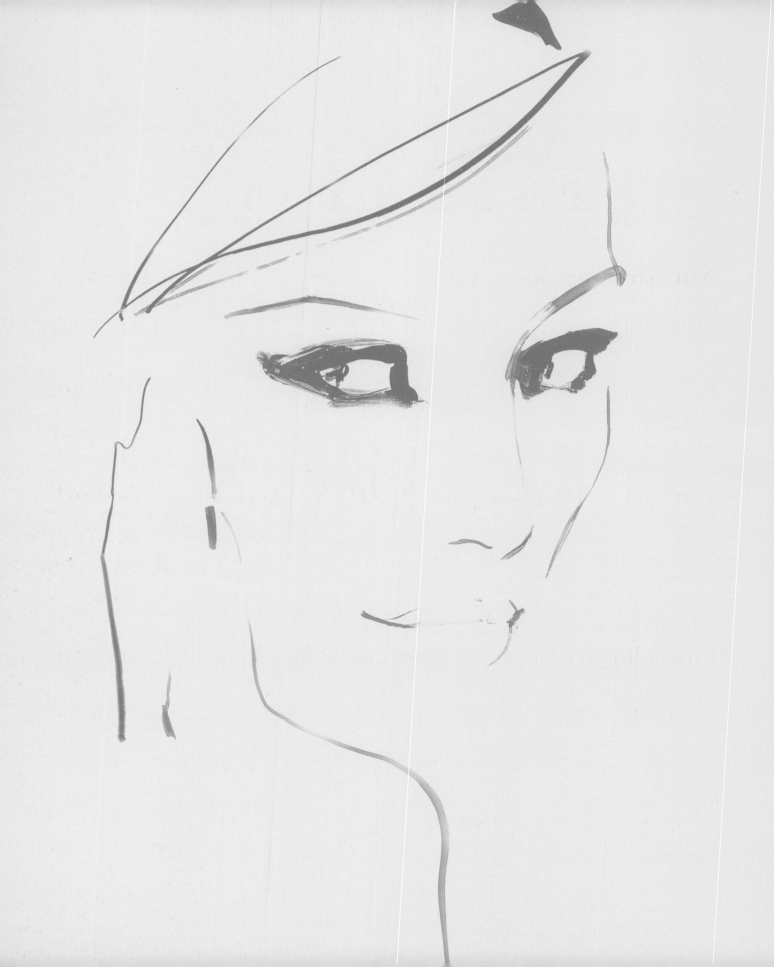

FAST FIXES

Not so long ago, the only true turn-back-the-clock option was cosmetic surgery. Drastic stuff. But today, new and faster **age-defying techniques** are booming. Actually, it's not so much about looking younger as **looking brighter**. From Botox to tooth bleaching – via high-tech facials, non-surgical facelifts and even **wrinkle fillers in a tube** – there's a huge choice of cosmetic tweaks available. (And plenty of delicious natural remedies you can use at home to **wake up a tired face**.) So if it's a fast fix you're after, set your stopwatch now...

SMOOTHERS AND SHAPERS

Laugh lines we love – the rest aren't so welcome. But nowadays we don't have to play hostess to most lines and wrinkles – and even puffiness can be coaxed away. Here's the lowdown on how to peel back the years – without resorting to the knife

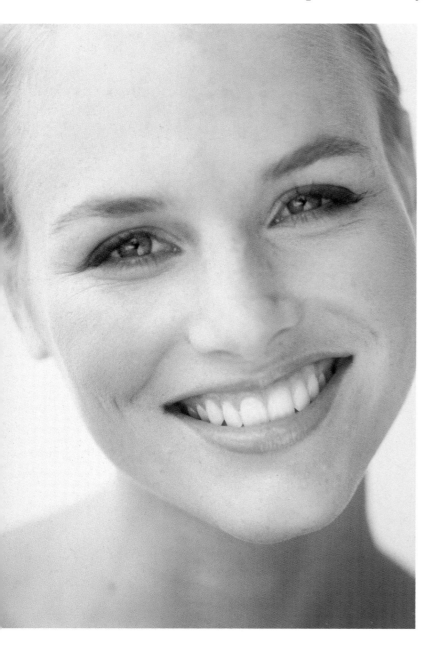

Botox® injections are undoubtedly the most talked-about beauty fix for their almost magical smoothing effect on forehead lines and crows' feet. Botox® works by paralyzing the muscles which make you frown and squint your eyes. It's also being pioneered as a treatment for the neck "cords" that come with aging. (Additionally, Botox® has a good track record for helping headaches and migraine and preventing underarm perspiration, according to London-based aesthetic plastic surgeon Dr. Andrew Markey.)

But things may be getting slightly out of hand. In some places, Botox® parties are the latest rage – kind of like the old Tupperware gatherings, except you buy an injection between courses instead of plastic food containers. In fact, it all sounds so much like choosing the latest lipstick that someone might just forget to mention that Botox® is actually a derivative of botulinum – a deadly plant toxin which is even used in biological warfare.

Doctors, however, swear that Botox® is incredibly safe, pointing out that it has been in use medically since 1980, when it was developed as a treatment for Bell's palsy and facial muscle spasm. The amounts used in medicine are so minuscule that the poisonous element is "virtually not present", according to doctors. Its cosmetic potential was discovered when a Canadian eye doctor, Jean Carruthers (who was using it for tics) noticed her patients were reporting that their wrinkles had improved. Her dermatologist husband, Dr. Alastair Carruthers, latched on to the possibilities – and the rest is history.

For crows' feet, Botox® is increasingly combined with laser resurfacing (as well as other 'filler' injections, more of which overleaf). In research carried out by Dr. Nicholas Lowe, this "double-whammy" approach has given significantly improved results over Botox® alone. As well as Botox®, there's now Myobloc® (marketed as Neurobloc® in the UK), another botulinum toxin which was developed to treat spasms linked to neurological problems. It seems to work in the very rare instances when the original Botox® doesn't. (If Botox® doesn't work, the likely cause is that it was either injected into the wrong muscle or was over-diluted so had no effect.)

Although doctors say that Botox® is completely safe – many of them use it on friends and family (and have it done themselves) – they emphasize that, like every other cosmetic procedure, you shouldn't have it just because your best friend did.

So our advice is: resist squeezing the Botox® in between the dim sum and the Häagen-Dazs, or dropping in for a lunchtime jab. Instead, consult a qualified dermatologist who has performed the procedure hundreds of times and can give you the best advice.

Below are the key facts. Ask questions of your expert then go away and think about it before you decide. And no, we wouldn't have it done but we know plenty of women – and men – who have, and most of them are delighted with the treatment. Newby Hands, Director of Health and Beauty at Britain's *Harpers & Queen* magazine, says she is 'a huge fan of Botox® as long as it's not over-done'.

BOTOX® FACTS

✳ Botox®, a safe derivative of botulinum toxin, is injected into lines on the forehead and crows' feet to paralyze the muscles.

✳ Botox® is not usually suitable for use on the lower half of the face because it may cause muscle droop, according to Dr. Nicholas Lowe.

✳ You can have an anaesthetic cream applied before the injection if you wish: ask the doctor (or nurse) who does the procedure. (Some doctors offer this as routine.)

✳ The injections take a few minutes but the results won't be apparent for three to eight days.

✳ The amount of Botox® used varies; many doctors prefer to start with a very small concentration so that they can gauge the effect on each patient.

✳ The injection sometimes causes a bruise, occasionally a headache and, very rarely, produces redness and blistering (a reaction to the human serum albumen in the injection cocktail, not the Botox®). Patients are advised to stay upright for an hour after the injection.

✳ Results last from three to six months. Some people find that after a course over, say, two years, their paralyzed muscles actually 'forget' how to frown, so the benefits may last much longer.

OTHER FILLERS

There is a range of other ways of plumping up lines and enhancing your facial contours – but, like with all forms of invasive treatment, it's a case of 'caveat emptor': let the buyer beware. You should be aware that (as with Botox®), the success of these procedures depends on the skill and experience of the surgeon (or nurse), so always look for someone with a good – and long – track record of this work. You don't want to be the guinea pig!

Artecoll® (formerly known as Arteplast®): microspheres of PMMA, a form of plastic, suspended in a collagen solution; useful for filling deep lines, plumping the lip outline, evening out the nose and filling depressions such as acne scars or grooves under the eyes. Not suitable for anyone with an allergy to collagen (you must have a sensitivity test first). This material doesn't leave your body and, in the worst case, may form unsightly lumps.

Autologous Fat Injections: the patient's own fat is syringed out of the thigh, abdomen or buttock and used to plump out deeper lines and wrinkles (not fine, shallow ones) and depressions such as sunken cheeks. It's also used for hands. It's your own fat so there's obviously no risk of allergy but fat doesn't always stay put, so the results are not totally predictable. It can also be quickly metabolized so the effects can disappear quickly. This is a less popular treatment nowadays because of all the other options available.

Collagen Replacement Therapy®: also known by the brand names Zyderm® (for fine lines and wrinkles) or Zyplast® (for deeper ones), these injections replenish the body's own collagen (responsible for plump, smooth, 'elastic' skin) as it dwindles with age. It's very effective but a sensitivity test four weeks beforehand is vital, as some people are highly sensitive to the purified bovine collagen. (Some people feel understandably squeamish about this after mad cow disease, although there have been no reported problems.) We personally know of a woman who had a very serious allergic reaction to her injections, despite having had the sensitivity test first, and she required many weeks of steroid therapy. Good for lines around the lips, crows' feet, frown lines, and the creases running from nostril to mouth (medically called nasolabial lines). Duration varies by individual, but between two to six months is usual.

Hylaform®: this is a derivative of hyaluronic acid, a lubricant found in human and animal tissue (and also used in skin creams as a moisturizer). There is little risk of allergy except for those who are allergic to chicken or eggs (the key compound comes from rooster combs) and it can be used on people who test positive against collagen. Hylaform® is used for frown lines and crows' feet (but Botox® is probably more effective), nose-to-mouth lines, acne scars and lip plumping, but not fine lines and wrinkles. (Also derived from hyaluronic acid are Perlane®, Restylane® and Restylane Fine Lines®.)

The success of these procedures depends on the skill and experience of the surgeon (or nurse), so always look for someone with a good – and long – track record

Silicone: one of the first and most effective fillers for all facial purposes (also, of course, used in breast implants) but now regarded as the most risky. The problem is that you can't remove silicone and it may migrate around the body causing inflammation and/or the formation of inflamed nodules. Breast implants have been linked to many illnesses. We don't recommend you try silicone.

WARNING

Pregnant women or anyone with an autoimmune condition such as rheumatoid arthritis or lupus or anyone who has an allergy should be extremely careful before having a treatment which involves any kind of foreign substance being introduced into their body. Always check with your own doctor.

SoftForm™: this is a permanent (although removable) filler used to enhance thin lips and/or plump out nasolabial lines; like its predecessor Gore-Tex, it's fed in and out of the area to be filled using a needle that's inserted via two tiny cuts. Looks and feel very natural, although it may slowly be being replaced by a material called Ultrasoft™, which performs the same task.

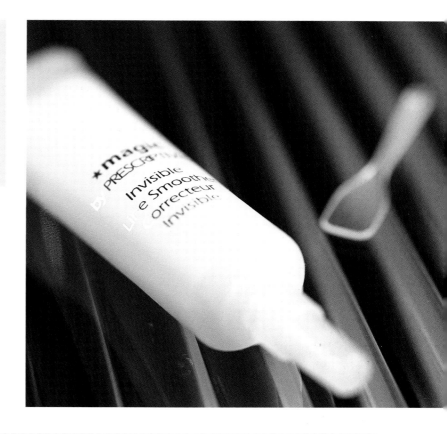

MAKEUP FILLERS

Before you embark on Botox®, collagen or any of the other invasive facial fillers, consider spending an iota of the price on one of the cosmetics industry's high-tech disguises for lines and wrinkles. Our favorites include:

✳ Prescriptives Magic Invisible Line Smoother: stroked on lines and deep wrinkles this silicone-based gel behaves exactly like spackle on cracks with the added bonus that it creates a soft-focus effect due to special 'optical diffusers' which bounce back light. Use before or after applying base, patting into crows' feet and furrows. Don't powder, though, or you spoil the effect.

✳ Lancôme Touche Optimage Line Blurring Concentrate: a creamy-gel product that does what it says. The gel helps fill in fine lines and the light-diffusing compounds visibly soften the area.

✳ Trish McEvoy's Line Refiner: not a filler but an eye-cream-in-a-wand, this streamlined product delivers moisturizing, light-diffusing ingredients to make lines and wrinkles look softer and dewier.

NONSURGICAL FACE LIFTS

Since the concept of nonsurgical face-lifts hit the market some two decades ago, we have seen a raft of different technologies launched. All are based on the same low-voltage electric current which recharges tired muscles, thus giving a temporary 'lift'. But most have kicked the bucket within a short time. One brand, however, has consistently been way out in front: CACI, otherwise known as Computer Aided Cosmetology Instrument. And this is the one we (and other beauty editors) recommend

CACI, like Botox® and many other cosmetic procedures, was pioneered for medical use – in this case on stroke and facial palsy patients. The original CACI system has recently been updated to the CACI Quantum. As before, the electrical current is introduced to your skin and tissue via cotton-tipped probes or adhesive pads applied to specific points on your face. The technology kickstarts flagging muscles by stimulating the fibers responsible for maintaining the tone, length and elasticity of muscle, and individual treatments can also be created to suit your skin. Additional features of the CACI Quantum include a Lymph Drainage mode, which helps reduce puffiness and drain excess fluid, and a Micro-mode which works on eyebags.

CACI Quantum softens lines and wrinkles, helps sags and bags, and gives a temporary face and neck lift, which may still show some effects after a week (though it's best within 24 to 48 hours). Additionally, the gizmo can be programmed to work on stretch marks and cellulite, and for bust enhancement. Many busy women swear that the hour or so's relaxation is one of the best parts of the treatment, and the new technology incorporates a heart monitor so that it works in time with your heartbeat. Ten to fifteen treatments are recommended, with maintenance treatments every four to six weeks afterwards. In practice, it can take longer to see a real change and upkeep may need to be more frequent: some women choose to go once a week (as their treat) and say that the effect is then marked. But if you're a 20– or 30–something with good skin, you may not see much of an effect. It's the ones most in need of help that will notice more of a difference.

FAVORITE FACIALS

Jo loves facials by Amanda Lacey, Eve Lom (herself) and the Dr. Hauschka facials at Sharon Devold at the Rye Sanctuary

Sarah is a fan of Jurlique facials (from Apotheke 20-20 in West London) and Dr. Hauschka (preferably from Grania Sims in London), also Anne Semonin (from Eva Berckmann at Claridge's in London)

Newby Hands, Director of Health and Beauty at *Harpers & Queen*, plumps for the Thalgo Velvet Collagen and Guinot Cathiodermie facials

Kathy Phillips, Director of Health and Beauty at British *Vogue*, is a devotee of the Vitamin C facial by Murad

Justine Cullen, Beauty Editor of *Marie Claire*, Australia, chooses aromatherapy-based facials by Aveda and Decleor

AND NOW FOR SOMETHING COMPLETELY DIFFERENT

When you think osteopathy, you don't think face lift. Well, we didn't until we discovered Vicky Vlachonis at the Integrated Medical Centre in London, who combines clunk-click methods with the extremely gentle shifts of cranial osteopathy and acupuncture to realign the body. One of the techniques she uses (which she learned, interestingly, from French obstetrician and water-birth guru Dr Michel Odent) is to release the muscles at the base of the tongue. Be warned: it can hurt – briefly but painfully. But the results on your face (as well as the trickle-down effect on your body) are extraordinary: any downward drift perks up and your contours seem redefined and, altogether, you look as if you have had a vacation and a face lift! Do be certain that you find a practitioner who has really learned this technique; again, you don't want to be a guinea pig. Jo, meanwhile, swears by amazingly 'lifting' and relaxing acupuncture facials from Yuki Umeguchi, which offer the bonus of an allover body tune-up!

FABULOUS FACIALS

Your skin and face show the results of stress – of all kinds – quicker than any other part of you. So having a good facial with a skilled practitioner can improve your skin temporarily, and having them regularly can make all the difference to your face – as well as ease your mind. What's more, going to a salon is a wonderfully pampering experience. So which one to choose? Well, we're not going to lay down laws about this because it is such a personal choice. However, we have listed, opposite, the ones we and some of our colleagues prefer. In general, we recommend that you go to a salon which uses products you know suit your skin, and try out different therapists. Facialists will use different massage techniques. In well-run salons, all will

work to a high standard – but you may find some personalities suit you better than others. When you find ones you like, stick with them: they're gold dust.

If you're on a budget, though, you don't need to pay a lot for facials; you can achieve wonders on your own at home – either with your favorite products or by using gorgeous natural recipes: see page 80 for facial oils and page 114 for natural face masks.

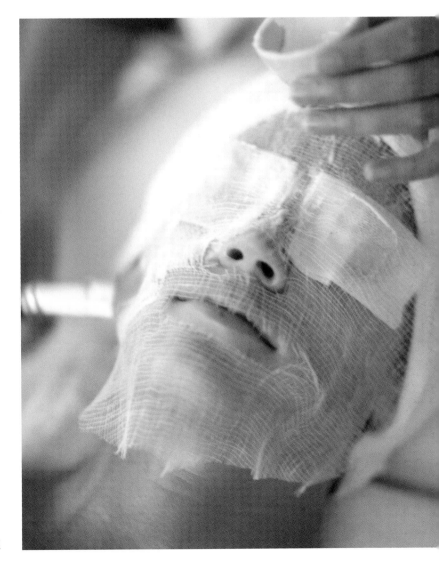

INSTANT FACE SAVERS – *Tried & Tested*

These are the lotions, potions, serums and complexion-boosting masks which are the equivalent of a facial-in-a-bottle, designed for times when true miracles are required. (Think: sleepless nights, hangovers, post-flu, post-op – or when skin's just plain got the 'blahs'.) Our testers tried a veritable mountain of products, but the consensus was: these are the ones that really do the business.

CLARINS BEAUTY FLASH BALM
8.8 points out of 10

The outstanding marks our testers gave this product confirm Flash Balm's place in the Beauty Hall of Fame. It delivers a firming film to skin – and is known to Clarins insiders as "Cinderella-in-a-tube".

UPSIDE: "I recently got married and after little sleep was looking like a less-than-radiant bride – this restored a nice, healthy glow!" • "truly believe that this should be every woman's beauty secret" • "it's become one of my must-haves – I'm not a cosmetic junkie, but this is fab" • "my face glowed as soon as the product went on" • "used it on combination skin and words fail me: I look and feel wonderful; I'm 51 – but it made me look 40!"

DOWNSIDE: "I'm just a little concerned about long-term use, as it could be drying" • "not entirely sure that it lived up to the hype".

CHANEL HYDRA SÉRUM VITAMIN MOISTURE BOOST
8.71 points out of 10

A mega-moisture boost, this can be used in emergencies or on an ongoing basis for thirsty skin; active ingredients include vitamins E and F (to help restore the skin's barrier function), as well as pro-vitamin B5.

UPSIDE: "Excellent – skin looked firmer, prettier and plumped-up for 4-6 hours" • "makeup went on very smoothly and skin looked bright underneath" • "a joy to use – just like velvet" • "like a mini face-lift – skin's peachy; I never had skin this good, even when younger" • "very luxurious – a treat for skin, which feels soft and velvety" • "used this on the day of my son's wedding – my skin stayed looking good all day and night; fantastic!"

DOWNSIDE: "Skin felt quite tight and dry after each application".

GUINOT GOMMAGE BIOLOGIQUE
8.5 points out of 10

In general, we're not fans of facial exfoliators – but this doesn't use granules (which can scratch skin), relying instead on enzymes to soften the links between cells before they're sloughed away. It also includes green tea extract and shea butter and, say Guinot, is good even for sensitive skins.

UPSIDE: "Skin much improved – sort of 'plumped-up'; loved this" • "I looked all rosy and attractively flushed; it's great it works so fast – really, a super-quick boost" • "face felt fresh for most of the day" • "felt like I'd had a facial – without the expense" • "a dream product and a must-have for a great pick-me-up" • "firmer, brighter, softer, smoother skin".

DOWNSIDE: Testers had absolutely nothing bad to say about this.

❀ AVEDA TOURMALINE-CHARGED PROTECTING LOTION
8.37 points out of 10

Although this is primarily marketed as a longer-term, anti-aging moisturizer, Aveda was confident enough about the instant benefits of this cream to ask us to test it as an "instant face-saver". It contains tourmaline – a crushed, semi-precious gem – along with antioxidants lycopene, beta-carotene and sugar extracts, and an SPF 15 chemical sunscreen.

UPSIDE: "11 out of 10 – this sent my eye bags into the next millennium and it seemed to lock in moisture and boost my sagging skin" • "skin felt very fresh – it soon wakes you up" • "brilliant – infused skin with visible life and radiance, restoring moisture balance" • "glided on beautifully; great for cheering up my winter-dull skin" • "skin looked even – and full of vitality" • "felt uplifted".

DOWNSIDE: "Not too good as a base".

DECLÉOR INSTANT DE BEAUTÉ RADIANCE LIFTING FLUID
8.22 points out of 10

Plant-based "tensors" create an "elastic film" over the skin's surface – for an instant firming effect – while borage oil and wheat germ replenish. This is designed to be used under your foundation.

UPSIDE: "Instead of feeling fiftyish, I felt fortyish – lovely!" • "a facelift at a fraction of the cost" • "a fabulous boost for one's looks and confidence – like an instant facelift!" • "used it when recovering from a bad cold and skin looked relaxed and radiant; a real find for days you don't feel so perky" • "a fantastic base for makeup; I felt positively glowing by the end of the day".

DOWNSIDE: "By the afternoon, my skin felt dry" • "extremely drying".

❀❀ JURLIQUE HERBAL RECOVERY GEL
7.88 points out of 10

An all-botanical, lightweight skin serum which scored well in our previous books for long-term benefits; this time, it's done brilliantly as a quick fix. This contains extremely potent antioxidants and herbal extracts from organic rose, licorice, marshmallow, calendula, daisy, chamomile and violet, plus oils from rosehips, evening primrose, carrot, macadamia nut and jojoba. It can be worn alone, or under moisturizer.

UPSIDE: "This product is magic – it makes my easily irritated skin look calm, smooth and well-cared-for and has people commenting on how great my skin looks" • "promised miracles – and delivered them; saved my day on New Year's Day as I'd drunk too much; it should be available by prescription!"

DOWNSIDE: "Fragrance not too pleasant, with a slight 'turned milk' note".

BEST BUDGET BUY
❀❀ NEAL'S YARD SPRITZER IN ZEST

7.66 points out of 10

Organically certified essential oils, together with a blend of Australian Bush Flower Essences, give the face-waking power to this 100 percent natural, preservative-free aromatherapeutic facial spritzer, designed for when skin needs extra 'zin'. (Good for planes and dry environments, too.) Though not cheap-cheap-cheap, it's definitely the best buy among the less expensive face treatments.

UPSIDE: "Felt awake – like a slap in the face, but much nicer!" • "excellent results; skin felt nourished/hydrated/refreshed – a real must-have-pick-me-up" • "zesty, reminiscent of a cooling gin and tonic, lifting my spirits and leaving me feeling revived" • "I also spritzed this on bedlinen, wardrobes etc. for a very refreshing, clean smell" • "a wake-up call for my skin – but also great for tired feet!" • "I used this after a severe bout of flu – a wonderful pick-me-up".

DOWNSIDE: "Good for cooling off – nothing more".

The lowest score in this category was 4.33 points out of 10.

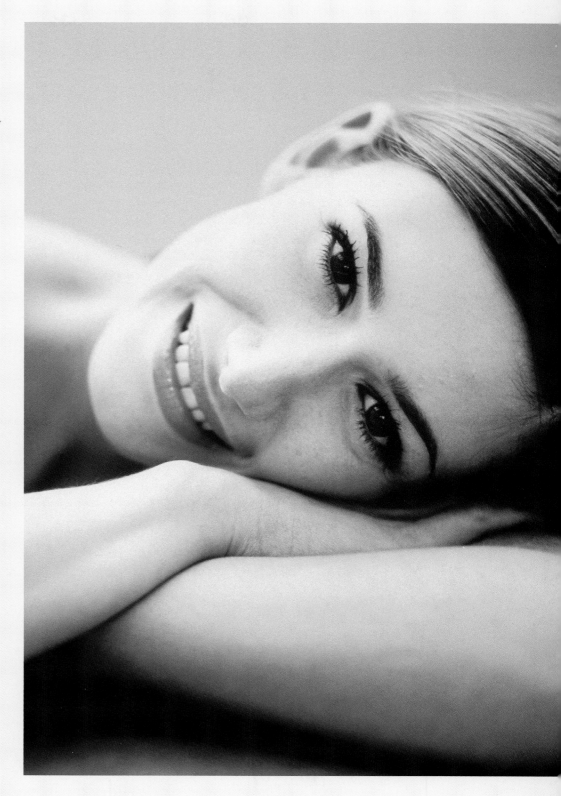

2-MINUTE FACE DE-STRESSERS

Your face is a prime place for holding tension, especially around the eyes, brows and temples, cheeks and jawline and the base of the neck. Banish the tension and your whole being changes. When you feel like your face is frozen in a mask, try this quick routine given to us by Susan Harmsworth, who founded the worldwide E'SPA line of aromatherapy products and spas. This can take two to five minutes – or as long as you like...

1 Take three to six long deep breaths: this will slow down your pulse rate and calm you.

2 If possible, pour a couple of drops of essential oil into your cupped hands and inhale them at the same time. Try orange, lavender or palmarosa to restore, peppermint or rosemary to energize, or ylang-ylang, frankincense or patchouli to soothe. (E'SPA makes blends of these oils or you can combine drops of each yourself.)

3 Now calm each area of your face in turn:

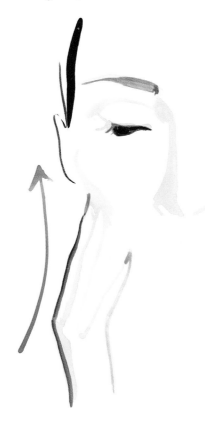

※ Take away negative tension from the temples: using the first two fingers of each hand, massage your temples in counter-clockwise small circles.

※ Relax your brow area: with a thumb below each eyebrow and index finger above, start in the center and slowly and gently pinch and lift along each brow right out to the temples.

※ Relax the eye sockets: with the three bigger fingertips of both hands (include your little fingertips if you can, although some find their hands are too big), circle all around the eye with a light tapping motion, starting at the top of your nose then working out, around and back.

※ Relax the forehead area: starting at the brow line, use the pads of your fingers to gently press and lift upwards, sliding up in ½in (1cm) steps, up and into the scalp.

※ Relax the cheeks: with your index, middle and ring fingers under your cheekbones on each side, lift and hold for a count of three; you may find you inhale naturally as you lift; then exhale slowly for a count of three, or six if you can manage.

✳ Relax the jawline: starting in the middle of your chin, with your thumbs below the jawline and middle fingers just above it, pinch, lift and hold the skin, working outwards to your ears.

✳ Supporting the back of the neck with your fingertips, stretch your neck gently forward; place the right hand over your head onto left ear and gently stretch your neck towards the right, then reverse the procedure. Then massage the base of your skull, just where it meets the neck at the back, and gently lean backwards if comfortable.

✳ Complete the relaxation with an eye-soother. Susan recommends damp cotton pads sprinkled with E'SPA Soothing Eye Lotion (or cold chamomile tea). Split one pad in half and mould the halves to each eye lid; tilt the head back, or lie down and cup the face and eye area with

AMANDA LACEY'S FACE DE-PUFFER

Stuffy sinuses are a key cause of face puffiness. Counteract them by lying down, then dip your ring fingers in a few drops of face oil – camellia, sweet almond or apricot. Starting with your fingers on either side of your nose, just in from your eye socket, tap out towards your temples. Repeat at least six times.

the palms of the hands to create a dark cocoon of peace. (Alternatively, try chamomile tea bags which have been infused in water and then left to cool in the fridge.)

QUICK FACE REVIVER

You know those mornings when you get up, look in the mirror and want to hide that tired, pale, wrinkly, blotchy face from the world? Don't panic; leading facialist Amanda Lacey has this remedy. Drink a mug of hot, pure, still water with a squeeze of fresh lemon in it. Now get some exercise to oxygenate your skin; go for a walk or a jog. Do some yoga (see pages 238–43) or simply dance around the house. At the very least, take six slow deep breaths. Look in the mirror again and you'll already begin to see a difference. Now clean your face with a good cleanser, then wash off with a face cloth wrung out in water as hot as you can bear, followed by a cold cloth to calm any redness; a good tip is to lean your head back when you use the cloth so that it lies on your face for a moment or two. Finish by pressing moisturizer into your skin with your fingertips – but don't rub or you'll start a blotch attack. Then drink at least 2 pints (1 liter) of water during the day.

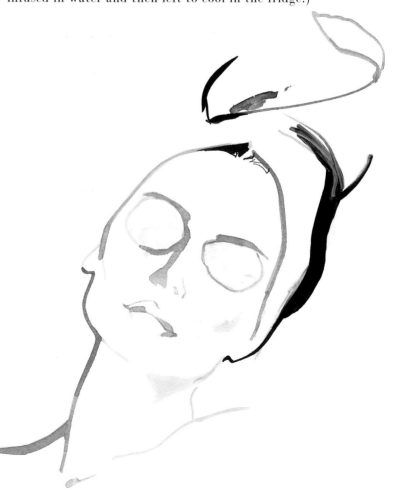

NATURAL MASKS

These good-enough-to-eat masks cost very little to make. So don't just pamper your face: use on hands, feet and back – if you can find someone to act as mask spreader

Aloe, rose and clay mask

This recipe was given to us by Margo Marrone, who has her own Organic Pharmacy in London. It is good for all skin types, especially sensitive.

1½ teaspoons of French green clay
½ teaspoon of bentonite (kaolin)
⁷⁄₁₀ fl oz organic aloe vera gel
³⁄₁₀ fl oz organic rose hydrolat (pure distilled rose water)
2 drops of organic rose essential oil

Mix the clay and bentonite together, then mix the aloe and rose hydrolat together. Slowly add the aloe rose mixture to the clay, stirring until all lumps are gone. Add the rose oil at the end. This will make two to three facial treatments, and will last in the refrigerator for 1 month.

Almond, honey, milk and aloe mask

Another Margo Marrone recipe, which is very hydrating for dry skin.

1 teaspoon organic powdered milk
1 tablespoon organic ground almonds
1 tablespoon organic honey, preferably Manuka
1 teaspoon organic aloe vera gel
2 drops neroli essential oil

Mix the milk with the almonds, add the honey and aloe and mix well. Finally, add the two drops of neroli. Smooth over the face. Leave on for 10-15 minutes. This will make two to three facial treatments, and will last up to two weeks in the fridge.

Amanda Lacey's Fridge Mask

Raid your fridge and revitalize your face. Simply mix one tablespoonful of live-cultured natural yogurt (room temperature) with one teaspoonful of natural runny honey. Apply to your face and neck for 20 minutes, then remove with a face cloth wrung out in hot water, repeating until it is all removed. For dry skin, use two teaspoonfuls of honey. For oily skin, add a few drops of fresh lime juice.

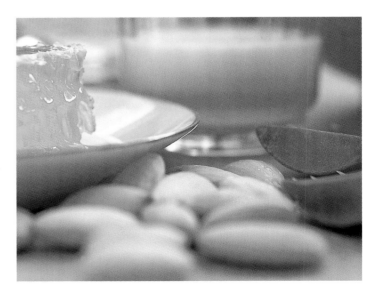

FACE MASKS – *Tried & Tested*

We asked manufacturers to supply us with products that were suitable for all skin types, although we should warn you that some of them have intensely moisturizing benefits and may prove too rich for oily skins (which tend to prefer oil-absorbing ingredients like clay or mud).

GUERLAIN INVIGORATING MOISTURIZING MASK

9 points out of 10

This contains mallow, renowned for its moisturizing properties. It should be left on skin for 10 minutes, once or twice a week, then washed or tissued off before applying makeup. It's more suitable for drier skin types.

UPSIDE: "Light and silky, with a tea-rose scent, it smoothed and relaxed, plumped, softened and moisturized" • "so light you didn't realize you had anything on your skin – but it left a lovely glow, with brilliant brightness" • "this product is heaven – and made my makeup last longer" • "skin felt like a baby's bum – soft and supple!" • "can be used instead of moisturizer before applying makeup" • "felt ten years younger – that's a miracle!".

DOWNSIDE: nobody had anything negative to say about this product at all.

ELEMIS FRUIT ACTIVE REJUVENATING FACE MASK

8.55 points out of 10

Elemis warn that a natural tingling sensation is normal with this mask, which should be left on face and neck for 10-15 minutes. Botanical skin-brighteners include kiwi and strawberry, while shea butter and macadamia nut oil have a nourishing effect.

UPSIDE: "High pamper factor – felt expensive and luxurious" • "total, blissful relaxation; my skin didn't need make-up next day and my husband remarked how sleek and silky my face felt" • "utterly rapturous!" • "I used it on Christmas Eve to restore a glowing complexion – great whenever skin is looking tired and dull" • "gave a lovely "porcelain finish" and a polished gleam" • "my skin glowed with health and was evenly toned" • "skin soft and smooth for four days".

DOWNSIDE: "Skin looked no different at the end of the day" • "quite hard to remove afterwards".

SISLEY EXPRESS FLOWER GEL MASK

8.5 points out of 10

Lily and iris give this a light, flowery smell, while extract of organically grown sesame helps deliver a moisture boost in just three minutes – for all skin types, but especially tired and dull complexions.

UPSIDE: "A miraculous product! After use my skin looked so good, I abandoned foundation for the evening in favor of tinted moisturizer" • "you could answer the door in this without frightening anyone – and love the fact that it only needs to be left on for three minutes, as time is my enemy" • "light, refreshing gel with a scent a little bit like cut grass" • "skin was "plumper" for a day or two" • "really gave a healthy glow for an hour or two; immediate enhancement of clarity" • "good before a big night out as skin looks instantly soft".

DOWNSIDE: "Slight stinging sensation".

SHISEIDO MOISTURE RELAXING MASK

8.44 points out of 10

A special massage technique, described on the packaging, is meant to turbo-charge the benefits of this moisturizing (alcohol-free) mask, which contains hyaluronic acid, 'phyto-vitalizing factor' (as with all Shiseido skincare), glycerine, thyme and tea-rose extracts. After leaving for 2 to 3 minutes, post massage, it can be tissued or rinsed off.

UPSIDE: "Results were near-magical – skin glowed and looked exceedingly healthy, and I'd give it 11 out of 10!" • "difference wasn't immediate but, used over a period of three weeks, the effects were visible – a smooth, healthy-looking complexion" • "light, fresh scent" • "skin looked rested and alive" • "hydrating, cooling, softening and radiance-boosting" • "soufflé-like texture – truly a delight to apply".

DOWNSIDE: "Product was so light and clear I couldn't actually see where I'd applied it".

BEST BUDGET BUY

✿ LIZ EARLE NATURALLY ACTIVE INTENSIVE NOURISHING TREATMENT

8.02 points out of 10

Another affordable winner from Liz Earle, this contains a "rich assortment of skin nutrients", in the form of rich-in-fatty-acids borage oil, shea butter, vegetable glycerine, St John's Wort extract, soothing comfrey and rose geranium oil. Like Liz's cleanser, it's best removed with a muslin washcloth and hot water (which, in fact, we'd recommend for efficient removal of any kind of mask).

UPSIDE: "Benefits seemed to last a couple of days after use – every time I used this, my skin felt like a soft, ripe peach" • "skin seemed more 'plumped-up'" • "really relaxing feeling" • "useful, too, for backs of hands in winter" • "skin felt calm and relaxed with a blushing bride tone – hooray!" • "skin looked altogether brighter and pores were tighter".

DOWNSIDE: "Felt more like applying a moisturizer than a mask – too greasy so skin didn't feel refreshed".

The lowest score was 4.2 points out of 10.

VEIN HOPES

Veins are essential to life: without them, the blood wouldn't get around our bodies. But they're our enemy when we notice a flare of red threads on our cheeks or legs. Here's the lowdown on making unsightly ones "disappear"

You have two options with veins: to conceal them with camouflage makeup or remove them with sclerotherapy or laser surgery. While makeup works well on the face, it's usually more difficult to conceal leg veins. Partly because the time you really want to camouflage them is on the beach! However, fake tan can help temporarily.

Camouflage makeup: There is a very good choice of camouflage makeup (which can be used for port wine stains and scars as well, of course). The general trick with application is to build up the cover gradually, so use your middle or ring finger to tap on thin layers then add to them, rather than piling the product on. One way of getting a small amount is to put the product in your palm first, which also warms it slightly, making for smoother application.

Laura Mercier Secret Camouflage: Another excellent coverup; each palette (it comes in several different tones) features two shades of concealer, so that you can blend your own skin-matching shade. Dab your finger in the product, blend on the back of your hand to get the color right, then apply in very light layers to the affected area, building up the coverage gradually so that it doesn't cake; set with a light coat of translucent pressed powder.

Dermablend: Again completely waterproof, this more medical product is available in 20 shades (including ones for women of color) and gives thick enough cover to disguise birthmarks and port wine stains, as well as broken capillaries.

Estée Lauder Maximum Cover: More a foundation-type product than a concealer, but offering high-density coverage perfect for broken capillaries (and opaque enough to make birthmarks disappear) and comes in five shades. Also waterproof.

Jane Iredale Circle/Delete: A concealer that you can blend to match your skin tone from a range of mineral-based, waterproof cosmetics, much favored by dermatologists and cosmetic surgeons after invasive procedures such as face lifts, as well as laser treatments.

JO'S TOP TIPS FOR BROKEN VEINS

Because I suffer from spider veins on my cheeks, I'm pretty much a world expert on concealers and foundations that are dense enough to camouflage broken capillaries without making me look as if I'm wearing a mask. The key is to always choose a concealer (such as the ones listed above) that is waterproof, so it won't budge during the day. I prefer to use a foundation that builds up to conceal my veins – my top choice is Lancôme Teint Idôle Hydra Compact. The best method of application, I've found, is to 'tap' the product lightly into the skin with my second finger, building up coverage and blending gently at the edges. I put the same product on other areas of my face where needed – but more lightly. One other product I love is Estée Lauder Idealist Skin Refinisher, a serum-like lotion that goes on before moisturizer. I've used it for over a year now and it has definitely taken the edge off the redness of my veins (and also makes a lovely velvety base for makeup).'

SCLEROTHERAPY AND LASER TREATMENT

First things first: we recommend that you always go to a qualified medical practitioner. We have both known beauty therapists who perform sclerotherapy (or micro-sclerotherapy) and now some are using flash-light sources which they claim work as well as lasers. But these are invasive procedures and, to maximize the chances of successful treatment, we believe they should only be performed under medical supervision.

Secondly, you want to proceed very carefully if you're considering sclerotherapy for your face, insists Dr. Nicholas Lowe, Consultant Dermatologist at the Cranley Clinic, London and Santa Monica, Senior Lecturer and Consultant at University College, London and Clinical Professor at UCLA School of Medicine. "I don't recommend sclerotherapy for faces, because there's a risk that the solution may track into veins leading to the eye." (Dr. Lowe tells us that this has led to cases of blindness.) He does, however, support its use for spider veins on the chest – or, most appropriately, the legs.

The general rule with legs is to have laser treatment for small veins and sclerotherapy for medium to large veins. Remember that both approaches may (although not invariably) take several sessions. Lasers don't do well with larger veins because, unlike sclerotherapy, they don't have the capacity to "close them down". Sclerotherapy involves an injection of an irritant solution which shrinks the veins using a sclerosing solution, which is used in a range of concentrations which your doctor will decide upon. There are very rare cases of allergic reactions and we advise you ask the practitioner for literature, which you should take home and read before you decide whether to opt for the treatment (although Dr. Lowe says it is, in general, very safe). A recent breakthrough with sclerotherapy is the development of a new light source – a "polarizing magnifying illuminator" – which allows the practitioner to see the veins clearly through the skin.

Lasers and Intense Pulsed Light (IPL) therapies are used for veins that are too small to get into with injection needles, and around the ankles where it is not safe to inject because the veins are too close to the arteries. There are several types of laser and IPL equipment, including the long-pulsed Alexandrite laser (which Dr. Lowe currently favors) and the ND:Yag. Others include PhotoDerm and Dornier MediLase SkinPulse. Only medical professionals should use these lasers. Dr. Lowe also cautions against the cheaper flash-light systems that are permitted for use by beauty therapists and, he believes, may have the potential to cause damage. In the future, bigger leg veins may be treated from within the vein itself, using electric diathermy wires or lasers; research is ongoing (mostly in the USA).

A word of warning: if leg veins are large – more than about $\frac{1}{5}$ inches in diameter – and blue and lumpy, they may be varicosed and need expert medical care. The safest thing is to consult your GP before embarking on any treatment for leg veins. To prevent any leg vein conditions from becoming more serious, Dr Lowe recommends wearing support stockings or socks if you are on your feet a lot.

TEETH TALK

*Caring for your teeth isn't rocket science, and it needn't take hours.
Give them simple daily TLC, with regular visits to the dentist and dental
hygienist, and they will reward you a thousand times over. Not only will you
never need dentures but you'll smile beautifully at the world. We asked Dr
David Klaff, past President of the British Academy for Aesthetic Dentistry,
and hygienist San Marie Botha for their advice*

✳ **Brush thoroughly twice a day:** before or after breakfast and before bed. For most efficient brushing – to get out the debris which causes plaque and to avoid damaging teeth and gums – use a battery-operated toothbrush such as Braun's Oral-B, which has a round head for 'cupping' teeth. (A battery-operated/electric toothbrush is like having an electric floor polisher instead of doing it all by hand; though we were initially skeptical, we're now avid fans.)

✳ **Make sure to brush the insides of your teeth**, particularly in the front; saliva is produced here and with it come minerals which can lodge in the teeth and form plaque.

✳ There's an ongoing debate about **whether or not to use fluoride toothpastes**. While fluoride may help protect against decay (although only one in six people are likely to benefit), it is also a highly toxic chemical which we prefer not to use. We like AloeDent Whitening Toothpaste, Urtekram Fennel toothpaste and RetarDEX, which is especially formulated to fight bad breath and remove stains caused by tea, coffee and red wine.

✳ **Floss once a day:** whenever it suits you. Flossing is the only way to eliminate the bacteria between teeth which cause decay and gum disease. Bacteria breed profligately and must be gotten rid of every 24 hours. Use a wide, flat floss which doesn't shred and then cause rough spots on your teeth.

✳ **Eat crunchy raw foods**, such as apples, carrots and celery which help 'clean' your teeth and gums. Avoid too many citrus fruits and juices (like orange and grapefruit), as well as coffee, which cause an acidic environment in your mouth and lead to decay.

✳ **Scrape your tongue** twice a week at least, daily if you wish. This ancient oriental practice removes bacteria which accumulate on your tongue. As well as looking unsightly, they can contribute to throat infections and bad breath.

✳ **Don't smoke** if you want to have sweet-smelling breath and healthy gums which will keep your teeth firmly in place. Smoking makes your breath smell horrible and contributes to loose, unhealthy gums.

✳ **Have a dental check-up once a year.**

✳ **See a dental hygienist every six months** to remove plaque and surface stains and give teeth a brightening polish. Make sure the hygienist reports any problems to the dentist.

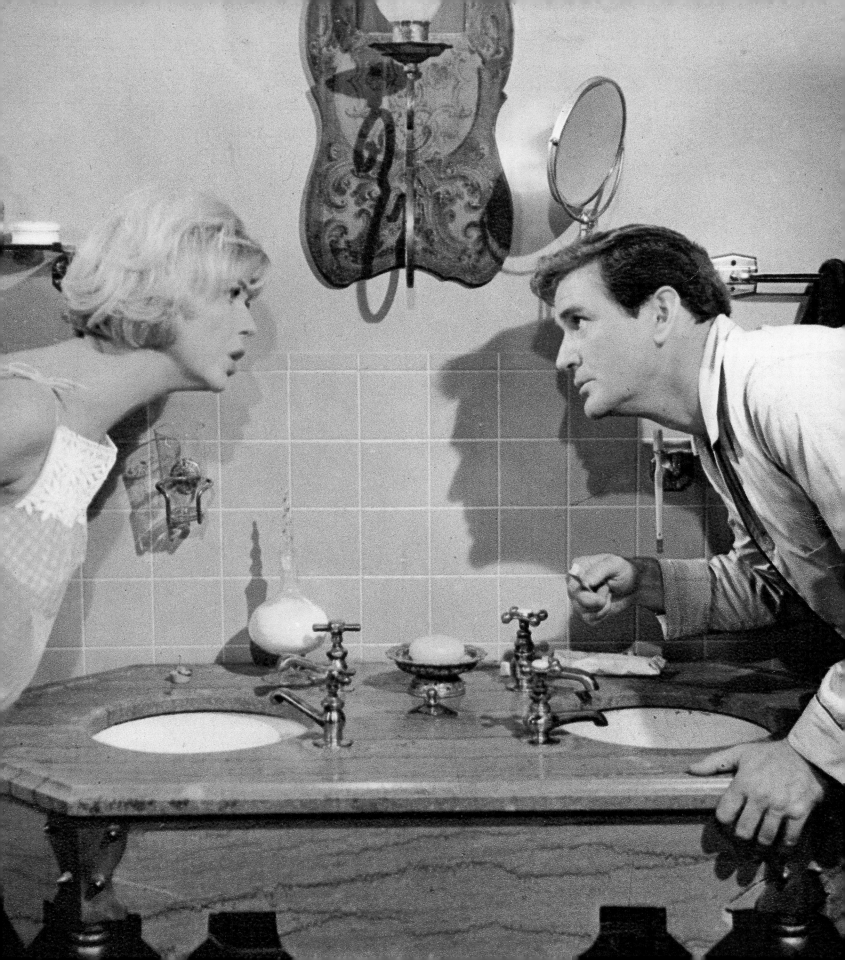

BRIGHT WHITE HOPES

So how do you get that Hollywood smile? Basically, there are three routes: whitening toothpastes, at home bleaching solutions and in-office bleaching at your dentist's.

The first and least invasive place to start is with a whitening toothpaste available at pharmacies everywhere. All toothpastes have mild abrasives to help remove surface staining but this new generation of products contains special chemical and/or polishing agents that are even more effective. Unlike bleaching agents, they do not penetrate into the tooth.

Your own dentist may recommend a particular product. If not, the American Dental Association (ADA) has put whitening toothpastes through stringent safety and effectiveness testing and given some products its Seal of Acceptance. These include:

• Crest Extra Whitening with Tartar Protection Toothpaste
• Crest Multicare Whitening Toothpaste
• Aquafresh Whitening Tartar Protection Toothpaste
• Colgate Total Plus Whitening Toothpaste, Paste
• Colgate Total Plus Whitening Toothpaste, Gel
• Colgate Tartar Control Plus Whitening Gel
• Rembrandt Extra Whitening Toothpaste

Bleaching is the other option. All bleaching solutions contain a percentage of peroxide – usually carbamide peroxide, which breaks down into the stronger hydrogen peroxide. This penetrates the tooth, breaking down pigment to remove color. Whether you opt for at home or in-office bleaching, consulting your dentist is undoubtedly the best route, especially if you have a lot of fillings, any kind of crown or veneer, or dark stains. (Or a medical condition, in which case you must seek advice from a qualified health professional.) Your dentist will be able to tell you whether bleaching is suitable for you and your individual situation.

You can buy home-use products from your dentist, which usually contain 10 percent carbamide peroxide (equivalent to about 3 percent hydrogen peroxide), though some contain more. The bleaching agent is delivered in a reservoir contained in a mouthguard. Your dentist can make a custom-fitted mouthguard that will fit your mouth exactly, avoiding the risk of the bleaching agent leaking from an illfitting one, and irritating the soft tissue of your mouth. (Bear in mind, you may have to wear this for a number of weeks, in some cases overnight.)

The ADA has evaluated the safety and efficacy of dentist-dispensed products containing 10 percent carbamide peroxide. Products that have passed the extensive testing required include:

• Rembrandt Lighten Bleaching Gel
• Nite White Classic Whitening Gel
• Opalescence 10% Whitening Gel
• Patterson Brand Tooth Whitening Gel
• Colgate Platinum Daytime Professional Whitening System

If your dentist does recommend bleaching, he or she will likely recommend a professional polish first because bleaching agents can't penetrate hard plaque. Most dentists also insist on carrying out any restorative work necessary, since unfilled cavities may allow the bleach to penetrate into the tooth pulp and cause permanent nerve damage.

The latest development in at-home technology is professional tooth-whitening strips, again available from your dentist. Rather than having to wear a bulky (and more costly) mouthguard at night, you simply put the strips on twice a day for 30 minutes for three weeks, or as recommended.

In recent studies, researchers at the University of Florida found that Crest Whitestrips Supreme were more effective in improving yellowness and caused less tooth sensitivity and gum irritation than customized tray whitening systems. However, the downside is that currently strips are only long enough to cover six to eight teeth so only your front teeth might get treated.

Like bleaching solutions, strips are available over the counter. With both options, we advise you to consult a professional. Remember, you will be using strong caustic chemicals in your mouth – it makes sense to get good advice.

The optimum route is to have your dentist bleach your teeth. Professionals use stronger and thus more effective peroxide solutions and should be experts at the procedure. This should take no more than an hour, including activating the bleach with a bright light or laser. (For stubborn stains, more treatments may be necessary and some dentists prescribe an at-home follow-up program.) Unless you have a reaction to the bleach, you should be fine immediately after. Teeth may be sensitive to heat and cold for a couple of days: this passes, but you may want to pass on the ice cream. Any discomfort can be treated with standard headache remedies.

So what can it do? Tooth-bleaching gives good results on stains from coffee, tobacco, wine, smoking or the general yellowing of teeth that goes with aging. However, it's easier to lift the color of stained teeth than improve on their natural color. Brownish stains from fluoride (fluorosis) or from tetracycline (which can cause teeth to take on a grey cast) can be treated, but that's likely to be a long drawn-out process – up to six months – and results are less predictable.

Some dentists don't consider smokers good candidates for tooth whitening, because smoking defeats the effect of whitening. There are also concerns that hydrogen peroxide plus smoking could exacerbate the tissue damage already caused by smoking.

How long will it last? Sometimes the first treatment doesn't work but a second or third will. In any case, your teeth will gradually become slightly more yellow again because of the natural process of aging. The rest depends on whether you smoke, drink staining drinks such as tea, coffee, soda and red wine, or eat acid-containing foods. In a study carried out by Ralph H. Leonard Jr. at the University of North Carolina School of Dentistry, Chapel Hill, the whitening effect remained stable for three years in 18 out of 32 people.

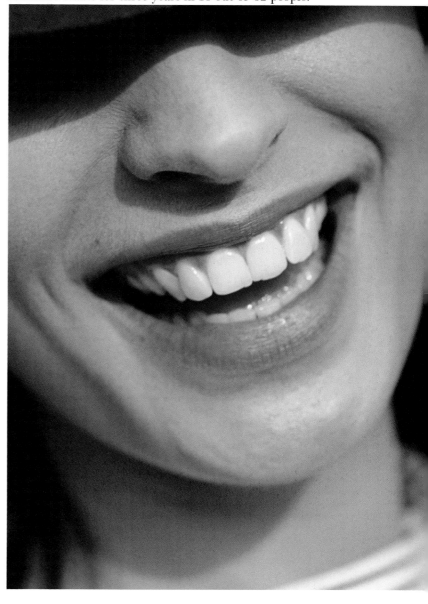

WARNING

• Pregnant or breast-feeding women should not have their teeth bleached.

• People with sensitive teeth should avoid bleaching as it can worsen sensitivity.

• Peroxide-based bleaches will only whiten natural teeth and will not whiten caps, crowns, veneers, or fillings.

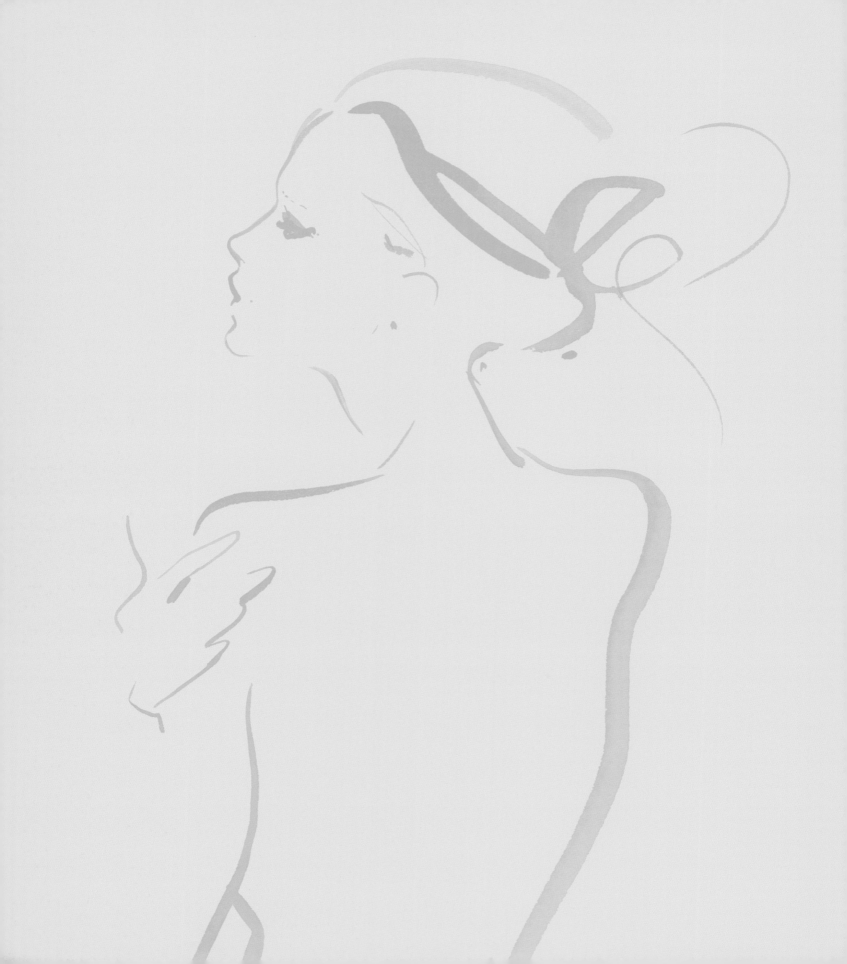

THE BODY

There's no such thing as the perfect body. (Even supermodels have their hang-ups.) But there's a lot we can do to make ourselves feel more gorgeous. (Including changing our mindset while we're working on our rear view.) In the 21st century, a great body is *your* best body. Just make it smooth, strokeable, healthy, energetic. (And with well-groomed extremities.) So here's the bottom line on achieving just that – without spending a fortune, or making it a full-time job. (Because who has time for that? Not us!)

GET GLOWING

The secret to smooth, soft, touch-me skin is simple: buff until beautiful!

Not to put too fine a point on it, the skin you can see with the naked eye is actually dead. As a result, it's often dry and dull. This surface layer also makes it harder for moisturizers and oils to penetrate. So while we believe in a softly-softly approach to exfoliating faces, we scrub areas like elbows, knees, ankles and upper arms regularly. For extremities and limbs that gleam with health, you should make body exfoliation a part of your beauty ritual. (Not just in summer, but winter too – when it's easy to forget everything below the waistline.)

Exfoliation is also essential before fake tanning – to smooth away the dead surface cells that self-tanners just love to cling to. (Which results in those telltale darker patches around elbows, knees, and ankles.) Just how often should you exfoliate? According to Susan Harmsworth, founder of ESPA, "The drier the skin, the more often you can exfoliate." She fesses up to dry legs, "so now I exfoliate them three times a week". Use salt scrubs and other body exfoliants on damp skin, Sue advises, except on areas with thicker skin like knees, elbows, and feet, where they can be used dry. (Be aware, though, as we've said, that sloughing away dead skin makes it a bit easier for ingredients – including chemicals – to be absorbed. Which is why we try to stick to natural-as-possible – best of all, organic – body lotions and oils.)

SCRUBS WE LOVE!

We admit it: we're a couple of old scrub fanatics. We are both somewhat obsessed with the skin-sloughing, get-your-blood-flowing power of salt- and sugar-based scrubs, used every few days on areas like upper arms, knees and feet – rather than all over. We have a long list of favorites (which admittedly result in a rather cluttered bathroom

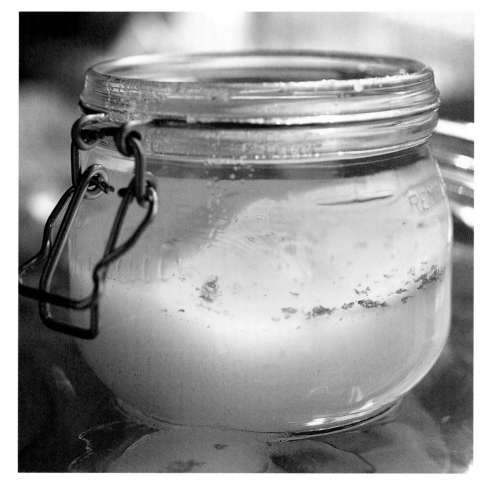

shelf): E'SPA Salt Scrub (both the Invigorating and Relaxing versions, which are hugely effective mood enhancers, too), peppermint-scented REN Guerande Salt Exfoliating Body Balm, Woodspirits Mountain Spruce Scrub and Fresh Sugar Bath Brown Sugar Body Polish, and E'SPA Exfoliating Body Polish.

Personally we like scrubs that use all natural ingredients and have often been known to create our own, using organically certified food ingredients, natural sea salt or sugar and essential oils. Sarah flings a tablespoon of sea salt (or any other) into a puddle of olive oil in a soup bowl to soften her scaly legs. And on the right, you'll find Jo's more sophisticated favorite recipe, which she packages in the kind of hinged fruit-preserving jars with rubber rims that you find in housewares stores. (Homemade scrubs make wonderful gifts – our friends and family love them! And you can even order your own labels, over the internet, from www.myownlabels.com.)

Jo's homemade scrub

Into a large jar, pour:
16 oz. brown sugar (for sensitive skin) OR salt (Jo likes Maldon sea salt – because it's grainy – but you can use any kind of rough or smooth salt)

Then add:
5¼ fl. oz. grapeseed oil
3½ fl. oz. sweet almond oil

Drop by drop, add:
25 drops neroli essential oil
10 drops sandalwood essential oil
10 drops sweet orange essential oil
10 drops ylang-ylang essential oil
5 drops patchouli essential oil

Put the lid on and shake well. Apply by the handful to problem areas on the body; you shouldn't need extra moisturizer afterwards. (And, of course, this can be made in smaller quantities.)

Noella Gabrielle, who is the aromatherapy genius behind Elemis's spa treatments, shared with us the recipes for Sea Salt Scrub and Green Tea Scrub (right) to help recreate the spa experience at home...

Sea Salt Scrub

2 tablespoons sea salt (exfoliant)
3 teaspoons grated ginger (warms the body and increases circulation)
finely grated peel of 1 lime (cleansing)
6 slices of cucumber, chopped (cooling)
½ fl. oz. almond oil (nourishing – a great skin emollient)

Blend together with a mortar and pestle or a food processor. It's great for the soles of the feet, knees, elbows – and the "orange-peel skin" (you know what we're talking about!) that can plague bottoms and the tops of thighs.

Green Tea Scrub

2 tablespoons green tea leaves (exfoliant)
1 tablespoon uncooked brown rice with the husk on (exfoliant)
1 teaspoon honey to bind the scrub (moisturizing and helps the mixture smooth over the skin)
½ fl. oz. sweet almond oil

Mix together with a wooden spoon; good for the bust, décolletage and delicate areas of the body.

BODY SHOPPING

Our prehistoric ancestors didn't need body lotions.
But then, they didn't have baths and showers...

Left entirely to its own devices, skin knows how to "rebalance" itself. But few of us are prepared to go without bathing for a month to allow it to do just that. So, for most women, body lotion has become a beauty essential, with many of us going through oceans of lotions in a year. If you're looking for truly effective body-quenchers, check out the creams and lotions on page 128, which impressed our testers. Meanwhile, here are some hints on caring for your largest organ (that's skin!)

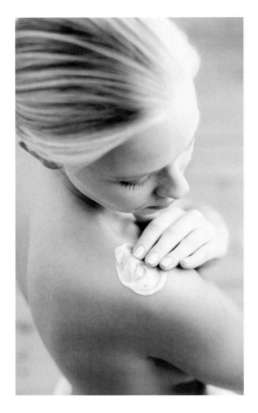

✳ Fact: moist air doesn't suck water from your skin – face or body – as readily as dry air does. So for anyone with dry skin, the higher the humidity level, the happier – and dewier – your skin will be. If you don't want to invest in a humidifier (the ultimate skin treat), balance a small dish or bowl of water on a radiator – or even on any flat surface away from a heat source. (So that it doesn't look like an abandoned bowl, try placing a few pebbles in the bottom. Very Zen!) You'll be amazed at how quickly the water evaporates into the air – moistening the environment around your skin, so that it won't be so dry in the future.

✳ Be aware that the moisturizing ingredient lanolin triggers sensitivity in some users – including Jo. (We also worry about possible contamination of this cosmetic ingredient with organophosphate sheep dip; some lanolin from non-organic sheep has been found to contain high levels of several different pesticides.)

✳ Ignore oft-repeated advice about "applying moisturizing lotion to still-damp skin". The moisture on your skin actually dilutes the cream, so what you're doing is applying a lighter film of moisturizer rather than the rich dose skin really needs.

✳ Do your skin (and the planet) a favor by limiting shower time to five minutes. Water rinses skin's own vital protective oils down the drain.

✳ It's a myth that you need to wash all over with soap – but it's one that has made soap-makers rich. Many soaps are highly processed and have had skin-softening glycerine removed, so look out for "handmade" soaps (we love Neal's Yard and Woodspirits, which still contain glycerine. In fact, rinsing with warm water gets everything except hands and feet clean enough. If you skip soap in the underarm area, you may find your "pits" aren't so prone to odor – which can be the result of bacteria frantically recolonizing, after you wash with soap.

✳ Itchy, flaky skin may actually be a signal that you're sensitive to something you're putting in your bath, especially if it's highly detergent. On page 208 you'll find bliss-inducing recipes for aromatherapy baths – including one for sensitive skins – but you could also try this tip from Julia Kwan, founder of the Orient-inspired cosmetics line Wu, which she learned from her mother. "Buy some sugar cane slices – available from Chinese markets – and half-fill the bath with hot water. Then put a couple of slices of sugar cane in the water, and leave them to 'melt'. Fill the tub with water and enjoy your bath."

✳ Applied after bathing (to a towel-dried body), the body oils on the right are wonderfully nourishing, all-natural alternatives to body creams that you can easily make yourself, at home. Preferably, decant into dark glass jars, and keep out of sunlight and away from heat...

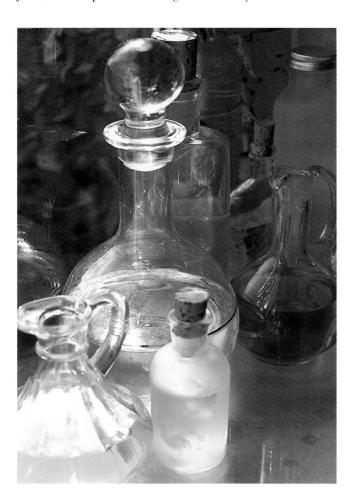

Nourishing Body Oil

Loredana and Mariano Spiezia, of Spiezia Organics gave us this bliss-inducing body oil recipe...

1¾ fl. oz. jojoba oil
1 fl. oz. almond oil
½ fl. oz. apricot kernel oil
⅛ fl. oz. wheat germ oil
18 drops ylang-ylang essential oil
10 drops sweet orange oil
6 drops lavender essential oil

Sensual Body Oil

From Michelle Roques O'Neill, one of the UK's leading aromatherapists, comes this get-you-in the-mood fusion...

1¾ fl. oz. peach kernel oil
10 drops grapefruit essential oil
8 drops ylang-ylang essential oil
4 drops West Indian bay essential oil
3 drops patchouli essential oil
2 drops myrrh essential oil

Revitalizing Body Oil

Another blend from Michelle. This one, she tells us, "is great to use if you're detoxing, and fantastic for drainage and circulation."

1¾ fl. oz. peach kernel oil
10 drops geranium essential oil
8 drops grapefruit essential oil
4 drops lavender essential oil
4 drops sandalwood essential oil
2 drops lemongrass essential oil

BODY MOISTURIZERS – *Tried & Tested*

If you're like us, you're constantly on the lookout for a moisturizing skin treatment to slather generously from top-to-toe. Because body lotions come in big sizes (and can be pricey), a mistake can feel super-wasteful, triggering a major guilt attack as we ditch a perfectly okay product. (Or forcing us to struggle through to the last drop with absolutely no pleasure factor.)

DERMOLOGICA BODY HYDRATING CREAM
9.2 marks out of 10

A high-scoring winner from Dermalogica's Spa Body Therapy range, which combines exfoliating hydroxy acids from sugar cane and apple, plus lactic acid, with essential plant oils (including lavender, tea tree and camomile) to smooth, soothe and moisturize. Lived up to all its promises, say our rhapsodic testers, several of whom gave it 10 out of 10.
UPSIDE: "Very quickly absorbed, smelt nice, almost like aromatherapy, no greasy residue and softer skin – full marks!" • "smooth silk texture, heavenly gorgeous smell that really awakened my senses, skin felt nourished and cared for, plus perfect pump-action dispenser" • "easy to apply even on slightly hairy legs!" • "worth the price!".
DOWNSIDE: "Required double doses on rough skin to see results but they were much improved".

❁ REN WILD YAM OMEGA-7 BODY CREAM
9 marks out of 10

Featuring Wild Yam (long used for menopausal women) to moisturize and help boost skin lipids, this popular product also contains Sea Buckthorn Berry Oil, a potent source of Essential Fatty Acids. Many women like to use a more natural product on their bodies and, while not 100 percent, this is trying hard. One tester gave it 11 out of 10!
UPSIDE: "Almost instantaneously absorbed, dry areas disappeared and my skin felt as smooth as velvet" • "my worst areas of dryness – shins and heels – were cleared up; I really enjoyed this product" • "light unobtrusive smell, generous-sized pump dispenser; seems to have banished late-winter scaly skin" • "all skin softer – even my husband noticed" • "I only had one ingrowing hair after waxing, while using this – normally I have loads" • "my new best product for my very sensitive skin".
DOWNSIDE: "deflating inner tube of dispenser looked sad…" • "not as effective on my scaly legs as the product I compared it with".

CLARINS RENEW-PLUS BODY SERUM
8.89 marks out of 10

Exceptionally good results (in a tough category) for this body "anti-ager", which features pro-retinol (a form of vitamin A) to enhance cellular renewal, along with plant extracts, gently exfoliating wintergreen, olive, cashew nut oil and Madagascan white lily – which is rich in vitamin C and (so Clarins trumpet) has an exceptional ability to retain water. Suitable for ages 30 plus, they say.
UPSIDE: "Glistening, dewy skin on first application with definite firming action, noticeably on thighs" • "a week improved texture, tone, faded stretch marks" • "body felt fresher, more alive, with thighs better toned after a week of using this perfect-consistency serum" • "skin felt like velvet and looked more toned and even – a definite 'pamper-yourself' effect" • "left attractive sheen on skin" • "a real miracle!".
DOWNSIDE: "Couldn't say it made my skin firmer – unfortunately!" • "extra needed on elbows and knees, and serum left hands lingeringly sticky".

JO MALONE LIME BASIL & MANDARIN BODY LOTION
8.83 marks out of 10

From the renowned London facialist whose cult brand was snapped up by the Lauder empire, this moisturizing and nourishing lotion is available not just in this zesty scent, but also several other Jo Malone fragrances.
UPSIDE: "Skin felt moisturized and fragrance lasted well all day" • "skin very soft and luminous, and a little goes a very long way – a real treat" • "made my dry skin tingle nicely after the shower" • "skin felt softer and smoother after a week" • "like putting silk on skin – my whole body smelt classy" • "immediately quenches dry skin" • "if I could afford this I'd buy it by the crate!".
DOWNSIDE: "Difficult to get the last bit out of the bottle" • "slow to absorb".

DECLÉOR SYSTÈME CORPS
8.66 marks out of 10

This light, creamy milk is suitable for all skin types but especially (so Decléor say) for dehydrated, dull skins or those recovering from pregnancy, weight loss or gain, or stress. The moisturizing ingredients include coconut oil, vitamin E and nourishing meadowfoam oil.
UPSIDE: "A great all-round product: super smell, quick and easy when you're rushing in the morning" • "dry patches gone from knees and elbows – loved this" • "smoothed and pampered, like I'd an invisible velvet coating on my skin – a dream!" • "left slight silky sheen on skin; softer skin on upper arms and fewer skin 'blips'" • "elbows instantly softened".
DOWNSIDE: "Consistency too thin – though that did help it spread".

OLAY TOTAL EFFECTS BODY TREATMENT
8.62 marks out of 10

From their mid-priced, turn-back-the-clock range, this stars Olay's unique "VitaNiacin" ingredient, designed to combat what they call the "seven signs of aging": dryness, roughness, lack of firmness in areas like arms, uneven skintone, fine lines and wrinkles. In some countries, they offer a money-back guarantee if you're not satisfied. N.B. One tester experienced a sensitivity reaction to this cream, so discontinued use.

UPSIDE: "Definite improvement in skin softness in about a week, especially behind knees, and the ankles" • "from day one, my parched, neglected skin was restored to softness" • "the best I've tried – after a few days I was happy to show my embarrassing heels in public again" • "skin looked less dry and wrinkly; crepiness diminished, flakiness gone" • "could be used in the morning before getting dressed as it absorbed quickly; wonderfully light-but-luscious".

DOWNSIDE: "Didn't like the smell" • "didn't change skin tone or texture or reduce appearance of stretch marks".

BEST BUDGET BUY
NIVEA BODY NIGHT RENEWAL CREAM
8.5 marks out of 10

Designed to make use of overnight skin regeneration, this new product from a tried-n-trusted company contains vitamins F and H to help repair and moisturize skin, particularly if it's dry, mature or damaged.

UPSIDE: "Oh I loved this – it's the miracle cream I've been searching for! I now have an unnerving habit of stroking my own so-soothingly-smooth skin..." • "thick, smooth, pleasant smelling, absorbed virtually straight away and left skin very soft with a nice sheen" • "really works on rough areas and has that lovely 'Nivea' smell" • "new skin in a pot! my husband said they should try it on crocodiles".

DOWNSIDE: "claim to help sleep is definitely dodgy" • "prefer pump to jar".

I COLONIALI DEEP MASSAGE BODY CREAM WITH MYRRH
8.3 marks out of 10

This velvety textured product combines influences from Italy and the far East with myrrh (resin from the tree) to tone, purify and soothe plus emollient oils. It features microspheres that melt into the skin to enhance moisturization, according to the manufactureres. (These may give it the initial slightly gritty texture commented on by some testers.) There was one sensitivity reaction.

UPSIDE: "Went straight in, felt sumptuous, smelt fabulous, exotic, and intense; made my skin silky smooth and gorgeously scented" • "I haven't needed to wear perfume at all while using it" • "a pleasure to use, felt very luxurious and smelt gorgeous" • "my skin immediately felt hydrated and softer and the delicious smell lingered all day" • "I could eat this out of the jar, noticed a vast improvement all over my body particularly on bust area".

DOWNSIDE: "My hands became red and sore followed by small blisters the first time I used this" • "smell was far too powerful and sickly".

❀ LIZ EARLE DAILY SKIN SMOOTHER
8.21 marks out of 10

This was the highest-scoring of the more natural products, and although not 100 percent natural, it features impressively generous levels of botanicals high on the ingredients list – including shea butter, avocado oil, echinacea, pro-vitamin B5, lactic acid and natural source vitamin E, together with essential oils of rosewood, orange, lavender and geranium.

UPSIDE: "Smoothed and made dry skin velvety" • "sensual, smooth, rehydrating, marvellous on rough skin" • "easily matches creams at the expensive end of the range" • "practically 24-hour moisturization – I could almost hear my body going 'aaaaaaah'".

DOWNSIDE: 'Let down by unglamorous bottle' • "immediate effect, but not long-lasting".

❀❀ BURT'S BEES CARROT NUTRITIVE BODY LOTION
7.7 marks out of 10

Specially formulated for sun-damaged skin, this moisturizing and protective lotion is 98.67 percent natural, according to the makers. One tester emailed immediately to say it treated her eczema better than anything the doctor could prescribe: it contains Balsam of Peru, an essential oil noted for treating eczema and chapped hands and feet. The antioxidant-rich carrot seed oil undoubtedly works well but some testers weren't keen on the smell or the fact that it may stain. (Sarah, who is a fan, suggests using it at night and letting it sink in for a few minutes before going to bed.)

UPSIDE: "Skin immediately felt soft and moisturized, looked dewy and healthy with a slightly silky shine" • "after two weeks' use I came to love this and now want more! It's the lightest effective body lotion I've ever used; you can even put on tights immediately, skin tone looks firmer and it leaves a healthy glow" • "even used it on my face and was good under foundation" • "wonderful product – it stopped the itching from eczema where doctor's creams did nothing" • "very good pump dispenser".

DOWNSIDE: "strange strong smell – stained clothes quite badly" • "loved everything except the smell but put up with that because it's so natural".

The lowest mark awarded in this category was 4.43 marks out of 10.

CELLULITE

More than nine in ten women say they have it, skinnies and fatties alike, and finally many doctors agree that cellulite isn't just plain old fat

Eat less and exercise, doctors used to say—and then, they claimed, we wouldn't have the familiar orange-peel textured lumps on thighs, butt (even arms and tummy) that can make getting into your swimsuit a nightmare if you're the least bit self-conscious.

Today, however, many conventional doctors agree that cellulite really is a bit different from ordinary fat – and needs a different approach. It's mainly the way the thousands upon thousands of fat cells are packaged that leads to the puckering and bulging. If the cell membranes are weak or damaged – as seems to be happening with cellulite, the fatty tissue doesn't lie neatly but forms lumps. Also, the strong fibers anchoring the fatty tissue to the layers of skin above pull at the pockets of fat, creating the button-back chair look.

The causes

Hormones: Cellulite is connected with women's reproductive hormones, principally estrogen, and forms in the areas where we are genetically programmed to store fat. Taking the Pill and HRT, both of which deliver added estrogen, is recognized as a big contributory factor to cellulite. The reason men don't get cellulite is because they don't have the same hormones. The male hormone seems to stop cellulite forming, whereas estrogen promotes it. Estrogen also triggers water retention, which is linked to cellulite: cellulite fat has more water in it than other forms of fat. (That doesn't mean women with cellulite should take diuretics or stop drinking lots of water.)

Junk food, additives and pesticide residues: According to Dr. Elisabeth Dancey, whose London clinic specializes in treating cellulite, it can be linked to eating junk food: some of the chemicals act as estrogen mimics and disrupt the smooth functioning of the body. This may explain why even rake-thin, superfit women – including Olympic athletes and supermodels – get cellulite. Also, lack of essential nutrients, particularly the antioxidant vitamins and trace minerals, is known to stimulate cellulite.

Sluggish digestion: Poor digestion and elimination of waste, due to lack of enough water, fresh fruit and vegetables and exercise, or conditions like Irritable Bowel Syndrome, candida and food intolerances, may also trigger cellulite.

Women store fat six times more readily on their lower body than the upper. But the lower body is far less eager to let that fat go.

Stress: Whether it's physical or mental, this can alter body chemistry and prompt the storage of fat.

Yo-yo dieting: Another big factor. Women store fat six times more readily on their lower body than the upper. But the lower body is far less eager to let that fat go. So if you lose seven pounds (or seven kilos), six go from the top and just one from the bottom. When you put it on again (as yo-yo dieters always do), six go to the bottom as one goes to the top. And the pattern intensifies if you go on dieting in this way.

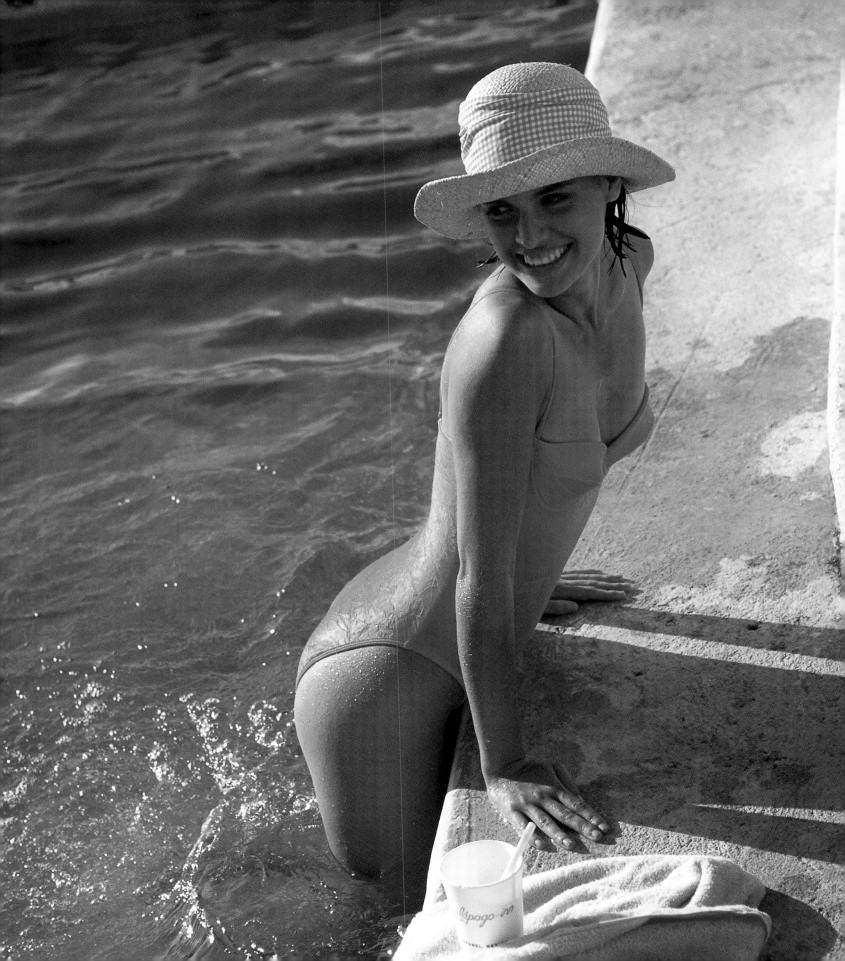

HOW TO TACKLE CELLULITE

Cellulite is such a stubborn problem that you have to treat it with a combination approach. And, as our testers found, even some commercial skin products can help

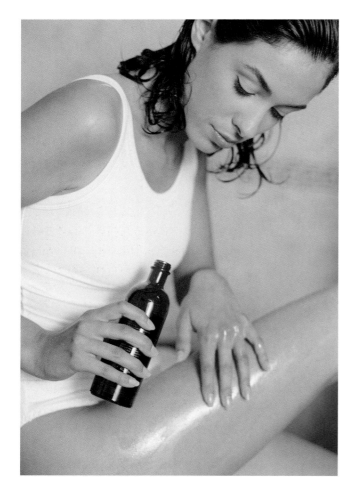

Let's be clear. You could spend a fortune on treating your cellulite and you might never budge it for good. However, there is no doubt that you can improve it greatly with lifestyle measures that cost little and will boost your health and beauty in general. You can then add in salon and/or medical techniques if you have the resources. Here we've listed the strategies we believe in.

Lifestyle

✳ Eat plenty of fresh foods, organic if possible; cut out processed, packaged and ready-made foods (see page 232).

✳ Make sure you eat some protein daily, particularly if you're vegetarian or vegan.

✳ Cut out fatty, sugary foods, which are stored as fat, mainly on your lower body.

✳ Cut down on dairy products, particularly cow's milk.

✳ If you have a blood sugar imbalance (you get shaky and depressed if you don't eat regularly), make sure you eat every three hours.

✳ Drink lots of still, pure water to help your body function smoothly; don't take diuretics or weight-loss pills.

✳ Exercise! Try to do at least four sessions of stretching, toning exercise like yoga (or dancing or swimming) four times weekly. Always do one stretching session a day (see our yoga section, page 238), and walk wherever you can.

✳ Relax... de-stressing will help your whole body. You can start breathing better now (see page 56). Also see our Well-being section for stress-busting ideas.

✳ Use a body brush to improve skin texture (see opposite) and use a good moisturizing cream.

Let's be clear. You could spend a fortune on treating your cellulite and you might never budge it for good. However, there is no doubt that you can improve it greatly with lifestyle measures that cost little and will boost your health and beauty in general. You can then add in salon and/or medical techniques if you have the resources. Here we've listed the strategies we believe in.

Supplements

✳ Take a good multivitamin/mineral daily.

✳ There is some evidence that vitamins C and E can help. New York dermatologist Dr. Karen Burke recommends taking 1 to 6g vitamin C daily, plus 400 IU natural vitamin E.

✳ Consider a calcium/magnesium supplement (400mg calcium with 200mg magnesium) to make up for reducing your intake of dairy products.

Therapies

These should be carried out in conjunction with the lifestyle remedies.

✳ **Manual Lymphatic Drainage massage (**aka **MLD)** – safe and effective. (You can also massage your body with anti-cellulite oils, but do it gently with long sweeping strokes; overly vigorous massage may cause more problems.)

✳ **Ionithermie, Endermologie and body wraps** – these salon treatments are generally accepted to have some effect; however they may not be lasting. (Endermologie has now been approved by the FDA for the treatment of cellulite.)

✳ **Mesotherapy** – a technique from mainland Europe, where it's well respected, in which tiny amounts of pharmaceutical drugs are injected into the cellulite deposits; needs a course of about 15 sessions; must be administered by a medical practitioner.

✳ **Electrolipopuncture** – pioneered in Switzerland over a decade ago; a gentle electric current is applied via very fine needles to the fatty tissue, stimulating the fat cells to activity which uses up their stored fat; it's not painful but must be carried out by a doctor or nurse; a course of ten sessions is recommended. (This is a much less painful alternative to cellulolipolysis – which was only effective in about half of patients in one small unpublished study.)

Surgery

✳ Various types of liposuction (where fat is sucked from the body in a syringe) may be effective. However, all surgery carries risks, is expensive and the results, overall, are not convincing for this condition. An absolute last resort. (If you really feel this is your only hope, please go via a recognized association of plastic or cosmetic surgeons. There have been fatalities, and near fatalities, with makeshift clinics. Don't believe that because you are paying a lot you are getting the best – check out the practitioners very carefully.)

Body Brushing

Body brushing undoubtedly helps combat cellulite by improving the texture of the skin. (We have also noticed that missing out on our daily body brushing has a marked negative effect after a few months.) Avoid too-stiff brushes that scratch the skin but remember that too-soft brushes won't work: test by whisking brushes across the back of your hand before buying. Brush before your bath or shower. Start at your feet and work up the legs and

CELLULITE CREAMS – *Tried & Tested*

When we tested the first batch of anti-cellulite products for our very first book, our testers were blown away by the improvements they saw in their thighs, hips and backsides. Then along came the European Cosmetics Directive – and suddenly, manufacturers were forced by law to list all the ingredients on the packaging.

So were some of those earlier wonder creams, in fact, acting more like drugs than cosmetics – and was that the secret of their success? Certainly, there was a massive scramble to reformulate – and it's fair to say that our testers have never again been blown away by the effects of these products.

We have now tested dozens of cellulite products on the market - and all tests were carried out over a period of months, on panels of ten women each. For comparison, we always ask testers to try their assigned product on one side of their body only, and to take before-and-after measurements.

The bottom line? Personally, we tend to believe that any diligent programme of massage and/or body brushing, combined with the use of a good body cream, will deliver comparable benefits.

YVES SAINT LAURENT LIGNE PURE
7.38 points out of 10

Active ingredients in this are bitter orange and caffeine – together with ruscus, yeast extract, marine plankton (and more). According to YSL, skin should be visibly toned and refined after just eight days of twice-daily massage.

UPSIDE: "Skin looked smooth and flawless; nice 'holiday' smell" • "skin felt very soft and nice – though I don't see a lot of difference in the dimples" • "noticeably less pitting" • "skin looks more toned and smoother".

DOWNSIDE: "Certainly not a miracle product – just a glorified body cream" • "I wouldn't wear tight trousers afterwards – the smell really absorbed into clothing".

❀❀ ELEMIS CELLUTOX ACTIVE BODY CONCENTRATE
7.3 points out of 10

For those who prefer a more natural choice, this is a 100 percent botanical product, in a base of almond oil, sunflower oil and vitamin E oil. (This also makes it more appropriate for nighttime use, when it won't mark clothes.) Active botanicals include juniper, seabuckthorn, lemon and sea fennel.

UPSIDE: "Very impressed; definitely firmer skin and orange peel has smoothed out" • "skin felt smoother, less rough" • "the oil sank straight into the skin like a drink, but you could get dressed straight away" • "cellulite looked smoother and less dimply" • "the top of the leg I used this on was slightly less lumpy than the other".

DOWNSIDE: "Cap on bottle a nightmare – really fiddly screw thread" • "no difference".

AVON CELLU-SCULPT ANTI-CELLULITE SLIMMING TREATMENT
6.81 points out of 10

According to Avon, it took a team of more than 50 people three years to create this cooling gel-cream, which contains active ingredients to help boost drainage and surface micro-circulation. According to the company's research, 96 percent of women saw an improvement in overall appearance after four weeks – and our testers were certainly generally impressed with the overall performance of this product, even if they didn't experience quite the inch-reducing effects they were hoping for.

UPSIDE: "After using up the bottle I can see a visible improvement in lumpiness – yes, I'm still big, but it does look better!" • "the thigh I tested this on looks much smoother and the product has made the contours more defined – this is definitely worth continuing with – on both thighs now!" • "skin felt decidedly softer, smoother and immediately better-conditioned" • "no difference in size, but texture slightly less bumpy – skin looks toned, and I like the way this cream makes it glisten, too" • "no difference in celllulite but it did soften a large, dry patch on my thigh" • "legs felt baby-soft".

DOWNSIDE: "No great change" • "measurements decreased by an inch but my stretch marks are more pronounced!".

The lowest marks awarded in this category were 2.5 points out of 10.

FUZZ BUSTING

Getting rid of unwanted hair may start off as a rite of passage in our teenage years – but the thrill soon wears off. So here's how to tackle one of beauty's most boring chores as effectively and quickly as possible.

There is a range of different solutions, temporary and permanent, for different areas of the face and body. If you have a serious problem with unwanted hair, discuss it with your family doctor, who may refer you to a dermatologist or an endocrinologist, as some cases may be linked to hormone imbalances.

Temporary

Results last several hours to several days, depending on regrowth rate:

✳ **Depilatories:** creams or gels which chemically dissolve hair (see our Tried & Tested survey on page 137) – suitable for face and body.

✳ **Shaving:** with manual razors or electric shavers – not suitable for face. Many women shave daily but results cn last several days at a pinch.

✳ **Tweezing:** suitable for face and legs (Jo loves tweezing her legs – then again she has about 20 hairs on each shin...).

✳ **Waxing:** hot wax is applied and ripped off with strips of cloth; do the same at home with hot or cold wax.

✳ **Sugaring:** similar to waxing but with a sticky sugar paste.

✳ **Threading:** a twisted thread is rolled across the skin catching hairs on the way.

✳ **Rotary epilators:** electric "whizzers" which grasp hairs and pull them out by the root.

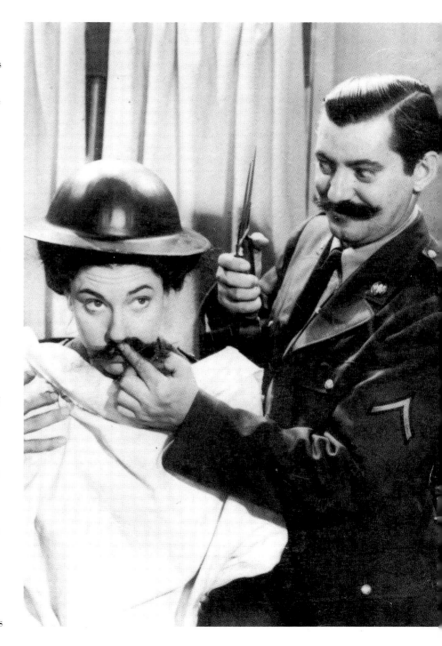

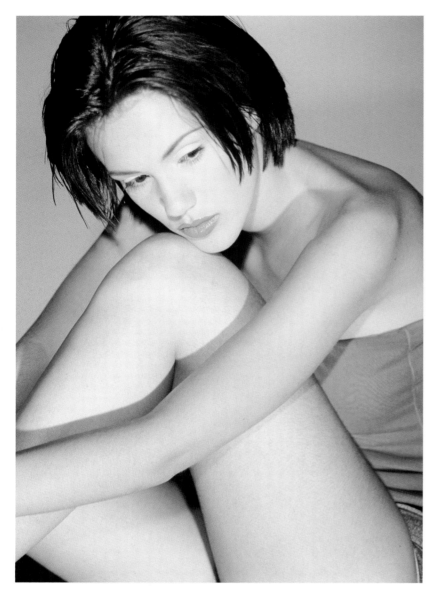

skin damage or infection. It may require several sessions to remove hair for good.

✳ **Laser:** pulsed light is aimed from a handpiece into the skin where it targets the dark pigment in the hair. So it's not as effective for blonde, red, gray, or other unpigmented hair and must be used with caution on darker skin tones and sun worshippers because it can affect pigmentation. It is a new therapy (developed within the last decade) with no longterm data on safety/effectiveness. It may work well but regrowth rates can't accurately be established, due to individual variables. So the FDA classifies this therapy as "permanent hair reduction" as opposed to sclerotherapy, which is declared permanent removal. Can be expensive. Must be performed by an experienced practitioner under qualified medical supervision.

General tips

✳ To prevent ingrown hairs, brush body vigorously and use Tend Skin, an over-the-counter lotion for ingrown hairs. Our favorite fuzzbusting website www.hairfacts.com (a mine of independent information) suggests exfoliating regularly (see pages 124–5). For a great kitchen cupboard exfoliator, use the sea salt and olive oil scrub, or one of the other exfoliating scrubs we describe on page 125. These leave your skin wonderfully soft – you might want to try them on your arms too. You can also try an exfoliating fruit acid (AHA) cream on your legs, if you wish, but remember to use sunscreen on your legs, because AHA's make the skin more sensitive to UV light.

Permanent

✳ **Electrolysis:** hair-thin needle (or probe) transmits electricity into a hair follicle to damage the root; used for over 125 years on face and body; safe and effective but can be painful; must be performed by a qualified, experienced therapist or may lead to hair regrowth,

✳ Trim bikini hair before waxing to save the tearing motion which can be so painful!

✳ A warm flannel placed on the bikini line before waxing can relax the area and reduce pain. If you're visiting a salon for waxing, ask them to do this first.

✳ If you prefer to wax but aren't happy with dark regrowth, try lightening hair with a reputable brand of bleach such as Jolen between waxing sessions.

✳ One thing we can tell you is: wax underarms and legs long enough – we've done it for a couple of decades – and the hair really does stop growing!

✳ Remember that waxing will remove self-tanner – so beware of stripes! (And don't use self-tanner on just-waxed skin, as it can be touchy – and you may have a reaction. Leave 24 hours before self-tanning – see page 146.)

HAIR REMOVERS
Tried & Tested

What women really fantasize about is a no-muss, no-fuss hair remover that will keep skin baby-smooth for months. For now, we can dream on. But here are three fuzz-busting products that impressed our tester panels – including an all-natural option, which earned high praise.

NAIR NO TOUCH GLIDE-ON CREAM
7.78 points out of 10
This features a built-in applicator for ease of use and contains vitamin E, baby oil and aloe vera to soften and condition skin. As with all depilatories, the regrowth tends to be softer and finer – unlike shaving where regrowth is invariably thicker and coarser.
UPSIDE: "Handy, quick, easy applicator does the job effectively – you don't have to be skilled to use it" • "skin was silky and smooth; lovely cucumber scent" • "unusually pleasant

scent for a product of this type" • "I was pleasantly surprised by this product, which was effective on my thick, coarse, dark leg hair" • "hair soft, smooth – and didn't start to regrow until eight days after use".
DOWNSIDE: "Faint unpleasant odor" • "hair returns fairly quickly and is stubbly".

VEET HAIR REMOVER GEL-CREAM
7.31 points out of 10
This pump-action, cooling gel formulation is infused with moisturizing jojoba to counteract the drying action some depilatories have.
UPSIDE: "Very quick – within seven minutes, hair was completely removed, leaving skin soft and not at all sore" • "easy-to-use – no mess and very quick; all over in ten minutes" • "left skin soft, silky and moisturized".
DOWNSIDE: "Gave me a slight eczema-like rash" • "rather stingy, uncomfortable sensation" • "disappointingly, my legs had that 'hedgehog' feel within 24 hours".

❀❀ AUSSIE NAD'S NO-HEAT HAIR REMOVAL GEL
6.78 points out of 10
This was originally cooked up in the kitchen of a Sydney mother, inspired by her daughter's unhappiness about her dark body hair. Based on the 'sugaring' concept, it features honey, molasses, lemon, fructose and vinegar and is 100 percent natural, melting with body heat. It can be used on any body area.
UPSIDE: "Brilliant on legs, bikini line, eyebrows – anywhere!" • "less painful than traditional waxing, no mess and water-soluble – wonderful!" • "great for my sensitive skin" • "the gel really is soluble – unlike wax; painful though!" • "fine stubble only returned after two and a half weeks".
DOWNSIDE: "Insufficient cloth strips provided – I ran out half-way through a leg" • "this product sticks to everything it touches!"

The lowest points awarded in this category was 4.6 marks out of 10.

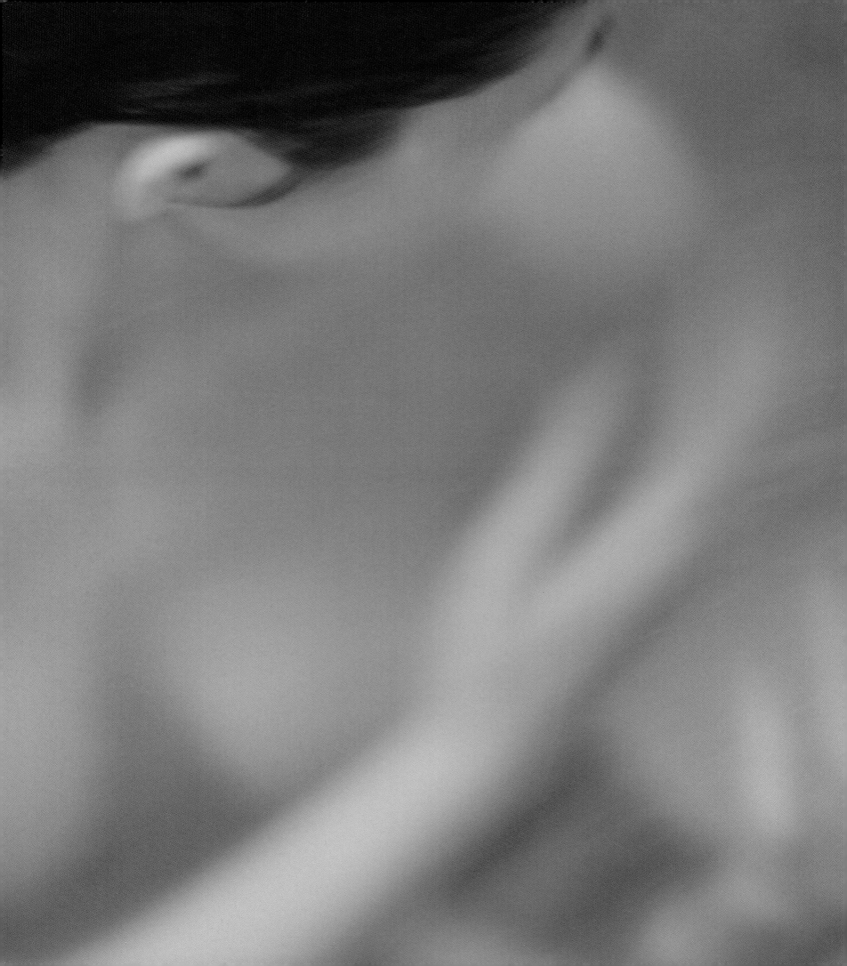

I Must, I Must Improve my Bust

*Some droop earlier and lower – others, usually the smaller ones,
stay perkier longer. But one inescapable fact of life is that
breasts head south as you get older!*

Half of Hollywood, of course, defies Mother Nature by going under the knife. But that's way, way too extreme for most of us. The good news is that there are plenty of noninvasive ways of enhancing your bosom. Surprisingly, perhaps, as you can see from our Tried & Tested survey of bust boosters (see page 140), some of our testers found these went some way to defy gravity.

Bras are the most obvious way of reversing the downward drift immediately – and a potent form of seduction. Do have your bosom measured professionally – at least twice a year – to avoid the dreaded "Double Bosom Syndrome" or, almost worse, "back bulges"... Once you've been accurately measured, try on plenty of

Exercise can't actually increase the size of your bust ... but resistance training with weights will strengthen the underlying pectoral muscles and give a more defined appearance

different options, advises London lingerie legend June Kenton of Knightsbridge undie emporium Rigby & Peller (bra suppliers to HM The Queen Elizabeth II – though she's not necessarily their greatest advertisement). "Move around, raise your arms up, touch the floor," June orders. "A bra shouldn't just fit when you're standing still in front of a mirror; it's got to work in real life."

If you can't find any bras that don't provoke lumps and bumps, under or over, try a "teddy" – those all-in-one underneaths that subdue unruly flesh into smooth curves. The downside is that you will have to deal with the inconvenience of buttoning and unbuttoning every time you want to pee. (Well, guys do it.)

If your personal poitrine situation is more akin to squashed fried eggs or even flat pancakes (usually due to breast-feeding), try subtle padding. Either go for a padded, underwire bra (as Sarah does, and very fetching it is too), one of the new "gel-filled" bras – or try implants; no, not surgical—the fake version. "Chicken fillets", as they're known in the fashion business, are silicone or gel-filled inserts that rest under your breasts, inside your bra, and feel surprisingly natural. Try Curves or the more economical Cleavage Enhancers by La Senza. Just don't leave them on your dressing table...

Exercise can't actually increase the size of your bust, or prevent sagging, but resistance training with weights will strengthen the underlying pectoral muscles and give a more defined appearance. Simply pressing your palms together just above chest level is one way. The other is to use light weights – a couple of cans of baked beans if you don't have the real thing – and perform what are known as Pectoral Flies. Lie on your back on the floor, legs bent, and grasp a can in each hand. Raise your arms perpendicular to the floor, palms inwards. Then with your elbows slightly bent, slowly extend both arms out to the sides, at right angles to your body. Contract your pecs and bring your arms back to starting position. Build up to three sets of 12–15 repetitions.

There are "bust care" sessions available at salons which will undoubtedly make your bosom feel cared for – at a price. A bracing alternative is to splash icy water on your boobs after your daily shower. Some beauty editors swear by this.

And finally, surgery: if you are set on augmentation or reduction, be aware of the risks: just because it's called cosmetic doesn't mean it's not the real thing and the jury is still out on safety issues. Start by consulting the American Society for Aesthetic Plastic Surgery at 1-888.ASAPS.11 or http.//www.surgery.org.

BUST BOOSTERS

Tried & Tested

The idea with these creams and serums is that they firm and tighten – though this obviously depends greatly on the size of your bosom. Manufacturers claim they're particularly good after weight loss or pregnancy (although not, of course, during breastfeeding).

For the most part, our testers were underwhelmed (which is why we've only featured the top three choices here, and even these only worked for some panellists), and we didn't feel that any of the budget creams – or the more natural versions – scored enough to warrant inclusion.

Frankly, we believe that any cream will help to improve skin condition and, for the rest, many of us could just be better off with a Wonderbra.

SISLEY BOTANICAL INTENSIVE BUST COMPOUND
7.5 marks out of 10
This lightweight gel is packed with plant and algae extracts, say Sisley, including horsetail, ivy, yarrow and red vine, and they recommend that it's applied morning and night in large, circular movements that also cover the base of the neck, shoulders and inner arms.
UPSIDE: "The product did seem to work – instantly firming, and my skin feels a lot smoother" • "seemed to work in lifting and perkiness – a good-textured gel that sinks in fast" • "skin condition was fantastic – very noticeable; visible sheen if wearing a low-cut top" • "definite difference in firmness and skin felt smoother" • "beautiful fresh fragrance".
DOWNSIDE: "No miraculous improvement" • "very disappointing".

PHYTOMER SEA TONIC TONING BUST GEL
7.12 marks out of 10
Based on thallassotherapy (marine therapy), the smoothing action in this gel is down to an extract of brown seaweed as well as chitin (from crustacean shells), said to help collagen regeneration.

UPSIDE: "Sustained improvement both in softness/smoothness and appearance" • "toned the bust, softened and increased suppleness" • "quite a bit of firmness – pleasantly surprised" • "breasts looked rounded, supple, "uplifted" and wonderfully smooth – a must for my bust!"
DOWNSIDE: "No difference – maybe my boobs are too small; nothing to lift!" • "not convinced at all".

CLARINS BEAUTY BUST GEL
6.18 marks out of 10
The best-known product in its category, this offers calming echinacea, anti-free-radical ginkgo biloba, ginseng, horsetail, mint and witch hazel, and should be applied in the morning for maximum "perking" effect.
UPSIDE: "Marked improvement – skin looked firmer like I'd had a 'mini-lift'" • "definite improvement: felt firmer, skin tone brighter – I've bought it again twice!" • "skin smoother, more toned" • "instant softening; made skin luminous" • "plus point is that it encourages you to check your breasts regularly".
DOWNSIDE: "No miracle-worker".

The lowest score in this category was 5.37 points out of 10.

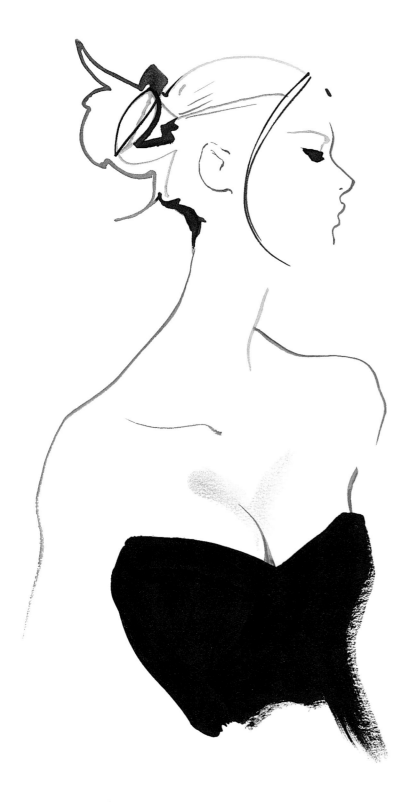

BUST BEAUTY

So nature didn't give you the cleavage of your dreams? Then fake it. According to makeup artist Robert Frampton, "You can use make-up to create cleavage just as you use it to create the illusion of cheekbones and pouty lips." (Although, he acknowledges, a push-up bra also helps.) So, dust off that low-cut dress and be prepared to flaunt it...

✳ "Smooth the skin in the bust and décolletage area first," advises Robert. "It's a sensitive part of the body, though, so use an ultra-gentle exfoliator – nothing harsh." We suggest buffing the area with a wet muslin cloth of the type we recommend for make-up removal – see page 58. If you prefer an exfoliant, use a sugar-based scrub – or a cream with gentle, rounded particles – rather than anything based on crushed nut shells or salt.

✳ "Moisturize well. Skin should be protected every day with an SPF 15 moisturizer, as sun damage shows up in this area first."

✳ "Use a mattifying gel to even skin tone, then smooth on a light application of foundation (the same shade as you use on your face). Brush a little blush on the area; use a matte natural color that blends well with your skin tone – nothing too dark and avoid red/pink tones. Also: nothing shimmery or shiny – if you're bony, there's nothing worse than a chest that looks like a sparkly xylophone. Apply extra blush or bronzer on the sternum, between the boobs, creating a 'Y' shape that curves out at the top (illustrated left). Build color up gradually until you get the right effect."

✳ "The final touch is to highlight the 'moons'. Apply a little shimmer (not sparkle) to the crescents of your breasts – but make it subtle: you want people to notice your breasts, not your makeup."

GOOD DAY SUNSHINE

For the last few decades, the suncare industry has been telling us about the importance of SPFs (Sun Protection Factors). But playing safe in the sun is more than a numbers game.

Most articles you've ever read about sun protection have probably told you that applying an SPF 15, for instance, allows you to languish fifteen times longer in the sun before burning than without. Or that an SPF 8 gives you eight times more sun time than you'd usually have before frying.

But in reality, according to leading experts including Dr. Lionel de Benedetti, Head of Research and Development at Clarins, "Sun creams give you somewhere between one-third and one-half of the SPF that's on the bottle." Explains New York-based dermatologist Dr. Karen Burke, "If you applied sun cream as thickly in daily life as they do in laboratory tests, you'd be covered in a thick layer of white cream. But when you massage that in, of course you get a lower level of sun protection – around a third of the figure quoted on the bottle."

This discrepancy is because the lab conditions in which SPFs are tested are quite, quite different from what we do when we actually hit the beach (or the pool). "In standard tests to establish a Sun Protection Factor rating,' Dr. Lionel de Benedetti explained, "we apply 2 m.g. of sun product per square centimeter of skin." That's a layer of white cream so opaque you can barely see the skin through it – bearing almost no relation to the way we might massage a sun cream into our skin in real life.

Most worryingly, according to Professor Brian Diffey of Newcastle General Hospital (who's published a paper in the *British Medical Journal* on the subject), this discrepancy between expectation and reality may be one contributing factor sunscreen use has been reported to be a risk factor for melanoma (the most serious – and

The lab conditions in which SPFs are tested are quite, quite different to what we do when we hit the beach

potentially lethal – form of skin cancer). Research is emerging that people who use sunscreens seem to run a higher risk of melanoma – at least in part because they've been spending much longer in the sun than they would have in the old pre-SPF days, when sunburn would have had them scurrying for the shade.

But this is certainly no reason to throw up your hands in frustration, toss out your sunscreen—and roast bare-skinned, turning your back on the whole notion of SPFs. Instead, according to Mike Brown, Scientific Suncare Advisor at Boots, in the UK, "to be on the safe side, you probably need a much higher SPF factor than you think

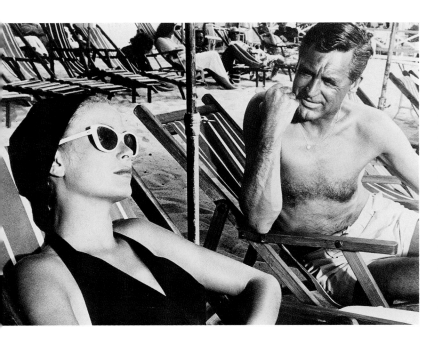

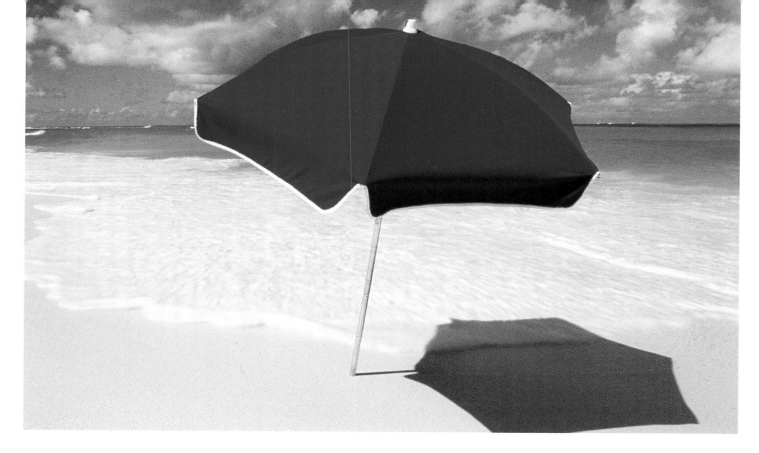

you do." Most crucially, "sun protection should be just one element of a safe sun strategy", says Professor Elaine Rankin, Chair of Cancer Medicine at the University of Dundee. (See page 144 for the savviest way to enjoy the sun.) We need to be slip, slap, slopping on sun cream much more generously than we thought – and more often. "Even waterproof suncreams aren't towel-proof," observes Mike Brown. "If you're turning over on your beach towel, you're rubbing product off, so you need to reapply regularly."

In order for sunbathers to get optimum protection, Professor Diffey would like to see users advised to apply sunscreen "generously or thickly". If you're applying it thickly enough, you'll get through an average 200ml (about 7 fl. oz.) sized bottle of sunscreen in just three or four applications. Use less than that and you're skimping.

What's also vital is to look for a sunscreen that says it's "broad spectrum" – so that it protects against both UVB (Burning) and UVA (Aging) rays. It should say this on the label or package insert, but if it doesn't – and it's a brand you buy from a beauty counter (rather than grab off the shelf) – you can ask a beauty consultant for advice.

NATURALLY BEAUTIFUL

Most sun protection today is based on chemical sunscreens such as benzophenones, benzene derivatives or cinnamates. Personally, we avoid them – in favor of "physical sunblocks" that include the minerals titanium dioxide and zinc oxide, which work by "bouncing" the light off the skin before it can do its damage. Chemical sunscreens can trigger reactions in those with sensitive skins like ours. What's more, studies indicate that by absorbing UV rays, these chemicals may actually encourage free radical damage in the skin – potentially fast-forwarding aging, and even damaging skin cells. (Research has even shown that some sunscreens may even mimic the effect of estrogen in the body, leading to a potential disruption of the endocrine system and other possible health problems.)

Weleda, Dr. Hauschka, Neal's Yard Remedies and Liz Earle Naturally Active Skincare all make suncare that is based on mineral sunblocks rather than chemical sunscreens. The only trade-off may be that you have to massage them in a little more vigorously.

SUN SAVVY

Even suncare manufacturers are encouraging consumers to regard protective lotions, creams and oils as only part of the safe sun picture. If you really want to stay safe in the sun, follow these guidelines...

✳ Remember, when suncare-shopping: the real SPF rating of your sun cream is likely to be between one-half and one-third of the SPF stated on the packaging. Buy sun creams that say they offer "broad-spectrum" protection or, better still, that have a Seal of Recommendation from the Skin Cancer Foundation. Look for suncare that features antioxidant vitamins in the formulation, too, which may help "mop up" some of the damage done to skin cells by sun exposure.

✳ Avoid sun exposure between 10am and 3pm, when the sun is at its strongest.

✳ The sun's rays are more intense in tropical and semi-tropical locations because exposure becomes more direct as you get closer to the equator, or at higher elevations. Extra protection for eyes and lips is necessary in both cases. Choose an even higher SPF in these geographical locations. (Log onto www.safesun.com for a "UV index" map of the world that helps you assess your risk.)

✳ Apply sunscreen 15 to 30 minutes before you go outdoors, and allow to dry and bond with the skin before dressing. Apply again as soon as you are at the pool or beach. (You can burn while you look for a lounger.) Protect yourself while swimming and reapply afterwards.

✳ Wear sunscreen on cloudy or hazy days; UV rays can penetrate these atmospheric conditions and cause sunburn. Cut down on exposure by spending time in the shade – but wear sun protection there, too.

✳ Wear a hat with a 4 inch brim (minimum) and sunglasses, which should also have broad-spectrum 100 percent UV protective lenses. And cover up. The more tightly woven clothing is, the better protection it will offer. Loose, tight-weave clothing – such as a long-sleeved shirt and palazzo pants – is best.

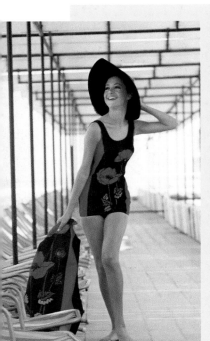

SAY NO TO SUNBEDS

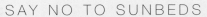

We say: don't go there. New medical research shows that regular use of sunbeds may damage skin for life, causing premature aging and increasing the risk of skin cancer. Most sunbeds emit 99 percent UVA rays and 1 percent UVB – and UVA is now known to be highly aging, even though the damage is invisible at the time. According to Dr. Julia Newton-Bishop, consultant dermatologist at St James University Hospital, Leeds, "People use sunbeds to make themselves look younger, but the irony is that doing so promotes aging." Insists Dr. Newton-Bishop, "There is no safe level of use." Most at risk are women with fair skin – who tend to use sunbeds the most in the hope of promoting a tan. Rona MacKie, Professor of Dermatology at Glasgow University, explains: "There have been four decent international studies in recent years that all essentially say the same thing: use of sunbeds, even for short periods, adds to your risk of melanoma." Don't say we didn't warn you.

SELF TANNERS – *Tried & Tested*

The goal: a can't-tell-it-from-real result – no streaking, no orange and preferably no hamster cage/cookie tin smell, either. As with facial tanners, exfoliate then moisturize first for best results and remember you will need to apply extra sun protection – even if it says SPF 15 on the label, it won't last longer than two hours. Most "tans" lasted for two to four days.

DECLÉOR AUTO-BRONZANT SPRAY EXPRESS HYDRATANT SPF 6
8.88 marks out of 10

Testers loved this new spray delivery, light milk and several gave it full marks. It's said to develop within one hour, but most women left it overnight for ease. The tanning agents are 100 percent organic mahakanni and DHA complex, plus protective Helioprotectine, Argan oil and soothing Aloe vera. It's suitable for face as well as body, say Decléor.

UPSIDE: "Lovely stuff: fantastic for a fake tan novice like myself" • "only had to stay undressed for five minutes tops!" • "realistic light golden tan" "second application gave a deeper still natural color" • "the best and least pungent fake tan I've tried, this one smelled fantastic like baby powder".

DOWNSIDE: "Spray can is a bit messy and unnecessary – pump dispenser would have been better".

LANCASTER SELF TAN SILK BRONZE MOISTURIZING MILK SPF 6 (MEDIUM SHADE)
8.77 marks out of 10

Another new one-hour golden wonder for body and face, using DHA plus Sweet Orange to naturally boost skin's own melanin plus watermelon and pineapple extracts to moisturize and exfoliate skin. Testers commented this gave a sunkissed effect, for deeper color you need to re-apply. (You could try the Intense shade for deeper color.)

UPSIDE: "I loved it, everything worked – color, texture, smell and the results were great on my body – and my face" • "excellent color, the best fake tan I've used and I have tried them all" • "only had to stay undressed a few minutes" • "I like the slow build up of color, lovely sheen on skin, not scary and easy for first timers" • "pleasant fresh smell".

DOWNSIDE: "Really poor instructions in tiny writing, texture too runny to control well".

ST.-TROPEZ WHIPPED MOUSSE
8.7 marks out of 10

The salon brand loved by stars including Elle McPherson, this superspeedy mousse includes aloe leaf juice and fruit acids to help achieve a deep rich tan. This too can be used on your face.

UPSIDE: "I left it overnight and by morning I was a lovely golden brown – non streaky and realistic" • "subtle and sweet smelling, thick but easy to spread and fast absorbed" • "I felt safe sitting on my sofa after 20 mins" • "I gave up sunbathing ten years ago and when I looked at myself in the shower after using this I immediately got that "feel good" factor".

DOWNSIDE: "Leave a good hour between moisturizing and putting on the tan or it may streak and be a paler color".

LANCÔME FLASH BRONZER MAGIC MOUSSE
8.13 marks out of 10

Light and airy but extremely hydrating – thanks to lashings of vitamin E – this mousse delivers a hint of instant color (so you can see where you've applied it), and develops fully within an hour.

UPSIDE: "Natural color and added a light tan" • "wonderful – no trace of fake tan smell; shimmery, glittery and perfect for an instant result" • "dried in 10 minutes, natural golden glow lasted for seven days" • "brilliant, easy-to-use mousse; the fact it's colored makes for easy application" • "glamorous and expensive-looking tan".

DOWNSIDE: "Tanner spluttered and dribbled out of spray" • "one coat gave a natural one-day-in-the-sun result – but a second coat just went orange".

❀ ORIGINS GREAT PRETENDER
7.88 marks out of 10

You can see exactly where you've applied this tinted shimmery body gel, which has a significant proportion of natural ingredients including natural sugars, vegetable-derived glycerin and essential oils of peppermint, orange and rosemary.

UPSIDE: "Absorbed into the skin very quickly" • "very nice pepperminty smell" • "pleasantly surprised by the nice golden brown result" • "smelt better than any self tan I've used and looked very natural on pale skin – golden and glowing" • "lovely shimmery particles which were great for evenings out – didn't last after initial application" •.

DOWNSIDE: "I would use it all the time but it did feel a bit sparkly for winter".

The lowest score in this category was 4.6 marks out of 10.

THE NO-SUN TAN

The secret of a can't-tell-it-from real glow is in the application. So follow these how-to guidelines and your fake tan will last longer. (And will really have your friends asking: "Where did you just get back from?")

✳ Now that many self-tanners come in a choice of shades, choose one that matches your natural skin tone – fair, medium, dark. (For a more bronzed effect, it's better to apply two coats of a paler shade than one dark coat.) Personally, we like tinted fake tans because it's so much easier to see where they're going.

✳ The day before fake tanning, exfoliate well. The smoother the "canvas", the more even the tan will be.

✳ Don't apply within an hour after bathing or showering; skin needs to cool to its normal temperature for foolproof application. Clarins founder Jacques Courtin-Clarins suggests a gentle shower foaming cleanser instead of soap, which is alkaline and can make a tan look yellower.

✳ Moisturize skin before you apply fake tanner, or else drier areas of the skin will soak up more of the fake tan.

THE ONLY SAFE TAN?

Most sunless tanners contain dihydroxyacetone (DHA) which reacts with the skin's amino acids to produce a darkened color in a couple of hours. Scientists insist that this sugar-derived chemical is entirely safe – but one thing's inescapable: the characteristic "biscuity" smell that develops along with your tan. For that reason, personally we're converts to Decléor Self-Tanning Hydrating Emulsion, which uses an entirely natural ingredient (an herb called Mahakanni) – and is non-smelly.

(For best results, try to allow an hour or two between applying body lotions/creams and self-tanner.)

✳ Warm the product in your hands and massage the self-tanner in, using long, smooth strokes and applying even pressure with your fingertips. Don't forget the back of the neck, sides of your waist, underarms, inner thighs and backs of knees. Apply more lightly where skin is thickest: elbows, knees, toes and fingers.

✳ Feet can be a real giveaway: to avoid streaks, work tanner around your whole foot, including between the toes.

✳ Gently swipe a damp cotton wool pad over elbows, heels and ankle-bones, where fake tan can go darker – or better still, massage a little extra body moisturizer into these "danger zones" to slightly dilute the product.

✳ Wash hands thoroughly – orange palms never fooled anyone. "And do your forearms, as well, surgical scrub-up-style," advises make-up artist Sara Raeburn. "Otherwise you can end up with streaky inner arms." To avoid the "white gloves" look, lightly swipe the back of your hands and forearms over your body after you've washed and dried them, to pick up just a little of the fake tan again. If you do end up with orange palms (for whatever reason), Estée Lauder's Dominique Szabo advises washing your hair. "The detergents fade color on palms."

✳ Relax while the tan "takes". If you're in a hurry, choose a gel formulation which sinks in faster and is less sticky. Don't swim or shower for at least two hours.

✳ Another good reason to relax: if you perspire immediately after application it alters the chemical reaction, which will also alter the resulting color.

✳ If you must get dressed right afterwards, wear loose clothes (and dark underwear). Bliss Spa founder Marcia Kilgore says, "Ideally, I'd wear a toga."

✳ When your tan appears (in up to four hours), repeat the entire application if you aren't as dark as you'd like. If there are any streaks, rub them with half a lemon, or slough with an exfoliant body scrub.

✳ It's now possible to buy after-sun products which contain low levels of self-tanner, to refresh a tan. Alternatively, mix half-and-half self-tanner with your regular body cream.

✳ Moisturizing diligently twice daily after using self-tanner will prolong a fake tan. (Its "life" should be three to four days – or up to a week with a salon application.

✳ Be aware that exfoliating or shaving while you have a fake tan will make your tan streaky.

✳ Many self-tanners are now being formulated with added Sun Protection Factors. Don't be lulled into a false sense of security: this protection is only active immediately after application, and has no longterm action. On the second day, the protective effect of a fake tan is basically zero.

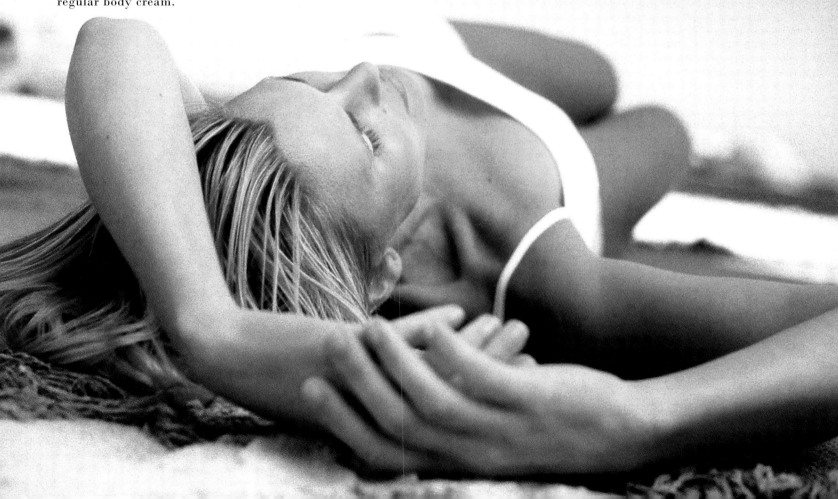

FACIAL FAKING

✳ Wear a headband to pull your hair off your face and dab a little Vaseline or Liz Earle Superbalm (which we prefer) over eyebrows and along the hairline, to act as a barrier and prevent staining.

✳ Perspiration can make fake tanner streak, so don't do this in a steamy bathroom.

✳ Remove earrings so they don't leave little white marks on your lobes, then wax (or use depilatory) on any facial hair that could become discolored.

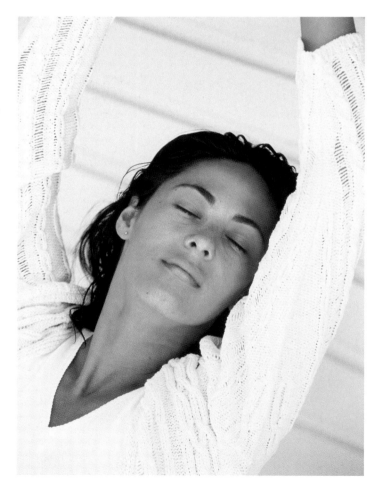

✳ The smoother the surface, the more even the color; cleanse your skin according to our advice on page 58, using a muslin cloth to remove any buildup of dead skin.

✳ Moisturize skin and wait at least ten minutes for the moisturizer to sink in (or preferably an hour, if you have the luxury of more time).

✳ Apply the cream to fingertips or palm – don't "dot" it directly onto the face – and smooth a thin layer into your face using circular movements. Be sure to go down the neck all the way to bra-level. If you're unsure how light or dark a new fake tanner will develop on your skin, mix half-and-half with your regular moisturizer in the palm of your hand. (We do this as a matter of course, preferring a light tan that can be replenished almost daily rather than a deeper tone.) For tricky areas such as the hairline or ears, use a cotton swab to "feather" the tan on.

✳ Be extra careful around the eye area. Rather than apply the tanner to lids, massage a dab of eye cream all the way round your eye socket; you'll pick up a little self-tanner from the cheek area and it should blend subtly.

✳ Swab eyebrows with a wet cotton swab and wash your hands thoroughly with soap and water. Keep your hands off your face for an hour (at least).

✳ Wait until the color has fully developed before you decide whether or not to deepen it with a second coat.

✳ After your tan has developed, avoid using moisturizers that contain AHAs (fruit acids) or vitamin A, as these speed up cell turnover and can make your fake tan fade faster.

FACIAL SELF TANNERS
Tried & Tested

Nowadays, most of us know not to bake our faces if we don't want to end up looking like a leather handbag. So the safe option is faking it with a fast-acting facial self-tanner. These are hugely improved from earlier versions: color is more realistic – gold rather than orange – and develops faster; the smell is much more acceptable – even pleasant; and some products, because they are tinted, give you more control over how much you put on. Several products are formulated with sun protection but this only works for about two hours after you've applied the cream, and no longer. You must still apply your usual sun prep if you're under rays. Every maker emphasises the need to exfoliate first for the most even coverage. There are no 'natural' winners in this category.

CLARINS RADIANCE-PLUS SELF TANNING CREAM-GEL
8.13 points out of 10
A light lotion, which contains skin-boosting vitamins and minerals plus kiwi to hydrate and soften. With the pleasant smell its makers claim, this took about four hours to develop a really natural "I've been in the sun" golden glow, which lasted two to three days.
UPSIDE: "Nice light easily spreadable texture" "didn't need makeup after, just concealer on thread veins" • "lovely product which left a glowing color and no tide marks" • "really natural sunkissed color – without a burned cookie smell; love it!".

DOWNSIDE: "Liked this but prefer a tinted moisturizer for the same effect more quickly'.

LANCÔME FLASH BRONZER INSTANT BRONZE GLOW FOR THE FACE
7.78 points out of 10
Voted "Best New Product" by *New Woman* magazine the year it launched, Flash Bronzer contains tinted pigments for an instant "sun-kissed" look (so you can see where you've applied it), plus skin-softening vitamin E. It's designed for darker complexions – fair skins should opt instead for Medium Color, which has less of the active ingredient (DHA).
UPSIDE: "After 45 minutes I had a golden glow; I loved everything about this – the smell, texture, color, and the tiny shimmering light-reflective particles" • "great for winter wanness – turns it into a healthy glow" • "pleasant smell – not chemical" • "loved the creaminess" • "if used daily, color builds up naturally and gradually" • "evened out skin tone, improved the texture of my skin".
DOWNSIDE: "A second application looked dark, patchy and unflattering" • "irritated my skin, unfortunately".

ESTÉE LAUDER GO TAN TOWELETTES FOR FACE AND DÉCOLLETAGE
7.6 points out of 10
Not so much tan-and-go as tan-on-the go, these are the fake tan equivalent of cleansing wipes. Individually wrapped towelettes, containing enough to do your face and neck, mean you can whip up a golden glow at your desk or even on the move in about an hour. Although this scored well, some testers were ambivalent, but all said it would be good for travelling.
UPSIDE: "Fantastic product – no streaks, lovely even color – so I looked very heatlhy. I used them before a wedding and they were excellent" • "good color, natural and even" • "really convenient and fun to use" • "color was great, very natural – thankfully".
DOWNSIDE: "Towel was difficult to use and dried up after a few minutes"• "faint fake tan smell that lasted all day" • "hands left slightly colored even after washing".

PHYTOMER BRONZE PERFECT
7.57 points out of 10
Has a "helioprotect" complex (with allegedly anti-aging and anti-inflammatory properties), along with oil of apricot, for nourishing. There's a low level of sun protection that's active just after application.
UPSIDE: "Effective and totally natural-looking" • "color was excellent"• "great – no stickiness, no shine, natural and even-looking color" • "nice, healthy glow still visible after seven days" • "natural color; left skin feeling very moisturized".
DOWNSIDE: "With my eyesight I'd have liked the instructions printed more clearly" • "smell and stickiness put me off the product".

The lowest mark in this category was 4.2 points out of 10.

AT YOUR FINGERTIPS

Whether you've got two minutes, five, or the luxury of half an hour for a truly professional manicure, giving hands a quick TLC fix is one of the fastest ways to look more groomed and glamorous

Supermanicurist Marian Newman has worked on the fingertips of everyone from Björk to Naomi Campbell and Nicole Kidman. A former forensic scientist (yes, you read that right), she believes "beautiful nails should be as common as stunningly cut and styled hair." Creating perfect nails for ad campaigns like Christian Dior's takes Marian hours. But she also understands women with time constraints – and gave us these tips to get you on the fast track to fab fingernails in three minutes (or less).

If you have just three minutes

1 "If any nails are uneven, file them with a very finely grained nail file – never metal – from the sides to the center, to even them out; never file from side to side because it encourages the nail layers to separate, and nails will start to peel."

2 "Wet the end of an old-fashioned white nail pencil (at pharmacies everywhere) and run it under the free edge of the nail. It whitens the tips more naturally than a French manicure ever could."

3 "Apply a dab of cuticle oil to each nail, rub in lightly, and use a chamois leather nail buffer to lightly buff the nails. The transformation is amazing!"

If you have just five minutes

1 File, as described left.

2 Apply an all-in-one base coat and top coat, or a base coat and a coat of quick-drying colored polish. (The base coat acts as a buffer.)

3 When nails are dry to the touch, apply a drop of cuticle oil (or any body oil) to the cuticle area, and lightly rub in over the nail surface. This sets the manicure super-fast while moisturizing cuticles.

If you have half an hour

1 Remove nail polish using a cotton wool ball with nail enamel remover and press gently onto the nail; if dark polish has gotten into the cuticle area, remove with an orange stick wrapped in a few wisps of cotton wool and soaked in polish remover.

2 File according to Marian Newman's instructions, left.

3 Soak nails in almond oil for five minutes. (Preferably, warm it lightly in a pan or the microwave. You can keep the oil in a bottle between treatments, and reuse.)

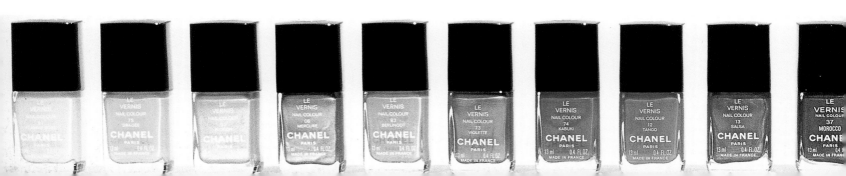

4 Gently push back cuticles with a rubber cuticle stick (much gentler on nails than an orange stick).

5 Clean under nails with an orange stick wrapped in moistened cotton wool.

6 Massage in hand cream (see our Tried & Tested results on page 152).

7 Scrub nails with a brush and soapy water to create a smooth, oil-free surface for polish to adhere to.

8 Apply base coat followed by two coats of polish. (See page 153 for nail guru Jessica Vartoughian's tips.) Ideally, leave at least one minute between each coat for optimal drying.

9 Wait three to five minutes and apply top coat.

10 When nails are dry to the touch, apply a drop of oil (as described opposite) and massage into nails.

NAIL NOTES

✳ Every time you apply balm to your lips, rub the excess goo into cuticles to keep them soft and pliable.

✳ Rosie Sanchez at John Barrett in New York gets rid of gunk on the rim of a nail polish bottle with a paper towel, soaked in remover, before screwing on the cap. "It cleans up mess and residue, and prevents glooping," she advises.

✳ If you clip your nails, use a small, easy-to-maneuver clipper, not a clunky, big one. (These are designed for toenails.) New York manicurist Jin Soon Choi advises: "Trim from side to side; nails can split if you start in the middle."

✳ Avoid acetone-based nail polish removers, which are drying; look for the words "acetone-free" on the label.

✳ Pale colors are much more "goof-proof" than dark shades, and are always best if you're short on time.

✳ We recommend taking your own polish to a salon for a manicure – so that you can use it at home, for between-manicure maintenance and touching up chips and scuffs.

✳ Top London manicurist Iris Chapple is so intent on clients not spoiling their perfect manicures that she escorts them to their cars and starts the engine for them! (It's worth asking if yours will.)

✳ Our advice, whenever painting nails, is to do so near an open window (or even outdoors, if weather permits), to avoid breathing the chemical fumes given off by polish.

TIP: A manicure should begin with the little finger of the right hand and it is always easiest to start outside and work in. (Start with the little finger of the left hand if you're left-handed.) The key to applying polish on your opposite hand is to keep your arm steady. A wobble-proof technique: put your elbow on a table, curl fingers towards you and use your other hand to put on the polish.

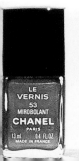
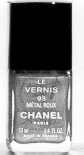
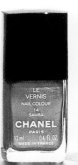
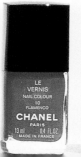
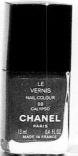
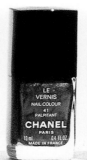
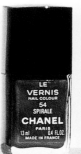
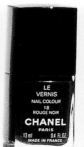
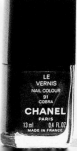
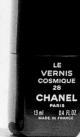

HAND CREAMS – *Tried & Tested*

Hand-cream heaven is a product that's rich and restorative – but doesn't leave hands too greasy to get on with life. We asked our testers to try these after any task that's particularly tough on hands – like gardening or washing up without gloves on. Two very natural creams performed exceptionally well in this category.

✤✤ CIRCAROMA ROSE HAND CREAM
9.1 points out of 10

A truly outstanding result for this natural cream from a tiny British aromatherapy brand (which will ship worldwide!), which basically handcrafts all their products in small batches to ensure optimum quality. It's based on organic rose water, organic geranium, organic rose attar and ultra-moisturizing shea butter.

UPSIDE: "Smells fantastic – real rose scent, not synthetic" • "very good on dryness, nails and cuticles, and seemed to have "brightening effect" – it has everything" • "perfect consistency; excellent product" • "I was so impressed I looked up their other products on the web" • "silky feel, sank in right away – a real treat" • "my hands look younger and brighter – the best hand cream I've ever used" • "scar on the back of hand less noticeable – and my hands are soft as cashmere and blissed out".

DOWNSIDE: "Fragrance far too strong".

CHRISTIAN DIOR PROTECTIVE NOURISHING CRÈME FOR HANDS SPF 8
8.8 points out of 10

Dior says this should "wrap hands in a voluptuous, protective cocoon", with its ceramide-rich moisturizing complex. It's designed to sink in fast, leaving hands velvety.

UPSIDE: "Skin felt very, very smooth immediately – "velvety", as claimed" • "smells gorgeous and really does leave skin velvety-smooth" • "nice, supple feel to hands – after a week of use, definite improvement visible, particularly on cuticles" • "skin looked fresh and young" • "elegantly packaged, and cream performs well, with a "powder-soft" texture; a little goes a long way" • "hands soft and silky" • "a slight sheen on hands improved appearance of skin; good conditioning effect on cuticles".

DOWNSIDE: "Not heavy-duty enough for gardening but a superb everyday cream".

LANCASTER SURACTIF AGE PROTECTION HAND CREAM SPF 12
8.8 points out of 10

This expensive hand treat aims to turn back the clock with a vitamin A derivative, together with vitamin E, glycerine and urea. It has an SPF 12 to shield skin against future damage, and also claims to fade age spots – but our testers were slightly less convinced about that particular action.

UPSIDE: "Very good on dryness and nails, and great after gardening" • "hands left feeling very smooth" • "improved condition of nails, while skin was soft and silky" • "I love it! Toned skin, protected in water and cold weather" • "loved this fragrance, which reminded me of chocolate bars" • "got rid of flaky skin on index finger" • "age spots are looking slightly lighter after one week; I'm using on arms, too – and they look great" • "excellent hand cream – I'd recommend it" • "a scar and burn mark seemed to fade in a week – very impressive".

DOWNSIDE: "Not particularly nice smell – chemical rather than floral" • "no change in age spots".

✤✤ JURLIQUE LAVENDER HAND CREAM
8.77 points out of 10

Alongside soothing lavender, this rich, non-greasy hand cream – said to be ideal for chapped, dry hands and cuticles – features rose, calendula, chamomile, honey, soy lecithin, macadamia nut oil and aloe.

UPSIDE: "Divine fragrance" • "very hydrating – and I have the driest hands in the world" • "hands felt fab! The best cream I've ever used" • "can't stop looking at my hands – they appear 10 years younger;" • "gave it to my daughter – a nursery nurse with dry, sore hands – she liked it very much, too" • "also made elbows beautifully soft" • "I loved going to sleep with my hands near my face, because the lavender sent me into a deep sleep".

DOWNSIDE: "I have dry, crepey hands and dry cuticles and felt this didn't meet its claims" • "no better than any supermarket cream".

BEST BUDGET BUY
ST. IVES COLLAGEN AND ELASTIN EXTRA RELIEF HAND AND BODY LOTION
8.1 marks out of 10

St. Ives claim that this collagen and elastin-rich cream should increase moisture by up to 200 percent - and here is the verdict of our testers.

UPSIDE: "Immediate softening effect that lasted" • "my daughter – who has outbreaks of eczema – tried this and within 48 hours there was a dramatic improvement; it's almost cleared up – amazing" • "lovely soft, herbal/floral scent" • "my manual worker boyfriend has adopted this as his hand cream".

DOWNSIDE: "My friend said this smells like furniture polish" • "fiddly packaging".

The lowest points in this category was 4.11 out of 10.

THE LADY VARNISHES

Jessica Vartoughian is a nail legend. When she opened her Beverly Hills salon 30 years ago, it was the world's first manicure boutique. The nails of actresses like Jamie Lee Curtis, Jodie Foster and Molly Ringwald score a "perfect 10" thanks to Jessica's manicures

Jessica calls her system "natural" nail care – not because her polishes and treatments are based on natural ingredients (they're not), but because to Jessica (and to us) false nails are a no-no. Great nails should be all about perfecting your own, even if that means cutting them off and starting over. (As she once did to Jo's. Which was quite an honor, actually, since the last manicure Jessica had personally given was to Nancy Reagan, about six years earlier!) Here's the nail wisdom she shared with us:

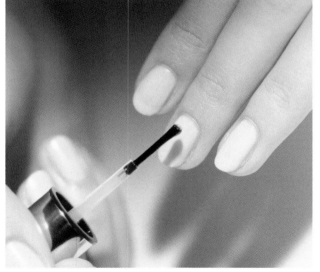

* "Use a nail file as if you were playing the violin slowly, using the whole length of the file in long smooth strokes, never in a sawing motion."

* "The perfect nail is strong but flexible. Massage oil into the nails on a daily basis, and only use nail hardeners for a very short time or they'll make them too brittle."

* "Use ten to twelve strokes to cover the nail with polish – most people think they can get away with three."

* "The secret of a long-lasting manicure is to 'seal' the tips, painting over them with base, varnish and top coat. And even on the underside of the nail, if it extends far enough from the top of your finger."

* "Redo your top coat two days after you have your manicure, then, three days later, add a new coat of color all over the nail, followed by top coat. Repeat that pattern and your manicure should last at least a week to 10 days."

* "Don't use nail varnish remover more than once a week; it's too drying. And always look for a formula that's acetone-free."

* "Exercise your fingers just as you would the rest of your body: stretch and tap them. It boosts blood flow and improves nail health."

* "Keeping your nails all one length looks best – even if that means cutting them all down when one nail snaps. It actually creates the illusion of length."

* "The shape of the nail tip should echo the natural shape of your nail base. If the base of your nail is square, a square tip will look best. Most women have a 'squoval' nail base – square with rounded edges – which should be reflected in the way you file and shape the tips."

* "Every six weeks, clip all your nails; just like hair, nails get 'split ends'. It encourages them to grow." This sounds like a dramatic solution – but it works.

MORE NAIL KNOWLEDGE

✳ After a manicure/pedicure, keep hands and feet above the water line if you have a bath that night. Submerging newly painted nails in hot water encourages peeling and dramatically reduces the life of a manicure.

✳ Cold air sets nail polish fast. If your hairdryer has a "cold" setting, give freshly painted nails a blast with the nozzle for a couple of minutes on each hand.

✳ The best time to push back cuticles is after a shower, when they're nicely softened. Use the corner of a towel.

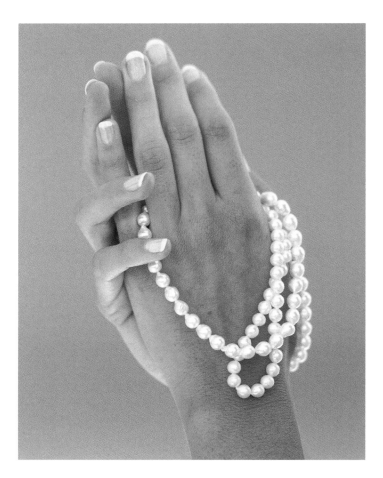

✳ Except in the case of a hangnail – which can catch, painfully, on clothing – we don't believe in clipping or nipping cuticles, ever, and refuse to let manicurists do this to us. Certainly, nippers should be soaked in sterilizing solution for 10 minutes between clients. At home, swipe before use with a cotton wool pad soaked in tea tree oil.

✳ For an ultra-softening treatment, slather hands in almond oil, lock in with a layer of rich hand cream and soak in a bath. Iris Chapple suggests exfoliating hands regularly – to keep them from looking dull—and suggests, "If you're putting on a face mask, slather some extra onto hands."

✳ Nutritionist Kathryn Marsden claims her nails are so strong "I could undo screws with them!" Sure, she has a great diet – but also believes in daily buffing with a Body Shop Nail Buffer. "One side of the buffer is gentle enough to be used over polish, without causing any damage; the friction with this side of the buffer stimulates blood flow to the nail area. I keep several around the house, so I can be reminded to use them during the day." (The Body Shop version is particularly gentle, but proceed with caution with most other buffers – which should only be used sparingly, if ever, on weak nails; they actually remove layers of nail, which is weakening in the long run.)

✳ Keeping polish in the fridge stops it from thickening but, to be honest, we like to keep all our manicure tools in one place. So just try to keep polish out of sunlight and in the coolest place you can find. (A bedside drawer is ideal.)

✳ Leading hand model Linda Rose advises: "Clever use of color can help camouflage hands that you're less than happy with: if you have short, wide fingers, avoid intense shades. Either very light or very dark colors are best for short nails. If you have large hands, the longer your nails, the slimmer your hands will look. Pale or natural-colored polish plays down the size of the hand."

✳ We're avid gardeners – but gardening and glamorous nails aren't terribly compatible. Experts advise wearing gloves, but these can be unwieldy. So we've discovered the best way to stop hands from becoming ingrained with dirt is to run nails over a bar of soap, then slip on a pair of latex surgical gloves (at pharmacies everywhere). These allow freedom of movement and let you feel plant roots through the soil. After slipping off the gloves, we scrub under nails with a nail brush – removing the soap, along with any dirt that may be buried under the fingertips.

✳ Iris Chapple advises women to "rediscover gloves" for winter as well. "Get your hands measured in a glove shop or department store and invest in comfortable, warm gloves. Nothing too tight – and don't just grab any old pair. The right gloves really do protect hands against the elements."

✳ If you want nice nails, be nice to them. They aren't staple-removers, for example!

✳ And at the very least, aim to moisturize your hands at least as often as you moisturize your face! TLC pays off.

LONG-LASTING NAIL POLISH

Tried & Tested

A truly long-lasting nail polish is one of the great beauty time-savers. We instructed our testers not to use additional top coat or quick dry, in order to judge the polish itself.

ESTÉE LAUDER PURE COLOR SHEER STRENGTH NAIL FOUNDATION
8.5 points out of 10

This neutral-toned polish evens and smoothes the nail surface, while light-reflecting pigments minimize the appearance of ridges and imperfections. Can be worn alone, for everyday protection, when you've no time for a manicure.
UPSIDE: "Very durable – made nails look very shiny and healthy; felt stronger to the touch" • "looked great; shiny, glossy and very durable" • "subtle, natural, chip-proof sheen" • "lasted well through various office duties".
DOWNSIDE: "Bottle quite heavy" • "too thin to use on its own – best as a base coat".

CHANEL LE VERNIS NAIL COLOR
8.25 points out of 10

Certainly the most stylish nail polish you can have on your bathroom shelf – and our testers raved about its staying power, too. Shades are constantly updated in line with catwalk trends – and there are often "limited edition" versions, too. Most testers used the word "rich" to describe color and coverage.
UPSIDE: "Touch-dry in 60 seconds – the easiest polish I've ever applied" • "just starting to chip after four days – impressive, after housework and gardening!" • "just one coat gave the "I've-made-an-effort" look for work; on vacation, it lasted a week without chipping" • "my mother commented her nails felt stronger after a few applications".
DOWNSIDE: no negative comments at all.

O.P.I. NAIL LACQUER
7.77 points out of 10

A celebrity favorite, packed with pigments for depth of color and cover, in a huge shade range updated to reflect fashion trends.
UPSIDE: "Lovely shine and richness; dried in 90 seconds, too" • "glorious color, good shine, excellent cover" • "lasted six days without chipping – the most durable polish I've tried" • "no need for top coat; lasted a good four days with typing, housework – brilliant!" • "one coat is enough".
DOWNSIDE: "Brush didn't apply color evenly – needed two coats".

BEST BUDGET BUY
REVLON NAIL ENAMEL
7.66 points out of 10

A moisturizing, fortifying complex plus a blend of resins protect against the drying effects of detergents. Enormous shade range.
UPSIDE: "Big brush made for even and easy-to-apply, one-stroke cover" • "Revlon was always tops for nail enamel and hasn't lost the expertise that made it famous" • "resisted typing, filing, etc." • "lasts a couple of days longer than most brands".
DOWNSIDE: "Lovely, glossy sheen and smooth finish at first but soon became dull".

The lowest score in this category was 4.27 points out of 10.

HOW TO BEAT FLAKING NAILS

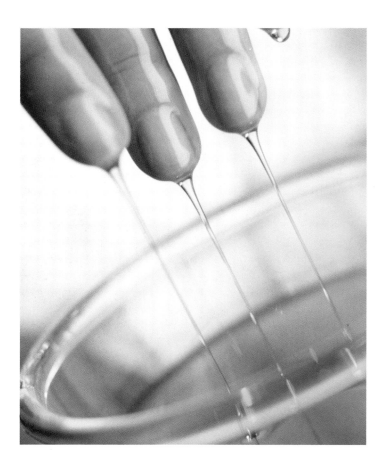

Weak, flaking nails are a common complaint – and strengthening them can be an uphill battle. Although nail products can help – as our Tried & Tested survey opposite shows – there's no doubt that your general health is a factor. Any period of illness or stress will affect your nails. In Traditional Chinese Medicine (TCM), weak brittle nails are associated with an imbalance in the liver and its partner, the gall bladder. TCM practitioner Dr. Jennifer Harper, author of *Nine Steps to Body Wisdom*, suggests taking a supplement of artichokes (such as Cynara

Artichoke by Lichtwer Pharma, to detoxify and tonify the liver and to strengthen the absorption of Essential Fatty Acids which are vital for nails, hair and skin. Nutritionist Kathryn Marsden always recommends oil of evening primrose for weak nails.

Dr. Harper also recommends the mineral silica for strengthening and smoothing ridged nails (it helps skin, teeth and hair too). Try a supplement for three months as a "cure" to stimulate your body's own silica processes and then take a month's break before starting another course if needed. Dr. Harper suggests Silicol Silica Gel by Saguna, or Dr. Hauschka's Delicious Siliceous with Pollen, a powder that you mix with water (some converts eat it directly off the spoon). The richest plant source of this mineral is the herb horsetail (available in capsule form from Solgar).

Along with internal supplements, nails respond to TLC from the outside. Our favorite unguent is Liz Earle's Superbalm from the Naturally Active Skincare line which, rubbed into nails and cuticles daily, has a marvelous effect on dry nails. Sarah, who grooms and rides her horse ungloved, covers her hands and nails in Superbalm first as protection – and it works fantastically.

We find that regular rubbing with a good lip balm also works well, giving nails a rosy pink sheen. Dr. Harper's favorite remedy is Neem Nail Oil by Dr. Hauschka, designed specifically to strengthen weak nails: just use one or two drops of the oil morning and evening, massaging gently but firmly into nail and cuticle. Tissue off any excess and, says Dr. Harper, "Wait for luscious, long nails to develop!"

The most important thing is to keep on keeping on with whatever remedy you try. Nails take weeks and months to improve, especially if they are splitting. You have to give any remedy at least three months' regular use – so don't give up halfway through.

NAILBITERS ANONYMOUS

The New York Nail Company (NYNC) is an expert at helping clients kiss their nibbling habit goodbye. NYNC's Maggie Callaghan tells us: "to give up successfully, you need a constant program of support and monitoring." Enlist a friend as a "buddy". Sign up for a series of "therapy" manicures – time to discuss your habit with a pro. And follow these tips:

✳ Establish the situation and reason you bite; it could be habit – when you're watching TV or reading a book – or nerves – when you're anxious before a meeting, say. Being aware will help you keep the habit in check in the future.

✳ Painting on something that tastes horrible may not work: you'll wash it off eventually or just stop using it. "It's all about discouraging yourself," says Maggie. "When you have a manicure, select a bright polish to draw attention to the nail, That will give you a strong visual wake-up call every time you're tempted to bite."

NAIL STRENGTHENERS
Tried & Tested

None of these are overnight wonders, so we asked testers to use them for a month or more. But do read the labels because using these for longer than prescribed may make nails over-hard and prone to snapping. (Though that advice only applies to chemical treatments rather than nail oils like Decléor's). We asked our testers to try the strengtheners on one hand, for comparison.

OPI NAIL ENVY
8.07 points out of 10

This celebrity fave contains hydrolyzed wheat protein, calcium and vitamin E to help weak, thin, brittle nails. Apply over bare nails as a base coat, or two coats alone. Use weekly as a base and/or top coat for maintenance.

UPSIDE: "Made a big difference to my nails; I'd recommend it" • "lovely clear, glossy finish; after using this for a month, my nails look rosy, healthy, buffed and smooth, with no flaking" • "easy to use – love this; an excellent top coat too" • "definite strengthening benefits after a week or two".

DOWNSIDE: "No difference at all in my brittle, splitting nails" • "made cuticles dry and cracked when it strayed there".

❀❀ DECLÉOR AROMESSENCE ONGLES STRENGTHENING CONCENTRATE
7.33 points out of 10

An all-natural, aromatherapy-oil treatment with essential oils of myrrh, lemon and parsley (to diminish pigmentation), in an oil base (castor/hazelnut/avocado). It should be applied daily to the base of nails and massaged into dry skin on hands.

UPSIDE: "Nails tougher – flexible, not brittle – and skin conditioned" • "nails now look pinker – maybe from frequent massage" • "easy to use; left unpolished nails with a slight sheen; good at stopping flaking".

DOWNSIDE: "Too much of a bore to apply" • "too greasy for my liking".

BEST BUDGET BUY
SALLY HANSEN DIAMOND STRENGTH PREMIUM NAIL HARDENER
6.8 marks out of 10

This was the best of the "budget" nail treatments that our testers tried. It works as a base coat and can be used to bond a broken nail or prevent future splitting, and features a "Micro Diamond" formula. According to Sally Hansen, it nourishes nails and promotes growth in just 5–7 days – but we have to say that while it impressed half our group of ten testers, the others were less-than-blown-away.

UPSIDE: "I was very impressed with this product – it gave a natural shine to my nails when worn alone, and does what it says on the label" • "nails noticeably stronger, split less easily" • "fantastic – in just a couple of months, my nails – which were weakened from having artificial ones applied – have been transformed in time for my wedding" • "amazing – nails seemed to strengthen from the very first use" • "my nails were not as brittle and dry as usual, and the polish made them look very feminine, with a pretty sheen".

DOWNSIDE: "Made nails brittle, not flexible" • "overwhelming nail varnish smell".

The lowest score in this category was 5.44 points out of 10.

HAPPY SOLES

We've said it before (and we'll say it till the cows come home): happy feet make a happy woman. But the happiest feet aren't just gorgeous — they're truly healthy!

Flip-Flops. Slingbacks. Mules. Slides. We love them – but we know plenty of women who stick to running or tennis shoes all summer because they don't feel their feet will bear close scrutiny. If a lifetime (or even just a winter) of neglect has taken a toll on feet, the mere thought of baring them may be – well, unbearable. But no matter how hard you've been on yours, it doesn't take much fancy footwork to get your feet in tip-top shape. (And in reality who's going to get close enough to notice tiny flaws?) Nobody can guarantee that a glass slipper will change your life, but you'll have the satisfaction of knowing that you're beautiful from head to toe!

The five-minute pedicure

1 Remove any polish.

2 Wash feet and dry thoroughly (including between the toes) with a towel.

3 It's a myth that feet need soaking before you exfoliate them; instead, buff them while dry with a foot file. The Body Shop's (which is a bit like fine sandpaper) is excellent, but our favorite is the somewhat pricey Diamancel Foot File (see Directory, page 246), which is made of metal. (And far less scary than it sounds.) If you regularly buff your feet in the bath at night with a pumice stone or a foot file, you'll be able to skip this step because that will keep hard skin at bay on an ongoing basis.

4 Pedicurist Elisa Ferri advises taking great care when cutting nails, to minimize the risk of ingrown toenails.

The trick is to cut the nail straight across and not too short – and Elisa suggests cutting with careful little snips, rather than all at once, which can cause the nail to split and break. After clipping, she carefully files the nail so that the edges are very, very slightly rounded, using long, smooth filing strokes – and then tests for smoothness by drawing a piece of old stocking across the top. "I'd rather discover snags that way than by catching my toenails on an expensive new pair," she explains.

5 Slip a toe separator between your toes and apply a thin coat of base coat and one of the new "quick dry" polishes which, we find, really do cover in a single coat, for an instant transformation. (The base coat buffers the nails so that the pigments don't discolor them.) You can walk around with the toe separators in until you're ready to put your shoes on.

6 Once polish is dry to the touch, lightly moisturize feet with a favorite body lotion to give them an instantly smooth appearance and softness.

7 Don't want to polish nails? Massage your toes with almond oil and use a buffer to buff your nails rosy; this boosts circulation and strengthens them.

If you have more time

1 Soak feet for five to ten minutes in a bowl of warm water to which you've added three drops of peppermint essential oil (to revive feet) or three drops of lavender essential oil (to soothe them). Or try this almond-and-milk

pedicure: simply dissolve a cup of powdered milk in warm water, then add a tablespoon of almond oil. Soak for fifteen minutes and feet will emerge kissably soft. (If that's your thing.) For a D-I-Y massage made in heaven, add a layer of marbles to the bottom of your bowl and roll feet backwards and forwards across them.

2 After soaking, gently push back cuticles with an orange stick swirled in cotton wool and dipped in tea tree oil. (The tea tree does double-duty: it moistens the tissue and is antibacterial, helping to minimize any risk of infection.)

3 Massage feet with a rich cream or balm. (Our favorites are Spiezia Organics Foot Balm, Circaroma Frankincense & Geranium Hand & Foot Balm and Liz Earle Intensive Nourishing Treatment – not originally devised for feet but wonderful.) Before painting, wipe moisturizer from nails with polish remover, which cuts through any greasy film or residue left over from foot soaks or creams; otherwise polish won't adhere.

4 If you're not in a super hurry, paint using a traditional varnish rather than the quick-drying versions – there's a wider range of shades to choose from and the finish tends to be glossier. (In our experience, Lancôme, Christian Dior and Revlon polishes are unbeatably long-lasting.) Apply a base coat and two coats of polish (allowing a minute between each coat), and start with the big toe since this takes longest to dry. Finish with a quick-drying top coat (Seche Vite, , is in a league of its own here.)

5 To erase smudges and smears on skin, manicurists like the precision control of an orange stick dipped in polish remover; simply press the tip on the smudge, and it should lift off without leaving a mark.

6 When nails are dry to the touch, apply a dot of oil – preferably a nail oil, but virtually any body oil will do – at the base of each cuticle, and massage into the nail. This keeps fluff from sticking to your pedicure and also – by preventing exposure to air – "sets" the polish super-fast.

7 It's still best to wait at least 45 minutes (longer is better) before putting on a closed-toe shoe – or slipping between the sheets. But if you can't, do what salons do and wrap feet in plastic wrap. Works like magic.

8 Pale, pastel shades compensate for poor hand-eye coordination. Every goof shows with a darker polish.

9 A salon pedicure might last a month or so – at which point you could be bored with the color. So Roxana Pintilie, manicurist at the Warren-Tricomi salon in New York, has this trick: "Start out with a light color, like a pale pink. Then a few days later you can put on a coat of something darker – say, an orange. Then three days after that, maybe a purple or a gold. That way, you're not stuck with the same color for weeks."

FOOT NOTES

✳ For swollen feet, add a handful of Epsom salts to a bowl of warm water and fill a second bowl with cold water. Soak your feet in each bowl for a couple of minutes (the temperature changes reduce puffiness). Dry thoroughly.

✳ Podiatrist Lorraine Jones recommends rotating shoes. "Never wear the same pair of shoes two days running; it takes 24 hours for them to dry out thoroughly. Damp shoes allow fungi to thrive" (encouraging athlete's foot)!

✳ Don't wear your highest heels for more than two or three hours a day. Vary heel heights. Simply changing shoes halfway through the day will help ease pressure. Orthopedic surgeon Francesca Thompson says: "My advice about heels is to treat them sparingly – like a hot fudge sundae. You wouldn't eat one every day."

✳ Never try to "break in" shoes. (Feet surrender first.) If possible, shoe-shop late in the day, when feet are at their largest. Get measured occasionally; if you were size six at age 20, you may not still be at 40. Feet grow as we age.

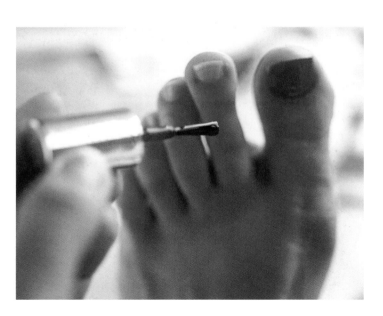

✳ According to the Chinese, cleansing the feet every night before bedtime is as important as washing the face. Dr. Hang Song Ke of the Asante Academy of Chinese Medicine in London explains: "During the day, toxins are excreted through the feet which can be reabsorbed at night." So, even if you don't bathe at night, get into the habit of foot washing before bedtime and, it's said, you'll have fewer colds and infections. (Jo swears by this.)

✳ Ever been caught in the rain and had your feet turn blue because your socks/shoes have run? Scrub feet as soon as you can, as some dyes are potentially carcinogenic.

✳ Because feet are so absorbent, when they are sweaty, we like to use an organic, cornstarch-based product like Neal's Yard Remedies Geranium Orange Body Powder.

✳ Or try this: brew two teabags in 1 pint (0.5 liters) of boiled water for 15 minutes. Add 4 pints (2 liters) of cool water and soak feet for 20 minutes. The tannic acid changes skin's pH level, banishing odor-causing bacteria.

✳ Without wanting to sound like a couple of germ-obsessed Howard Hugheses, we have both initiated "no shoe" rules at home. Going barefoot is blissful. Our feet "breathe" better, don't get calluses of any kind, and outside germs tracked into the house stay by the door, making for a healthier (and much less grubby) home.

✳ Ponder this, though: many hotels routinely spray bedroom carpets – and especially bathroom floors – with pesticides, to keep bugs (sorry, we're talking cockroaches here) at bay. By all means go barefoot at home – but pack your slippers when you're going away to avoid exposure to these chemicals!

FOOT REVIVERS

Tried & Tested

The best thing for weary feet is to put them up (preferably with someone massaging them!). Next best thing is foot treats packed with invigorating ingredients to boost blood flow while soothing and softening built-up hard skin. For a double whammy, slather these on, then lie on the bed, facing the wall; raise feet to a 45-degree angle to the body, legs straight, and rest them on the wall (putting a pillow between your feet and the wall to avoid getting gunk all over it). Just five to ten minutes works like magic. We like to use natural products because feet are so highly absorbent.

❀ AVEDA FOOT RELIEF

8.8 points out of 10

This cooling cream contains alpha-hydroxy acids (salicylic and lactic acid), to slough off dead cells, plus lavender and rosemary oils to help deodorize. The softening action is down to jojoba and castor oils.

UPSIDE: "Really, really good refreshing smell; feet instantly tingly and less achey and sore" • "needed a lot of rubbing in which helped sore points" • "considerably improved cracks on feet" • "even my bunions are less painful and red" • "the best I've used – send up to Fred Astaire, please!" • "I'm on my feet all day and they didn't throb as much after using" • "reduced tenderness after wearing high heels, used on legs it took away that heavy feeling".

DOWNSIDE: "Needs to be rubbed on bare feet, not applied through tights".

BEST BUDGET BUY
❀❀ WELEDA FOOT BALM

8.1 points out of 10

An outstanding result from this small natural health company, which grows its herbs biodynamically. Free from any synthetic ingredients at all (bravo!), it features antiseptic calendula, disinfectant/anti-fungal lavender, rosemary and myrrh, along with invigorating rosemary and zingy sweet orange. Works as an antiperspirant deodorant for sweaty feet, too.

UPSIDE: "I loved this – it absorbed really fast, leaving no greasy residue – the best" • "made me feel like I had new feet – reviving and refreshing" • "cracks on feet vastly improved by this" • "uplifting, tangy non-cloying smell – loved this" • "liked the fact you could put tights on immediately" • "feet felt 'lighter'".

DOWNSIDE: "A bit like antiseptic cream".

L'OCCITANE SHEA BUTTER FOOT CREAM

8 points out of 10

This rich lavender-scented cream was a very popular entrant. Several testers liked it as a hand cream too.

UPSIDE: "Heaven after a hard day; delicious smell for feet, minty, lavender, rosemary – top marks for refreshing-ness" • "best on hard skin on heels and under toes" • "immediate relief and definite improvement to post-high heels aching" • "this product was pretty perfect – a little even went a long way" • "I found this two years ago and can't live without it; great for long-haul flights to banish swollen ankles and heavy legs".

DOWNSIDE: "Took forever to soak in so feet very slippy for ages".

CRABTREE & EVELYN FOOT & LEG THERAPY WITH PEPPERMINT OIL

7.88 points out of 10

A light creamy lotion infused with peppermint oil and shea butter aims to leave your feet feeling fresh, tingly and rejuvenated within minutes of application. It scored highly with testers who had medical conditions, including varicose veins and one deep vein thrombosis.

UPSIDE: "The fresh cooling feeling was wonderful and lasted a long time" • "instant refreshing feeling that made feet comfortable and really took the heat out and tired ache away" • "I have weak veins due to DVT and this eased the ache in my bad leg – a great product that eased tiredness in legs and feet".

DOWNSIDE: "Took a long time to sink in".

KIEHL'S INTENSIVE TREATMENT AND MOISTURIZER

7.62 points out of 10

This thick, rich, emollient cream isn't designed so much to refresh as to soften very dry skin or callused areas. (So it can be useful for elbows and knees, too, or for cracked skin around the nose after a cold.) Avocado oil and shea butter, cocoa butter and vitamin E appear on the list of moisturizing ingredients.

UPSIDE: "Excellent, heavy-duty intensive moisturizer that worked well on my sensitive feet" • "slather on, then put on gloves and socks overnight; when I did this, my hands and feet felt ten years younger next morning" • "reduced soreness on heels and the balls of my feet".

DOWNSIDE: "Had little effect unless applied in large quantities" • "took forever to sink in".

The lowest score in this category was 4.85 points out of 10.

SPA ETIQUETTE

Two of the world's top spa gurus – Bliss's Marcia Kilgore and Tova Borgnine (founder of a Hollywood spa and eponymous signature cosmetics line, Tova) – share insider tips on making the most of visiting a beauty salon or day spa.

Visiting a day spa can be one of the most therapeutic experiences going – or it can be the opposite, if you lie there worrying whether you've breached the (un)dress code, or thinking about all the other things you ought to be doing, or wondering what on earth the therapist is doing to you. So here's how to make the most of your longed-for pampering treat...

MARCIA'S SPA ETIQUETTE

✳ "Leave your fears in the locker room. So what if you have a moustache? Who doesn't? If you want to get rid of it, just SAY something. If you've booked for a Brazilian bikini wax but you're not sure what it is because you've never had one before, ask your beautician. If you're worried about blackheads on your nose, say so. You'll get more out of your treatment and leave feeling satisfied."

✳ "If you're unhappy about anything at all, speak up. If you dread having your scalp rubbed, for example, but you don't say anything about it, it's unlikely that your beautician will pick that up through ESP, and you'll spend your time on the table enduring, rather than enjoying."

✳ "Leave the evening open, if you possibly can, in order to get the maximum out of this expensive treatment you're paying for. For me, there's nothing worse than when I'm giving a facial, and my client keeps telling me not to do parts of the treatment because she's going out for dinner and doesn't want to: 1) be too flushed; 2) look greasy; or 3) mess up her hair. Personally, I'd trade a good scalp massage, a blackhead-free nose, and a hot cream shoulder and arm massage for a rescheduled dinner any

day. If you don't let your technician give you 'the works', you're not taking full advantage of your spa time."

✳ "Don't obsess about your flaws! Some people approach their spa services with an overwhelming insecurity; they are so worried about what their massage therapist or esthetician might think of their legs, their pores, or their mountainous PMS pimple that they can't relax. Always remember: not only do spa service providers see breakouts, lumpy legs, and large pores all day long, they've often got them. They're not in the spa business to judge you, they are in the spa business to help you!"

TOVA'S SPA WISDOM

✳ "If you feel guilty taking time off to pay a visit to a beauty salon or a spa, choose a date like a birthday or an anniversary for your appointment; then it's sometimes easier to tell yourself you deserve it."

✳ "Leave plenty of time to get to your appointment so you don't arrive late and stressed. Otherwise you'll be lying there obsessing about the time you've wasted, and trying to slow down your beating heart."

✳ "Try not to drink coffee or other caffeinated drinks such as cola before an appointment; these can give you the jitters and make it harder to relax."

✳ "A good therapist will tell you to take a few good, deep breaths before your treatment. When you arrive at the salon or day spa, start breathing properly, from your abdomen, and it'll calm you right down."

✳ "You should feel comfortable at all times. If you don't like the music or the scented candle they're burning, tell the therapist. If you're not comfortable taking off your underwear, explain that you'd feel happier keeping it on – although shoulder massage, for instance, will be less effective with your bra straps in the way. But it's about you, and what makes you happy."

✳ "If you're really short of time, find a salon where they can combine treatments so you get, say, a pedicure and manicure – even a shoulder rub – at the same time."

✳ "If you have trouble justifying a visit to a spa because it seems too self-indulgent, think of – say – a lovely flower garden: if you don't care for it, it won't look its best. Women are the same: it's vital to make time for the personal maintenance that will bring mind/body/spirit into balance, and ensure you keep going. We need that sense of well-being that comes from recharging our batteries in order to take care of others."

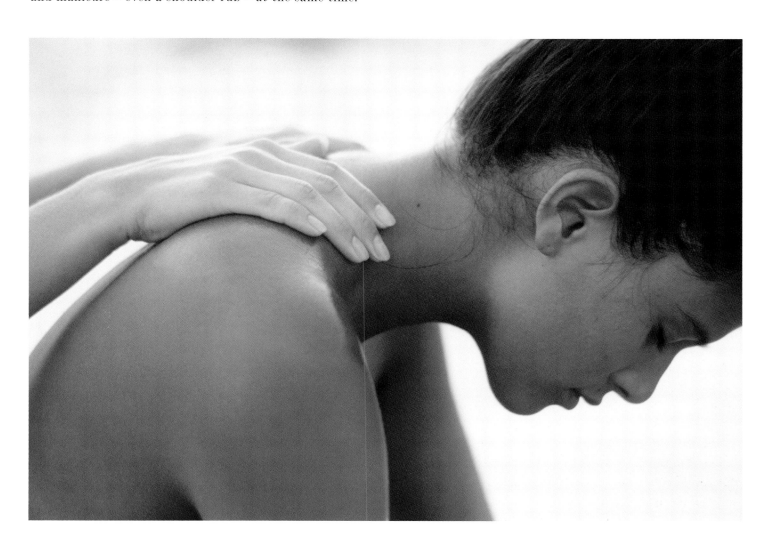

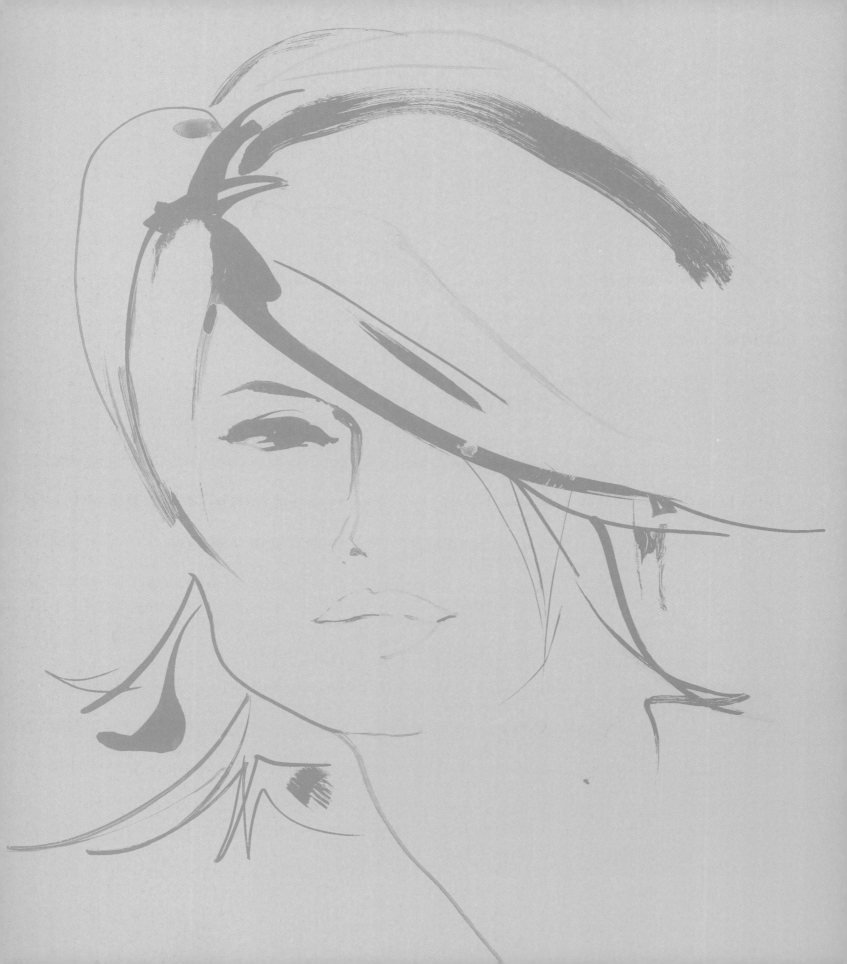

HAIR

Hair affects how we feel – big time. Bad Hair Days have a tendency to become bad days no matter what. But when your hair is **shiny, bouncy** and does what you want without a fuss, confidence is turbo-charged. Few of us have the time to get our hair done every week (let alone keep two hair appointments a day – which, insiders tell us, is the secret of Catherine Deneuve's enviably perfect coiffure). So here are **real-life secrets** for women who want beautiful hair with minimum maintenance. Hair products that really work. And cut, color and blow-dry wisdom that turns every day into a **Good Hair Day.** (Promise!)

GREAT HAIR

*Having beautiful hair isn't rocket science and you don't need a Ph.D or even
big bucks. Here's the lowdown on head-turning hair*

Cut, Color, Condition. In an ideal world, you want them
all perfect but if we had to choose one to start with, we'd
opt for condition. Here's the thinking: shiny, glossy hair is
lovely in its own right, even if the cut's a bit off, but even
a perfect cut can't disguise limp, lackluster hair. And you
can have the best hair color in the world but if your hair's
a haystack, that's all anyone will notice. So we say:

Start with... condition

As ever, think from the inside out. What you put in your
body affects your hair, just as much as what you put on

it. If you're healthy, your hair and scalp will show it.
Hair's main enemies are poor diet; not enough exercise,
relaxation and/or sleep; physical illness and any form of
stress; head and neck tension (which can affect blood flow
and nutrition to the scalp); pollution of all kinds; overexposure to sun, salt air, wind and chlorinated water; air
conditioning, and central heating; some pharmaceutical
drugs (including the Pill, thyroid drugs, antibiotics,
sedatives, tranquilisers and barbiturates, amphetamines,
cortisone); over-processing – too much perming,
bleaching, tinting; use of curling irons, heated rollers,
blow-drying at a high heat, brushing with a sharp-bristled
brush. And smoking...(please don't).

Prescription for healthy hair

Firstly, eat well. Hair is made up of a protein called
keratin (as are your nails), so be sure to include protein-
rich foods even if you are vegetarian or vegan. Choose
lean meat, poultry, fish, eggs, cheese (goat's or sheep's,
not cow's), plus nuts, seeds, legumes, and whole grains.
Strong hair begins in your scalp so also look at the
dietary recommendations we make for Skin (page 96).

Great hair foods (and drinks) are fresh, natural and
preferably organic. Try to include fish, seaweed, and other
sea vegetables; almonds (full of veggie protein); Brazil
nuts, figs, dates; natural goat's or sheep's milk yogurt and
cottage cheese; plus a wide range of colorful antioxidant
fruits and vegetables from dark to light green through
red, orange and yellow to pink and purple. LA stylist
Philip B.'s favorite "hair food" is avocado, which is rich in
unsaturated fat, vitamins, and amino acids.

Cut down on red meat, fried foods, and cow's milk

SHINE ON

Hair's natural shine comes from sebum, an oil produced by the
sebaceous glands (these are all over the skin). Sebum protects
the whole hair shaft, smoothing the cuticle and helping the hair
to be elastic and strong. Too much sebum – from a hormonal
imbalance, for instance – and your hair will be greasy; too little
and it's dry. Each hair has three layers: the cuticle or outer layer,
which has lots of tiny overlapping scales; the cortex, which
consists of fiber-like cells that provide strength and elasticity;
and the medulla in the center, made up of keratin cells. The
ideal is to have everything in balance with the cuticle scales
lying flat and overlapping neatly so that your hair shines and
looks silky. If the cuticle scales are damaged, the hair becomes
brittle, dull and tangly. If you have wavy or curly hair, you need to
pay even more attention to condition because it won't reflect the
light as much as the flat surface of straight hair.

products, caffeine (coffee, tea, and cola), alcohol, chocolate, sugar, salt, saturated, and hydrogenated fats, and processed foods.

If your hair is dull, try these supplements: Vitamin B complex, essential fatty acids (good fats/oils, including flaxseed oil, fish oil, and gamma-linolenic acid – GLA), antioxidants including vitamins C, E, and beta-carotene (the precursor of vitamin A), plus the minerals selenium and zinc (you'll find these in a good mineral complex).

When it comes to shampoo, conditioner, and mask, go for high-quality products that suit your hair type. Manufacturers spend a lot of time and money developing products for specific purposes and their descriptions are pretty accurate. The main categories are normal, dry, oily or combination hair (greasy at the roots but dry at the ends); anti-dandruff; colored or chemically treated hair; thickening or volumizing.

Choose protein shampoos and conditioners for flat dull

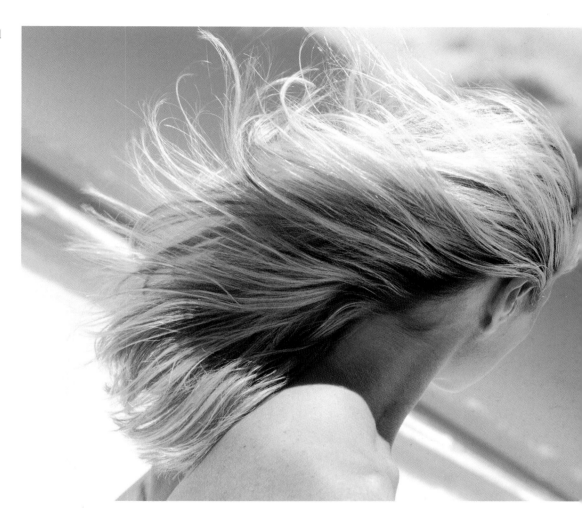

hair to improve elasticity and shine, moisturizing products for dry or frizzy hair. Don't use a protein product on frizz as it will kink up more. (See Shampoo Savvy, page 168, for more on hairwashing.)

Don't stick to the same product all the time: hair develops a resistance to some ingredients after a while, so use two or three bottles on a rotating basis. Get to know what works for your hair in what condition, and "self-prescribe".

Give your hair a condition-boosting treat with a mask once or twice a week and a really good scalp massage (a great relaxer if you're tense, too). See our Tried & Tested Hair Masks (page 169) for the most effective products.

HAIR RAISING FACTS

- Your hair grows about ⅜ inch (1 cm) per month, faster in the summer.
- Women tend to lose about 20 percent of their hair between the ages of 40 and 50.
- Hair becomes drier with age.

SHAMPOO SAVVY

We may have washed our hair all our lives, but that doesn't mean we did it right.
Here's how to get the most out of shampooing...

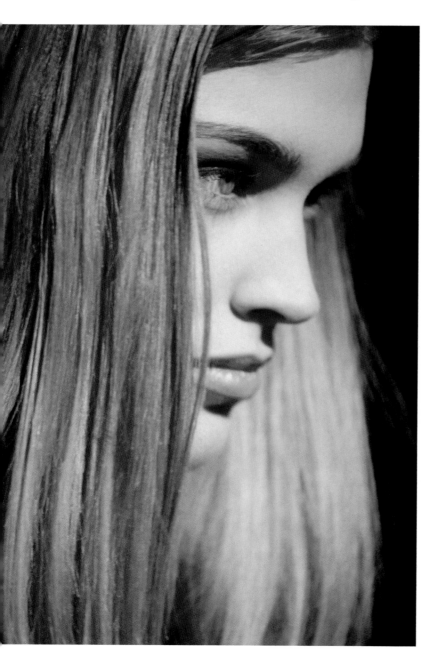

Brush your hair first to detangle, and loosen grime and dead skin cells. Wash and rinse your hair in the shower. Dirty bath water won't get your hair clean. But a fiercely hot shower isn't a friend to hair: try warm rather than hot water and turn down the pressure if you can.

Use about a soupspoonful of shampoo, less for short hair, more for really long. With the pads of your fingers, massage it gently but firmly into your scalp right up to the hairline, then work through to the ends. Spend a couple of minutes on this or you won't make the most of a good shampoo.

Rinse thoroughly. "The major cause of dull hair is too much shampoo or not enough rinsing," says London hairdresser Paul Windle. "That dollop of shampoo takes about four minutes to rinse out properly. So use less and rinse much, much more."

HOW OFTEN SHOULD YOU WASH YOUR HAIR?

Enough to keep it clean but not strip it of its natural oils is the ideal. In other words, whatever works for your hair and your circumstances. City living often means that hair needs washing every day or every other day, using a gentle shampoo formulated for daily use followed by a light conditioner. If you can leave it on longer, do. Washing is often not as much of a problem as heat styling. If your hair tends to dryness and you want to wash it frequently, condition sensibly and let it air-dry as often as possible.

TIP: Some intensive conditioners and masks (there isn't always much difference) are designed to be left in overnight (or all day) so comb through dry hair then twist into a knot or tie back.

HAIR MASKS
Tried & Tested

Masks are increasingly used as a weekly boost particularly for dry scalp and hair, for 'the frizzies' and for anyone who's had chemical treatments like coloring (that's us!) and perming. (Women with oily scalps may find masks too rich and weighty.) Our tip: slather on generously, comb through and leave as long as you can.

TIGI SELF-ABSORBED MEGA-VITAMIN CONDITIONER
8.2 marks out of 10

Most testers loved this mega-vitamin formula, which claims to pump hair full of body and shine. However, it didn't suit everyone so, as with most things, it's down to individuals.

UPSIDE: "Delicious smelling – my husband said how gorgeous my hair smelt; hair looked extremely shiny and was a lot easier to comb through and style" • "very simple to apply, no tangles, easy to brush, less frizz" • "after I left it on for five mins, my hair had a "just stepped out of the salon" feel" • "fantastically shiny hair, really easy to comb through" • "hair looks healthy shiny and sleek and I feel well-groomed" • "excellent for my long, fine-ish hair; I get through loads of conditioner and this one really stood out".

DOWNSIDE: "I needed more moisture content" • "need to squeeze the bottle hard to get product out" • "average product – hair lank again after two days".

REDKEN ALL SOFT HEAVY CREAM
8.05 points out of 10

This high-scoring product is "ideal for very dry, thick, wiry, coarse hair in need of moisture and control". Our straight-haired testers also found it fabulous (and fairly weightless). The gloss-boosting ingredients in this 5–15-minute hair pack include avocado oil, glycerine, and wheat proteins.

UPSIDE: "The best product I used – just fantastic; my straight hair was silky and light" • "hair looked healthier – brighter..." • "my hairdresser says it's one of the best conditioners he's used; superb de-frizz factor" • "instant gloss earned me compliments" • "nice, clean scent".

DOWNSIDE: "Ends still a bit dry" • "weighed down my hair although it improved condition".

❀ PHYTOLOGIE PHYTOCITRUS MASK
8 points out of 10

This product – crammed with natural ingredients including sweet almond protein, grapefruit extract and shea butter – is designed to "revitalize hair left dry by coloring and perming" and help keep color from fading.

UPSIDE: • "Made my recently colored hair feel thicker and glossy; it also looked brighter" • "only needed a 'dime-sized' dollop" • "my thick, long hair was smooth and controllable".

DOWNSIDE: "Left hair too floppy to style properly" • "comes in a jar which is tricky to open with wet hands".

MOP C SYSTEM RECONSTRUCTING TREATMENT
8 marks out of 10

A citrus-infused vitamin blend from a loved-by-the-stars brand designed to give intensive help to dry tired hair, containing organic alfalfa, papaya and organic elderberry (though overall, it's not quite as natural as those ingredients might suggest). One tester gave it 110 marks!

UPSIDE: "By the end of winter my hair usually feels lacklustre, dry and brittle, after this treatment it feels like HAIR again – as good as having a professional treatment" • "an excellent product that leaves hair glossy and manageable" • "a life-changingly good conditioner – truly amazing; I was having a nightmare coping with new gray hair trauma and this fixed it – will buy ALL their products and shares in the company!" • "love the cheeky orange packaging".

DOWNSIDE: "Looked good on the day, but next day my long thick colored hair was a haystack no matter how much I put on".

BEST BUDGET BUY
L'OREAL ELVIVE NUTRI-CERAMIDE DEEP REPAIR MASQUE
8 marks out of 10

This deeply nourishing mask contains a concentrate of micronutrients that claims to repair even very dry, damaged hair and restore it to gloss, smoothness and manageability. Our testers were impressed.

UPSIDE: "Within one hour of using this product, my hair looked as if it had been expertly styled (it hadn't) and stayed that way for over three days" • "aromatic smell of lemon, grapefruit and pineapple" • "hair felt incredibly soft and manageable after drying; movement was lovely" • "reduced the static in my hair"• "used for two weeks now and the condition of my hair is great – what a shine!"

DOWNSIDE: "Disappointed that my hair didn't look smooth or have a lot of shine" • "seemed to make my hair more curly".

The lowest score in this category was 5 points out of 10.

RESCUE REMEDIES

*Your hair and scalp need as much TLC as your face and body.
Here, LA hair guru Philip B. shares recipes for his homemade treatments*

Think of a dry sea sponge: rough, porous, dead. "That's your hair," explains hair-guru-to-the-stars Philip B. "Even after soaking in water, the sponge will eventually dry out as the water evaporates. But if you imagine the sponge saturated with oil, it'll still be soft and pliant to the touch, one hour, two hours, even three days later." That's the philosophy behind his best-selling hair treatments. Women literally fly halfway around the world so that Philip can rescue their tresses. (They definitely think it's worth the "hair miles".)

His advice is: "Hair and scalp should be treated with the same TLC as your face and body. Give hair deep treatments in addition to regular shampoo and conditioning – up to twice a week for extremely damaged or dry hair. For maintenance (for all hair types), deep treatments should be given anywhere from once a week to once every two weeks. In addition, treat hair a day or two before having color, a perm or a relaxer, to minimize potential damage and help deposit the chemical evenly."

Philip also has some tips for perfect conditioning technique: first, squeeze out extra moisture from your hair with your hands, then blot out any residue with a towel – rubbing or wringing wet hair may damage it. Apply the recommended amount of conditioner to your hair (not your scalp) for the recommended time. Comb through with a wide-tooth comb, then massage in. Rinse thoroughly. Finish off with cool or cold water if you can stand it. Blot hair dry with a towel then wrap round in a turban with a second – dry – towel and leave for a few moments to absorb any more moisture. Then dry and style – as often as you can, air-dry rather than blow dry.

Here are Philip's recipes for at-home treatments. "But at a pinch, you can make an emergency mask with a mixture of gently warmed olive and sesame oils," he says.

Vanilla-Rum Cocktail

Rum, explains Philip, is a marvelous remedy for oily deposits found on hair and scalp. This weekly treatment for oily hair should leave it baby-fine and soft to the touch.

¼ cup white rum
½ cup beer (not 'lite' beer)
2 whole eggs
½ teaspoon lemon extract
½ teaspoon vanilla extract
½ cup warm water

In a blender, mix all ingredients on medium speed for twenty seconds. Massage mixture through hair right down to the scalp; it will foam slightly. Leave on for up to five minutes; rinse with warm water and follow with regular shampoo and conditioner. This makes enough for at least a couple of treatments, but store in the fridge and discard after five days.

Sesame-Coconut Protein Conditioner

Both sesame and olive oils provide a moisture seal in this thick, luxurious hair conditioner. They nourish and rehydrate the scalp and hair and restore luster and shine to dry, brittle (and colored) hair.

2 tablespoons olive oil
2 tablespoons sesame oil (not toasted)
2 whole eggs
2 tablespoons coconut milk (canned is fine)
1 teaspoon coconut oil (optional)

In a blender, mix all ingredients together on a low speed for thirty seconds or until smooth. (It will foam up a bit because of the eggs.) Shampoo as usual and rinse. Then apply mixture to hair, massaging it in with fingers or a comb. Leave on for five minutes, then rinse very well with warm water. May be used daily and left on for longer for more intensive conditioning. (Cover and refrigerate any leftovers immediately; discard after five days.)

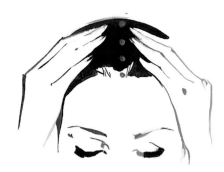

SCALP MASSAGE HOW-TO

You may not be aware of it, but you probably carry a lot of tension in your scalp. Just try moving your scalp over the skull; if you're like most busy, stressed women, it will be tight and immobile. Regular massage, however, makes the scalp move much more flexibly – and increases blood flow to the follicles, boosting hair health. Philip B. and Lois Dengrove (the Chief Treatment Specialist for Philip B.) gave us these smart scalp moves.

"All movements should be firm," advises Philip. This massage can help ease many hair and scalp conditions – from dry, damaged hair to flaking and psoriasis, hair thinning and loss – but is great for healthy heads, too. "The main focus is on maximizing the flexibility of the scalp and releasing tension so the follicles stay open. Tight follicles can't promote healthy hair growth."

1   Place the palms of your hands flat on either side of your scalp, fingers pointing up. Slowly and firmly push your palms upwards without lifting your fingers. Take a deep breath in, and exhale slowly.

2   Place your palms flat against your head, one at the back of the skull and one at the front, above the hairline. Follow the same movements as described in step 1.

3   Find the very highest point on your scalp, on your crown. Using both your middle fingers, press down on this shiatsu point; your other fingers should be resting lightly on the sides of your head. Now move all the fingers lightly over your head towards your hairline – press at intervals (see above), then once at the hairline itself. Repeat these movements backwards over the crown and down to the base of the skull, pressing at intervals and when you reach the very base of the skull.

4   Make circular motions with the pads of your fingers, using strong pressure. Start at the base of the neck, then move on to the sides, top and entire front and side hairline. Lift your fingers up and move them each time; don't drag them over the scalp.

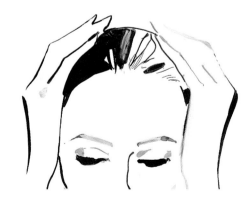

✳ For more great hair and body recipes, we recommend Philip B.'s book *Blended Beauty: Botanical Secrets for Body & Soul*.

CUTTING COMMENTS

Every time a woman goes to her stylist she is hoping for something magical. As British TV star Nigella Lawson puts it: "A haircut is never just a haircut, it might always be THE cut." Our experts, New York-based John Barrett and Marcus Allen of Aveda in London, help you get the cut you really want

Before you embark on a relationship with a new stylist, always ask for a consultation – which should last 10 to 15 minutes – so that you can discuss the points here. Remember – your hairdresser should be on your side: if he or she doesn't show interest and empathy, walk away. Give the low-down on your daily routine, a list of the products you currently use and, most importantly, a scrapbook of pictures of hairstyles you like—at least ten. Be realistic and pick hair that's similar to yours and women who look (vaguely) like you.

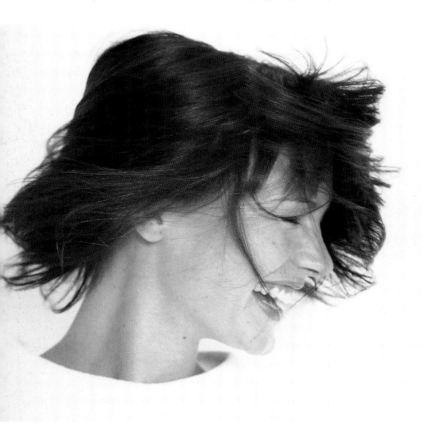

10 POINTS TO DISCUSS WITH YOUR (POTENTIAL) STYLIST

✳ **Your existing style:** what don't you like about it? Why doesn't it work for you? How long will it take to change to another style? If that involves growing it out, what can you do meantime?

✳ **Your face shape:** a good hairstyle creates an optical illusion of balance – that is the secret of attraction. See our illustrated guide to styling your hair for your face shape on pages 174–6.

✳ **Your best feature:** John Barrett's philosophy is always to play up the best feature – eyes, cheekbones, great jawline, beautiful forehead, pretty ears. Everyone has at least one, often two, he says, and your hairstyle should make the most of it. The style can not only expose that part but create a line towards it which the onlooker's eye follows naturally. As well as accentuating the positive, you want to disguise the negative: if, for example, you have a narrow pointy chin (as Sarah has), don't get a cut that falls to chin length and curves in, so that the eye travels straight to it – the line needs to lead away from it. Equally, if you have a square chin, round it out with a curve of falling hair.

✳ **Body Structure:** don't just discuss your face and hair; they are part of a bigger whole, including neck, shoulders and chest, then the rest of your body. You want to avoid, for example, a pinhead on broad shoulders and a tall body, or big flouncy hair on a big curvy figure.

✳ **Nature of hair:** the texture and thickness of your hair is a powerful governor of what style you can realistically have. With your stylist, you need to decide whether it is fine, medium, or coarse-textured, thick or thin; straight, wavy or curly – you can change these last (by perming, straightening etc.) but remember that these involve expense and upkeep and also affect the longterm condition of your hair. Always work with nature, if possible.

✳ **Maintenance:** how much time do you really have to tend to your hair? Can you wash it every day? Spend 15 or 30 minutes blowdrying it? Or do you have 5 minutes maximum? Also: how often can you get to the salon to have it cut? (And colored? See page 178.)

✳ **Your personal style:** what sort of look do you like? Talk through the pictures you have brought. Think about your clothes – they are potent indicators of your "look". Do you veer more towards classical/elegant? Or funky/trendy? Many women mix, say, blue jeans and Armani but usually there is one dominant theme. Your hair and clothes need to complement each other, so remember the attraction of opposites. Big curls on your head along with ruffled tops or big collars are overkill. If you want to wear big clothes, or frou-frou of any kind, choose sleek, smooth hair. If you want big hair, wear lean lines. Remember, however, that sleek hair goes with everything, you can then add the accessories: big earrings, ruff collar, lace, wacky handbags – the works!

✳ **Your mannerisms:** do you play with your hair – push it behind your ears, push back your bangs, twirl it geisha-style with your pen, pull and prod it all the time (which makes hair greasier, incidentally)? Anything like this needs to be taken into account – no good having wispy bangs if you go *insane* when it gets in your eyes.

✳ **Color:** if you are contemplating having your hair colored, the stylist should involve the colorist in your discussions. The lines and details of almost every cut can be enhanced with good color, and problem hair can be transformed. If everything is working against you – say you have dull flat straight hair which never really looks good – a delicious rich color can make you feel reborn.

✳ **Other chemical extras:** this means perming (rare nowadays) and straightening (AKA relaxing). The best method for the latter, according to our experts, is Yuko Hair Straightening Systems from Japan, which bombards the hair with protein to make the cuticles lie smooth. Stars who've been Yuko'd include Julia Roberts and Madonna, but it's not for African-American hair (see pages 196-9). The process takes several hours but results last about six months. (Many women love Yuko though some stylists think hair ends up looking a bit like the synthetic hair on dolls...)

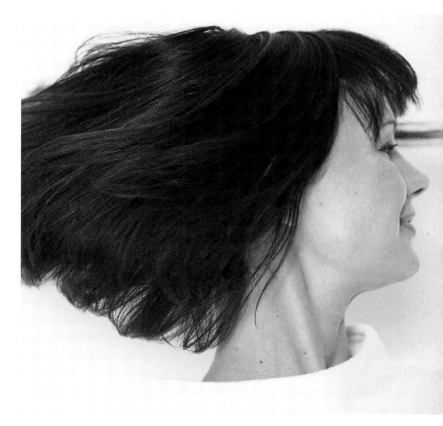

FIND THE HAIRSTYLE TO SUIT YOUR FACE

Most of the problems with haircuts are due to the style not suiting the shape of your face. There are a few simple guidelines which can make all the difference and help you to decide what style will really suit you. Start by tying your hair back so that you can see the proportions of your face—and, crucially, your jawline—in the mirror

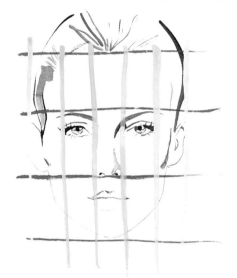

IDEAL PROPORTIONS

Curiously, perhaps, lots of research has looked into "ideal" facial proportions. It's basically about a look that feels harmonious and balanced. According to experts, the ideal face can be divided horizontally into three equal sections: from the hairline to the eyebrows, eyebrows to just under the nose, and below nose to base of chin. It divides vertically into five equal sections, widthways from ear to ear, as you can see in the drawing. Very few of us have these naturally lovely proportions but we can use our hair to frame our faces in a way that fools the eye into thinking we do.

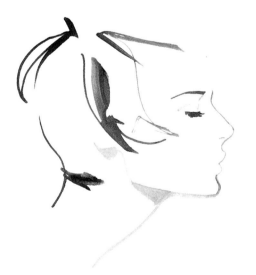

WHY YOUR JAWLINE MATTERS

Überstylist John Frieda claims your jawline is the deciding factor in the length of your hair. If the distance from your earlobe to your chin is short (see left), and you have a sharp angle where the jaw turns, you can wear almost any length of hair or have it swept up. But, if your jaw is long and sloping, you should avoid really short hair which exposes your jaw and nape, and not draw it back into severe styles.

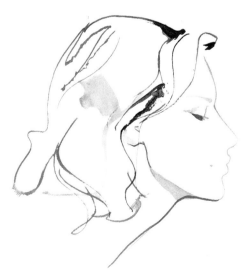

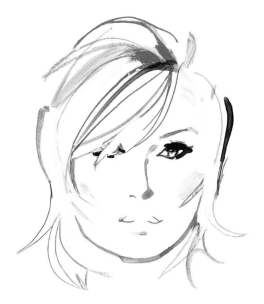

ROUND FACE

If you have a round face, choose a soft, choppy style rather than flat/sleek or curly/wavy. Try getting some layers cut around your cheeks to shade them and narrow the face. A domed look on top will add height, with graduated bangs cut on an angle and falling to below the cheekbone. Choppy hair at the neckline can break up a plump, thick, or short neck.

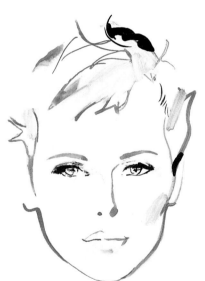

TIP: Be aware that layered haircuts are usually much more high-maintenance than straighter cuts. "If you want a choppy look, be prepared for the time you'll have to spend styling it," says Marcus Allen. "It's important your stylist knows your lifestyle and how much time you have before giving you a cut, otherwise it may not look great again until you next go back for a trim."

CLASSIC OVAL

This is the perfect face shape which can pretty much get away with any haircut. With all other face shapes, you are trying to create that oval look. A short cut like this is also great if you have a beautifully shaped head.

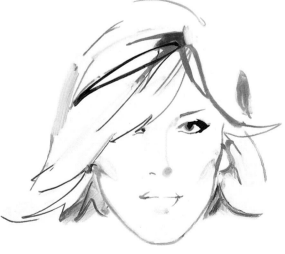

LONG FACE

Long faces can be made to look shorter with bangs, but think wispy and see-through—not Cleopatra or Coco Chanel. A chin-length cut is good, and if you have thin hair, let it flip out to add width. Avoid long straight bobs. Keep fullness behind the ears and have it soft and low on the crown. For a thin face, try tucking hair behind the ears to add width. If you have a pointy chin, don't have your hair curving in towards it, but get it sweeping up and away.

SQUARE FACE

Avoid short crops, symmetry, or anything geometric which emphasizes the squareness; go for soft curves and swings which will soften the jawline. Aim for a slightly pointy look at the top of the head to break the square outline. Choose light, see-through bangs, or longer graduated ones. If hair is short, try tucking some behind the ears but let some pieces fall forward to break the line. Have it graduating at the bottom, not blunt cut. If hair is long, make sure there is fullness at the top and upper sides to balance the jawline. Avoid hard sleek lines, but don't go nuts with waves and curls – aim for soft curves.

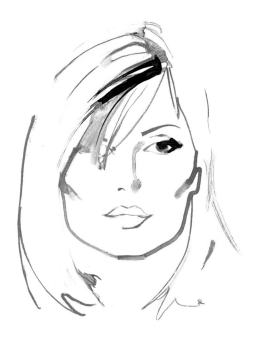

PRETTY EARS

If you have pretty ears, let people see them! Tuck hair behind them, or scoop hair back into a pony tail, braid or chignon. This look is also good for adding width to a narrow face.

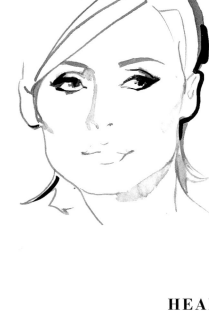

TIP: If your hair is chopped too short, say exposing too much chin and neck, you can correct the look by wearing a high neckline, which closes the gap between hair and flesh. And remember – it will grow...

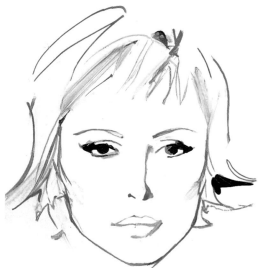

HEART-SHAPED FACE

If the face is very narrow at the bottom and wide at the top, hide the hairline with soft graduated bangs or a fall of hair, and a choppy, kicked-out style – not necessarily long – which gives volume around the bottom of the face.

If your face is shaped like an upside-down heart, narrow at the top and heavier on the jaw, make sure there is fullness at the top of your head to balance the chin and jawline. Disguise a narrow forehead with bangs that are graduated and sweep down and back at the sides.

ROLL BACK THE YEARS

If you want to turn back the years, emulate the look that gives babies, children and most supermodels their charm...

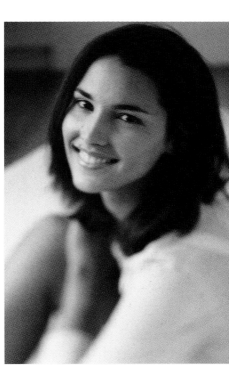

Openness is the one simple secret to taking years off your face, according to top stylist Marcus Allen of Aveda in London. "The face is fresh, clear, uncluttered," he explains "with a wide forehead, and you can see the eyes and lips." He's not rigid about this – we're not talking pulled-back ponytail (or shaven head). But try simple tricks like tucking wisps of hair behind your ears, having a side part so that you can sweep your hair back on one

If you wear specs a lot of the time, wear your hair off your face to avoid a cluttered look

side, or having wispy see-through bangs instead of a solid "shelf" so that the light can pass through it and give your forehead and eyes the illusion of openness. Have your hair cut so that the line leads back from your temples, widening the eye area. It's not just the face you want to open up, it's the neck and bosom as well. A turtleneck, tight scarf, or choker shortens the face/neck area, thus reducing the openness – and focusing all attention on your facial features (not great when you're feeling less than your best). You can counter that with an open-necked shirt, V- or low-necked top, or even off-the-shoulder numbers.

When it comes to age and hair length, conventional wisdom used to be that you should chop off your hair in middle age. Now there are simply no rules. Lots of women choose to grow their hair as they get past 40-something, and even 50-something. "It can soften the face wonderfully," says Marcus Allen. And twirling medium to long hair into a knot, pleat or chignon opens up the eye area and emphasizes cheekbones, while longer, soft bangs – which you can sweep to the side, or even back sometimes – are good for disguising forehead lines. Also remember that long hair can camouflage a thickening neck or a thinner one – both of which can happen with age. So just play around with your options.

GROWING IT OUT

Growing out an old style can be one long succession of Bad Hair Days but the trick, says Kerry Warn of John Frieda, is to ignore it. "Don't fuss about it. Wash and condition it regularly, get a box of bobby pins and pin the strands back – particularly that bump on the side of your head that comes when you're growing out shortish layers. Don't bother to hide the bobby pins, be gutsy. Have your hair trimmed every eight weeks, and when it's long enough to do a twist, pin it up. Then one day you'll wake up and voilà! you'll have long hair. Same with bangs: don't spend hours – and drive yourself bonkers – trying to blow dry and style it. Clip it back – cheap and chic."

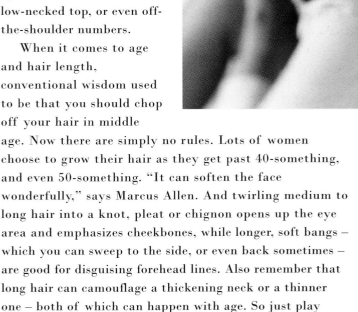

COLOR

Over the last decade, coloring technology and expertise have improved by leaps and bounds. It used to be that color dried your hair and often looked unnatural. Today's color can condition and even thicken as well as enhance the cut – and turn heads!

In the 21st century, cut and color go together like peaches and cream. Even the most conservative women don't think twice about having grey covered, and highlights are a matter of course. Despite that, it's still possible to make mistakes – both at home and in a salon. But, although the results can be magical, the process isn't – if you understand the basics. So here's the information you need to know.

Before you start, ask yourself one question: does the color I have really suit me? If the answer is yes, stop right there. The gods have given you a gift; don't mess with it. We, however, are immensely grateful for the gifts from our colorists.

If you're intent on color, talk to the experts. Even if you intend to color your hair at home, go and have a consultation with a couple of good colorists – someone who specializes in color, not a stylist who colors on the side.

Most good practitioners will give you a 5-minute consultation free (though make sure to ask what time is convenient for them). As with cuts, take along pictures of looks you like. Describing a color is difficult; what's light brown to you may be dirty blonde to a colorist.

While you're at the salon, try on wigs and hairpieces, if possible. You can do this in a department store too. Don't worry about the fit or style, just look at the general effect of the color.

"Always, always, always, check how much maintenance your color would need," says Susan Baldwin of John Frieda. "If you can only get to the salon or touch up at home every six months, you don't want a procedure that needs attention every two or three." Also consider the cost – good color isn't cheap.

COLORING OPTIONS

It's helpful to understand the (very wide) choice of products available when you're deciding whether to color your hair at home or in the salon.

Color-enhancing shampoos: give a hint of a tint; good for boosting natural shade or color maintenance.

Temporary colors: colorants in styling products such as mousse; last 1 to 3 washes on non-colored hair; don't use on colored, permed, or straightened hair.

Henna: unlike modern vegetable-based rinses, henna is a permanent metallic stain which you will have until it fades and/or grows out. You can't lift it out, color over it, or perm or straighten hennaed hair.

Chemical dyes: there are four types – progressive hair dyes, which gradually darken your hair; temporary hair dyes which wash out with your next shampoo; semi-permanent dyes, which last 6 to 8 shampoos, or longer-lasting ones—12 to 20; finally, there are permanent dyes/tints, which last 2 to 3 months – though the roots will need touching up within 4 to 6 weeks, particularly if the color is many shades different from your own.

The main difference is that with permanent dyes, the color penetrates the hair shaft with the help of compounds called PPDs, activated by another compound, usually hydrogen peroxide (see Is Hair Color Safe? on page 184). The other shorter-lasting methods simply coat the hair with color.

SALON COLORING TECHNIQUES

David Adams, Creative Director of Aveda, London, describes the most popular salon methods.

Highlights and lowlights: fine or thick strands of hair are weaved out (a few strands lifted out with a comb) and placed in foil. Colors may be soft or strong: highlights are lighter than the natural or existing color (see All-over tinting below), lowlights darker. Needs to be redone every 2 to 3 months, or more frequently depending on how near or far the color is from the natural base.

Balayage: colors are painted on (never through) the hair, in the direction of the cut – it's meant to look sunkissed, so positioning is all-important. Grows out well, and is relatively low maintenance.

Chunking: half the section of hair is taken out and wrapped in foil. Like highlights but a lot bolder and chunkier. Needs redoing every 2 to 3 months.

Allover tinting: this is whole head coloring where the hair is tinted with one or more solid colors. Highlights, lowlights, balayage, or slices may be added. Needs redoing every 4 to 8 weeks, depending on hair growth.

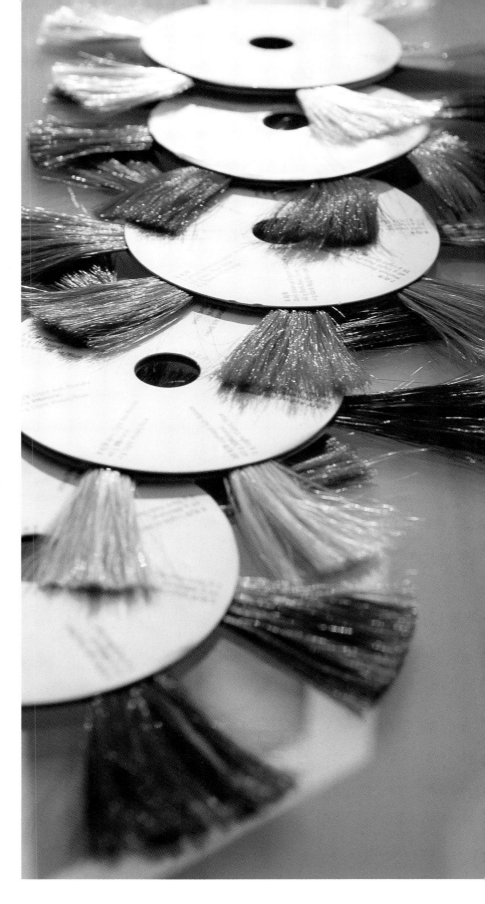

CHOOSING YOUR COLOR

Now you know the basic options, you need to think about what will look best on you. There are two main issues to consider – what color will suit your skin tone and what you can do with your natural color

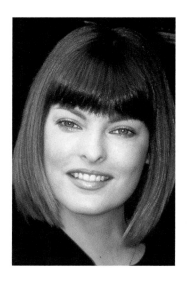 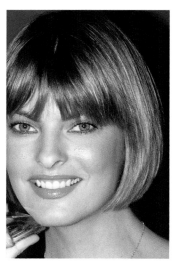 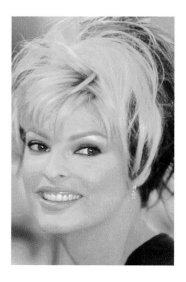 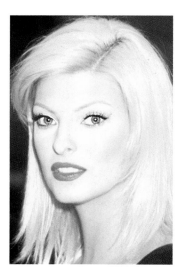

There are a few women – like supermodel Linda Evangelista, for example – who have the creamy ivory skin which can take any hair color. Most of us can't: too-yellow tones make a pinkish complexion scarlet and the hair brassy. Too deep a red/brown on sallow skin can make you look drained. Stick to our simple guide (right), and always insist that your colorist look at your skin and hair tone in full daylight...

SKIN TONE AND HAIR COLOR

Pink neutral tones – ash blonde, ash brown or dark brown (avoid red, blue/red or yellow blonde)

Yellow/sallow – dark rich tones with blue notes, like burgundy or deep auburn, to counteract the sallowness

Olive – stay dark; it's a perfect combination; add interest with a few rich burgundy lowlights

Pale white/ivory/cream – any color you like from ash blonde to auburn to dark brown or black

NATURAL SHADE AND ADDED HAIR COLOR

Natural

Added color

Black/very dark brown

Allover tint: one or two shades darker or lighter
Balayage: dark brown, copper or burgundy
(a single shade usually looks more elegant)

Dark to light brown

Allover tint: black, mocha, toffee, caramel, dark honey, auburn, copper
Highlights/balayage: toffee, caramel, dark honey, auburn, copper, mid gold through to strawberry blonde (can use 2 or 3 shades)

Dark to light blonde

Allover tint: warm shades of light chestnut, light honey, wheat, apricot, pale blonde; darker shades of milky coffee, copper, honey, dark chestnut
Highlights/balayage: as above, using 2 or 3 shades

Blonde to gray

Allover tint: pale icy blonde, pale ash brown, copper brown, beige, milky chocolate

Red/auburn/chestnut

Allover tint: dark brown or different shade of red, for example chestnut, auburn, copper
Highlights/balayage: similar shades, either lighter or darker, plus lighter golden tones (can add 2 or 3 shades)

HOME HAIR COLORING TIPS

According to experts, most problems arise because people don't follow directions – and heed the warnings – on the package insert. It's up to you: care and planning can give you good results, while not making that extra effort can mean not only a Bad Hair Color Month or so, but a potentially serious allergic reaction

These suggestions apply to both permanent and semi-permanent coloring.

✳ Don't go for a dramatic color change first time.

✳ Read – and follow – the instructions and warnings.

✳ Do your skin and strand tests well beforehand, as outlined in the directions. Allergic reactions can take 48 hours to appear so allow enough time with your skin test.

✳ At the start of your coloring session, put an old towel around your shoulders for protection.

✳ Remember to splatter-proof your bathroom if your walls are painted rather than tiled.

✳ Take off all your jewelery so you don't make holes in the plastic gloves.

✳ Smear around your hairline with Vaseline to keep the color from staining the skin.

✳ If the gloves provided with the kit are too loose, secure them at the wrists with sticky tape or a wide rubber band to prevent them from slipping and color from seeping down your hands.

✳ Use a timer or an alarm clock (there's usually one on cell phones) to tell you when time's up. It's all too easy to lose track of the minutes.

CONDITIONING COUNTDOWN

Louis Licari, owner of the Louis Licari Color Group in New York, advises women to plan ahead if they want to achieve the best home haircoloring results. Here is his conditioning countdown to perfect color – with maximum shine.

One week before coloring: Treat hair with a deep conditioner or hair mask; this strengthens the hair but allows enough time for the product to be fully rinsed out, ensuring that your hair color will "take" evenly.

On the day: Don't shampoo just before coloring. The natural oils secreted by your scalp protect and hydrate it during the coloring process.

One week after coloring: Deep condition with a hair mask once a week from now on. When it comes to day-to-day haircare, preserve your color with shampoos and conditioners specifically for color-treated hair. (Louis Licari, like many other top hairdressers around the world, swears by the gloss-restoring Phytologie range of shampoos, conditioners and hair treatments, from France).

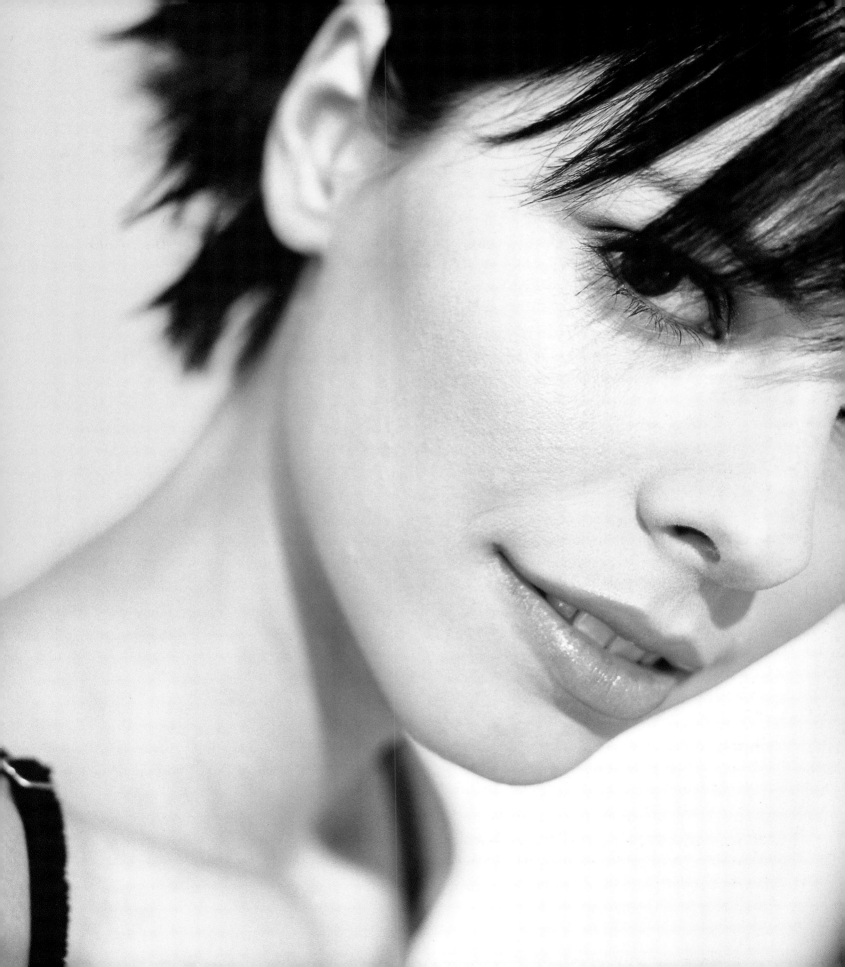

IS HAIR COLOR SAFE?

Over the years, fears have arisen about the safety of hair dye, despite the stringent testing carried out by manufacturers

A couple of years back, the European Commission (EC) published a report on hair dyes stating it cannot deem them safe on the basis of current evidence provided by manufacturers. This does not necessarily mean that they are dangerous, but scientists working on the EC report believe that consumers should know the risks.

The synthetic chemicals most likely to cause problems are a group called PPDs (para-phenylenediamines, also referred to as p-Phenylenediamine) which come from coal tar (a known carcinogen). They are commonly used in hair color in the USA and in the UK, particularly in permanent and semi-permanent colors as dark brown or black dyes. (They're also referred to as "black henna" although they have no chemical relationship with henna.) They are usually activated by hydrogen peroxide.

According to former research chemist Dr Stephen Antczak, co-author of *Cosmetics Unmasked*, allergic reactions are the most likely potential problem – and you'll see copious warnings on the package insert about this. The challenge with these allergic reactions is that they can occur without warning after years of trouble free use and are often dramatic.

To be safe, we should all do a patch test every single time we have our hair colored, whether this is at home or in a salon. Apply some of the fully mixed product (not just the colored part) to an area where your skin is thin, for example on your upper arm or behind your ear. If there is any sign of redness, soreness, swelling or irritation over the next 48 hours, do not use the product. You should also have a patch test when your hair is colored at the hairdressers, advises Dr Antczak. London-based hairdresser Daniel Field offers this to clients routinely.

Aside from possibly causing skin irritation, which can be severe enough to need hospitalization, PPDs can trigger asthmatic reactions, and are very dangerous if they get into your eyes. (Because of this, brow and lash-dying are now illegal in many countries and carry heavy warnings in Europe.)

In the long term, PPDs have also been linked to various forms of cancer. While there is no direct proof of cause and effect, they have been shown to affect the reproduction of cells (the basis of cancer) and epidemiological studies have shown links. The National Cancer Institute has recommended that the industry look for substitute ingredients.

The risk period is while the dye is on the head, so the more regularly people dye their hair with products containing PPDs, the greater the risk. However, Dr Antczak's view is that we are probably far more at risk of developing a chemically induced cancer through smoking, drinking alcohol or inhaling chemicals from dry-cleaning fluid, paint fumes, aerosol deodorants and the many other household products that contain synthetic chemicals.

Also worrying for many people are environmental concerns: PPDs are very toxic to aquatic life. Ammonia, commonly used in dyes and perms, is also a culprit here. Even tiny amounts of these chemicals are extremely poisonous and may cause long-term damage in rivers and waterways.

Progressive hair dyes (which cover grey gradually) may contain lead acetate or bismuth citrate – both very poisonous substances. Never use them on broken or damaged skin and always wash your hands thoroughly.

HOW TO HELP PROTECT YOURSELF

Dr Paula Baillie-Hamilton, author of a wonderful book called *The Detox Diet* (see Bookshelf, page 251) has spent four years researching environmental chemicals. Although she believes that we should all eat organically as much as possible and reduce our toxic load in every way we can, she still has her blonde hair highlighted – a less risky procedure than permanent allover tints. But to help minimize the potential damage from all kinds of hair-coloring chemicals, she recommends the following supplements, to be taken in addition to your regular daily supplements:

"I would suggest taking an extra 1g of vitamin C, 400 IU of vitamin E, and 3g of psyllium husks about half an hour before your appointment, plus another 500mg of vitamin C as soon as you reasonably can afterwards," she says.

"The scalp acts very much like a sponge when liquids are put directly on it. These supplements work to protect our body from any chemicals which may sneak in. The vitamins will increase the ability to neutralize the increased level of damaging free radicals which tend to be released as a result of our exposure to toxic chemicals, and the soluble fiber will help soak up any chemicals which have breached our defenses – then carry them out of our bodies."

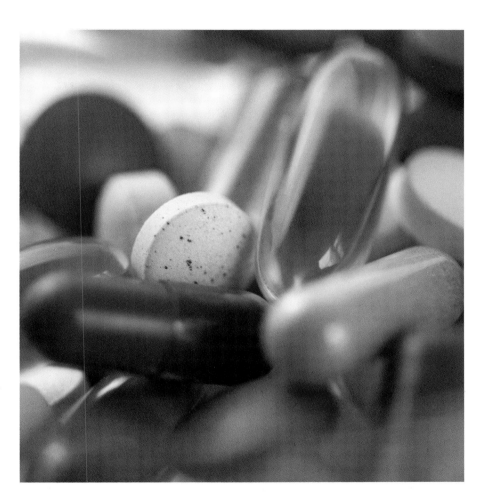

WARNING: ALWAYS STORE HAIR DYES OUT OF THE REACH OF CHILDREN

BLOW-DRY KNOW-HOW

A truly great hairstyle is one you can recreate at home. Many women, however, find the art of blow-drying fiendishly tricky – and very time-consuming. So—between salon appointments—theyre disappointed with their cut. But it is quite possible to achieve salon-perfect results at home, provided you have the right tools, the right product and the right brush for your hair

Here are our experts' tips on a great blow-dry:

✳ Squeeze hair to remove excess water, wrap it in a towel to remove as much as you can and then stroke hair downwards with a small absorbent towel to get it as dry as possible.

✳ If you're using a styling product, get hair as dry as you can before applying, otherwise you're just watering it down.

✳ Talk to your stylist about what product to use if you're unsure; see Our (Very Basic) Guide to Styling Products, page 188.

has 1810 watts of power, a directional nozzle and a really long cord.

✳ If your hair is prone to frizz you may want to try a diffuser, although it takes longer to dry hair because the air flow is slowed.

✳ Tip your head upside-down and ruffle hair while you blow-dry initially. It invigorates roots and builds body.

✳ When hair is just beginning to feel dry, start using a brush to style. Before that, you're wasting your time.

Style the front of the hair first; that's the part everyone notices. If you're in a real hurry, you can stop there

✳ Spread a tiny amount of styling product, if used, in the palms of your hands and massage it through hair from roots to ends.

✳ Use a powerful hairdryer with a directional nozzle. When most people get a new dryer, they throw away the nozzle – but it's the most important part of your drier. The more powerful the hairdryer, the quicker the results. Look for 1600 watts minimum. More wattage is better. Our experts recommend the Turbo Power Parlux 3000, which

✳ Style the front of the hair first; that's the part everyone notices. If you're in a real hurry, you can stop there. Otherwise it's generally front, sides and top, with back and underneath last (unless you have a short upswept style, in which case you may want to go from the front to the nape then do sides and top).

✳ Before you start styling, it may help to use clips to "section" off hair you're not working on, particularly if it's medium to long.

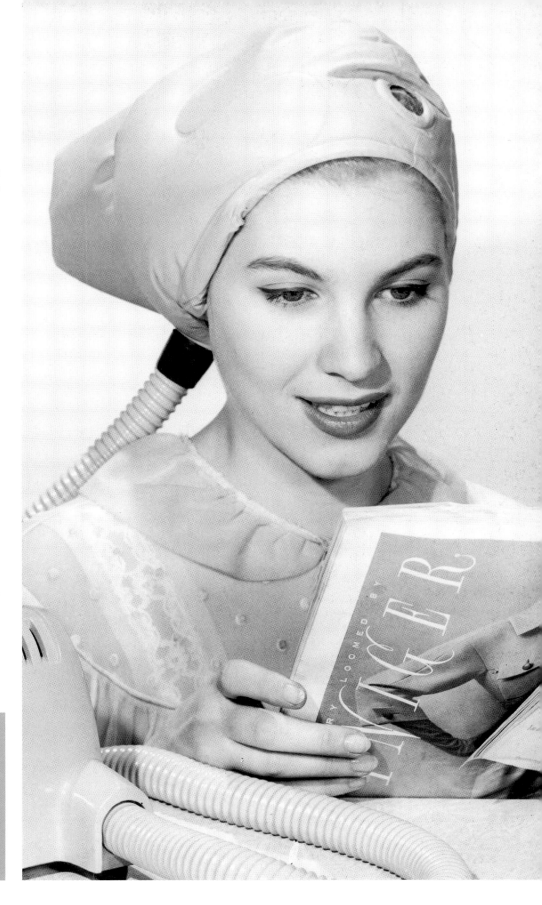

✳ Blow-dry down the grain of the hair, towards the ends. It makes the cuticle lie flat, so hair looks shiny and your style will keep its shape longer.

✳ If you want extra body, put in large Velcro rollers – one or three in the crown is very effective and saves you getting arm cramps holding the drier above your head; leave rollers in while you do your makeup.

✳ Give hair a final blast of cool air to fix the style. And a quick ruffle with your fingers, because the last thing you want to look is "set".

✳ Use a little bit of wax (we love John Frieda Sheer Blonde Spun Gold Shaping and Highlighting Balm, which gives a gold gleam) to separate hair and give a final gloss; or use a spritz of spray shine. If you want shine plus hold, spray hair spray on a brush and brush through hair right at the end.

TIP: Überstylist Nicky Clarke says "Styling is all in the wrist action. Try switching the hand you hold the dryer in – you'll find it easier to make both sides look symmetrical, if that's what you're after. It's tricky at first but practice soon makes perfect."

DIFFERENT STROKES

Today there's a daunting selection of brushes: bristle, cushioned, wooden, plastic, vent, paddle – and more. If you're baffled by brush-speak, here are the facts

"When you're choosing a brush, two factors count," says James McMahon, top photographic session stylist, "your hair type and the type of brush you enjoy using. Choose a brush that's easy for you to handle, gets through the hair easily – and is right for the task."

For blow-drying short or bob-length hair, choose a vent brush, which lifts hair at the roots, allowing air to get in and add volume. If you want to achieve smoothly curved ends, you should also have a radial (round) brush.

For curly or coarse hair, combination bristle/nylon brushes will ease through tangles to the scalp – or again, use a vent brush, which won't disturb the hair or create unwanted frizz. (Mason Pearson's popular nylon/bristle brush is the choice of many leading stylists.) Natural bristle brushes can make longer hair static and cause flyaways, while combination bristle/nylon brushes reduce friction. For long, straight hair, blow-dry using a brush like Denman's Classic Styling Brush, which lifts hair without adding kinks or tangling, then finish off using a paddle brush to smooth. Aveda's wooden Paddle Brush is a pleasure to use.

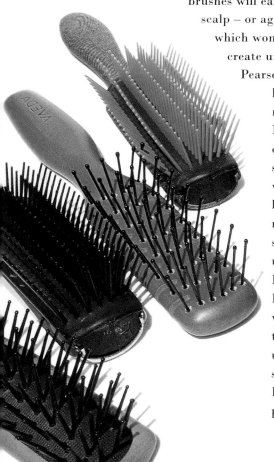

To add a curl, wave or a flip to straight hair, choose a radial brush. The shorter your hair, the smaller your brush should be. If you've got different lengths – bangs, say, or layers – you'll need more than one brush. Generally speaking, the brush should be just big enough so you can get it well into the hair without wrapping the hair around and round it.

If you find a full radial brush too bulky to handle, try a smaller, half-radial brush. Radial brushes with a metal interior are a great choice: the heat from your blow-dryer makes them act like heated curling tongs.

OUR (VERY BASIC) GUIDE TO STYLING PRODUCTS

This is one of the most overcrowded and confusing areas of the beauty market. We try and use the minimum because, mostly, we think it's overkill. But some are really useful, particularly when you have a touch of the frizzies or flyaway hair.

The best way to decide whether you need a styling product is to talk to your hairdresser. They'll tell you what they use and why – and you'll be able to see the results. Ask for samples from the salon brand and then practice on your own time.

Read the packaging carefully to make sure the product does what you want – the variations are endless. Most come in different strengths and for different hair textures. Remember to use a tiny bit – the most common mistake is using too much. Always start at the back of your head, where it won't show if it goes ape, and spend some time practicing.

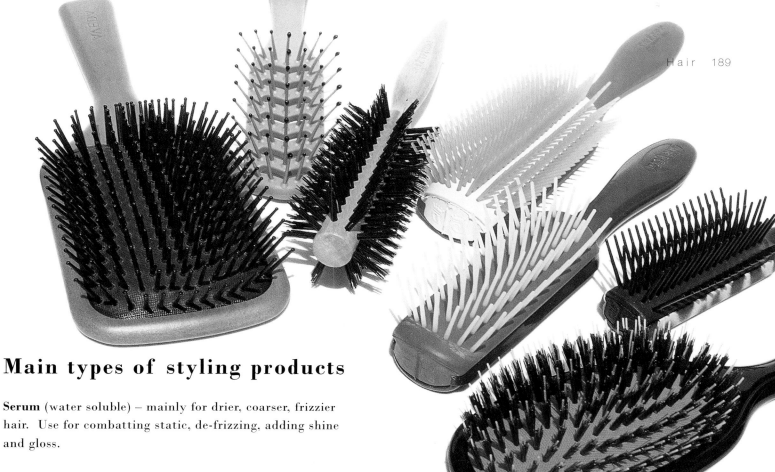

Main types of styling products

Serum (water soluble) – mainly for drier, coarser, frizzier hair. Use for combatting static, de-frizzing, adding shine and gloss.

Mousse – mainly for finer, flyaway or flattish hair. Use for blow-drying, scrunching, diffuser-drying and finger-drying. Provides natural, flexible hold and body, in much the same way as traditional setting/styling lotions. (Sarah refuses this at the hairdresser because her hair looks great for a day then goes flat the next and it seems to temporarily alter the texture.)

Setting or fixing lotions (AKA sculpting spray, molding mist, heat-styling lotion) – mainly for finer, flyaway or flattish hair. Use for setting, scrunching, blow-drying and air drying.

Thickening/volumizing lotions – alternative to mousse/setting lotion. Use for doing just that...

TIP: Brushing removes dead skin and debris from the scalp, stimulates circulation, "feeds" the hair with each stroke of the brush – and, done with a gentle rhythm, also relieves stress.

Finishing touches

Wax (also pomade, cream, clay, gum) – use for dressing, controlling frizz and static, slicking back, defining, molding, and building body. Good for conditioning and separating hair, giving it a "piece"-y, more casual look. Wax is also good for bringing down hair that has been overstyled and got too big.

Gel – use for accentuating shorter styles, dressing, texturizing, slicking, and molding.

Hair spray – use for holding, shaping and adding shine (you can buy shine-only products).

QUICK FIXES

Every woman has looked at her hair in the mirror and felt like putting a brown paper bag over her head. Take heart! Our experts have lots of nifty tricks for solving problems up top

BAD HAIR MORNINGS

On those mornings when you've woken up and your hair's a disaster zone, don't despair. Here are suggestions from hair whiz Peter Forester, who has worked on commercials all over the world, and our other experts.

If you have a straight bob and it's gone flat, spray the top layer with a plant mister filled with water, and blow-dry just that section, rather than everything underneath. If hair's curly, mist and scrunch the wave back into your hair to revive the look in minutes OR put in Velcro rollers, blitz with the dryer then let it cool down. Look for the new-generation Velcro rollers, which have metal interiors so they heat up more efficiently.

No rollers? No dryer? If you're having a flat-top day, or a kinky-bangs moment, you just need a brush and about five minutes. Make tracks for the bathroom (or the kitchen), dampen the roots in the problem area only and lift the hair with a brush until it's dry. You can do the same with any part of your hair, including the sides.

If your hair is dry and lifeless, and you have no time at all, give it a quick boost with a couple of minutes of scalp

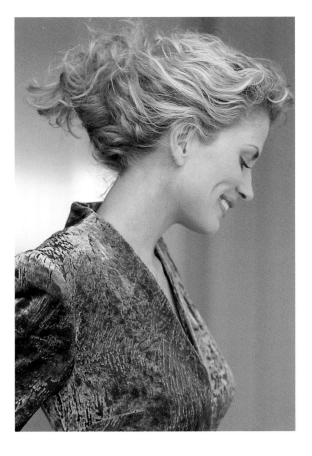

massage. Using your fingertips, simply rub your scalp vigorously from your front hairline to your nape. It wakes up your hair, gets the sebum out to give it a bit of shine, plus it's great for waking up your mind (and for a headache). It usually looks best if you don't brush it out, but you could hang your head upside down and give it a quick brush or a ruffle through with your fingers.

For short, spiky styles, dampen hair, work some grooming cream in the palms of your hands and slide them through your hair, then leave to dry naturally. (Kiehl's Creme With Silk Groom is ideal, although we also like John Frieda Sheer Blonde Dream Creme Instant Silkener.)

If you've been to a smoky party and your hair smells like an ashtray, spritz a favorite fragrance in front of you and walk through the "cloud".

Put some of the body back into longer hair by misting it with water, putting it up in a scrunchie or a big clip, then shake it out when you get to work. If you're going out that night, leave in the scrunchie all day for added oomph.

If your bangs have lost their oomph, just blow-dry them again and style with an appropriate brush (see page 188).

DAY INTO EVENING

A few nifty tricks can transform your daytime look into evening glamor. With five minutes in the bathroom, a styling product and an accessory or two, you'll be ready for the Ball (or hot date or whatever), says Kerry Warn of John Frieda. The key is to keep it as simple as possible; you don't want to be worrying and fussing all evening.

Kerry's suggestions:

✳ Use a styling product, such as John Frieda Frizz-Ease 5-Minute Manager, to boost and give a bit of bounce. Spray it just on problem areas, then brush your hair into place.

✳ Tuck your hair behind your ears, exposing cheekbones and drawing attention to the eyes. Redo your bangs if necessary (see opposite). Pop in a clip, pin or comb on either side. Make up your eyes and cheeks, gloss your lips and put on glam earrings.

✳ If your hair is dirty or greasy, just go with it. Use a little gel to give a slightly wet look then push it back. If it's short, give yourself a side part – always more dramatic – and make up your eyes to be big and smudgy. If it's longer, comb back tightly and twist your hair into a ponytail or knot or chignon. Add a flower. Pull a few pieces down around your face and gel into tendrils. It looks incredibly confident and glamorous. Add a jeweled clip or two, or a great pair of earrings.

✳ If the cut's grown out and it's medium to long but – quite frankly – a bit of a mess, make it *more* messy. Put it up with some barrettes, a bulldog clip, or a big slide. Don't even try and tuck the ends in; just fan them out and fix with spray if necessary.

✳ Push most of your hair behind a hair band ("thin," says Kerry emphatically – "those thick decorated ones can look like Chanel on acid"). Pull some tendrils out and let them hang around your face, take a few back over the band and grip or pin in place. Either let the hair hang loose at the back, gather it in a knot or chignon, or put it up in a messy twist. And don't worry if the pins or bobby pins show; decorate them with pretty accessories – see below.

HAIR ACCESSORIES

Here are some ideas for your Box of Hair Tricks – buy these whenever you see pretty ones, advises Kerry.

Bobby pins – different colors

Clips/barrettes – all kinds, all sizes

Combs (antique Victorian paste as well as modern)

Pins with flowers

Thin hair band (clear plastic, metal, black grosgrain, antique)

Black scrunchies

Jaw clips (tortoiseshell is chic, or clear, or metal)

Fresh flowers

STYLING PRODUCTS

Tuck small sizes of your favorite products into your makeup bag:

Serum

Gel

Thickening lotion

Shine spray

Fixing spray

Styling wax with gleam in it

DOWN WITH FRIZZIES

Fluffy may be fine for kittens and omelettes, but certainly not for hair. So Michael Gordon, founder of top Manhattan salon Bumble and Bumble, has these tips on how to cope with hair that turns into Medusa's as soon as the humidity level rises

✳ Consider a shorter style for summer. Shorter hair is easier to groom and control – as well as being much cooler. If you still like longer hair, learn to pile it casually on top of your head or tie it up and back in a loose ponytail.

✳ Hair picks up incidental sun damage as we walk around, so protect it with a spritz-on sunscreen, which helps it from drying out – which leads to the frizzies – and ensures color stays true. Scarves and hats are great, too.

✳ Use a leave-in conditioner, which coats the shaft and gives a tiny bit of extra weight – then let hair air dry rather than using a hairdryer.

✳ While hair is wet, rub a blob of silicone gel, cream or serum between your palms and smooth down the length of hair to seal the cuticles. To make sure every strand is coated, pin up the top layers of hair and smooth gel or serum onto the bottom layers first.

✳ Although Bumble and Bumble makes terrific thickening products, Michael advises avoiding them when it's humid as they make the problem worse by adding extra volume. Instead, groom hair with de-frizzers (see our Tried & Tested, opposite) and waxes. "Put the tiniest dab in the palm of your hand, rub in well – and skim over hair."

FOR NATURAL FRIZZIES

Keep hair long past the shoulders, suggests Kerry Warn of John Frieda (who tames Nicole Kidman's frizz), "to give it weight. It gives you options and you can always pin it back if it starts to take over your life."

If you're blow-drying naturally frizzy hair, use a large, round, natural-bristle brush (Kerry swears by Mason Pearson) with a comb for the very short pieces around the hairline: "Lock the comb into the hair and direct the nozzle down."

On days at home, he advises putting some corrective styling gel in front (John Frieda's bestselling Frizz Ease is his choice) and combing it back into a little ballerina knot. By the end of the day, it will be smooth with just a lovely natural bend. For longer frizzy hair, Kerry suggests changing the shape by styling just the hairline, where the hair is always finer and thus frizzier, and surface layers. "Put your part where you want, then take a larger curling iron and start altering strands around the face and on the top layers, but leave the natural curl underneath."

With a styling procedure such as curling or flat-ironing or adding product, start at the back so that you can practice. By the time you get to the front – where it shows – you will be an old pro.

HAIR DEFRIZZERS – *Tried & Tested*

About 30 percent of women have dry, frizzy, unmanageable hair. So womankind should be grateful for frizz-defiers, which can make a curl do what a curl oughta do. We asked testers to rate these products on improvement in shine, gloss, de-frizz, curl defining and enduring manageability. Our consumer testing brought a line-up of top products, all of which scored highly.

❀ AVEDA LIGHT ELEMENTS SMOOTHING FLUID

8.8 points out of 10

From Aveda's Light Elements line (plant-based like all their products), this is based on organic lavender water, with organic jojoba oil to help moisturize and condition. Several of our ten testers – not all with dry and/or frizzy hair – gave it full points.

UPSIDE: "The best product I've used on my long, highlighted, fluffy hair – really lives up to its promises, hair soft, manageable and bouncy, smoother and glossier" • "incredibly easy to use, gorgeous smell" • "excellent for use with irons" • "no residue" • "good for defining layers in straight layered hair" • "light, serum-like consistency is easy to spread on wet or dry hair, came up trumps on all my family's different sorts of hair – the best styling agent ever".

DOWNSIDE: "I need a stronger product for my thick, very curly hair".

KERASTASE OLEO-RELAX DISCIPLINE SERUM

8.78 points out of 10

This pump product contains a "unique Nutri-Huile complex" from Shorea Oil and Palm Treat Oil, also UV filters, to give control, gloss and smoothness.

UPSIDE: "Very good de-frizz factor – hair softer and smooth than ever before" • "fantastic for my fine, flyaway hair" • "my curly colored hair used to frizz a lot in wet weather but is now so well-behaved!" • "immediate shine – great for fitting into busy schedule" • "my new miracle hair product for my thick curly hair".

DOWNSIDE: "Slightly grim fragrance" • "made hair a little greasier than usual".

BEST BUDGET BUY
GARNIER FRUCTIS SLEEK & SHINE WEIGHTLESS SMOOTHING SERUM

8.3 points out of 10

From another range targeted at coarse, dry rebellious hair, this relies on micro oils from apricot kernels and avocado plus vitamins to nourish and soften hair.

UPSIDE: "Fantastic – my long, naturally wavy, slightly frizzy hair felt smooth, silky and looked sleek, excellent for styling with dryer" • "I'm a big fan – better value than similar ones and turns frizz into curls" • "superb for my very coarse, curly, frizzy, graying, colored hair; will definitely be changing to this".

DOWNSIDE: "Smell overly fruity, artificial" • "have to be careful how much you use".

BEST BUDGET BUY
ELVIVE SMOOTH INTENSE SERUM

7.77 points out of 10

With a silicone derivate plus camelina oil to treat dry coarse and rebellious hair, this product claims to make dry difficult hair soft, easy to manage, sleek, smooth and shiny...so read on!

UPSIDE: "Excellent – my slightly wavy long hair was shinier and sleeker, with very little frizz" • "my highlighted, quite dry, frizzy hair stayed smooth even in damp conditions" • "much easier to straighten hair with irons, even better used with matching conditioner".

DOWNSIDE: "Hair felt more manageable but less clean!" • "packaging is off putting and cheap looking" • "texture a bit gluey".

BEST BUDGET BUY
ALBERTO ADVANCED V05 SILKY SMOOTH MIRACLE MIST

7.77 points out of 10

The only blurb to emphasise that no product (even if it contains a blend of real silk extracts and five vitamins like this spray) is a magic bullet; a good diet, enough down time and looking after your hair (they suggest a satin pillowcase...) are vital too. Some testers loved this, but it didn't suit all.

UPSIDE: "Fantastic product – gave my chemically treated hair its life back" • "really helped smooth my thick curly hair, also good with ceramic straightener".

DOWNSIDE: "Overpowering smell" • "results were only good when I blowdried my curly frizzy thick hair – otherwise really fluffy!".

The lowest score in this category was 4.4 points out of 10.

SERUM SECRETS

The art is not to overdo it. Even if you have long or thick hair, start with a tiny amount – no bigger than a dime! (Or, for liquid product, no more than five drops.) Apply to one palm, rub together and smooth through hair. Start at the back, so that you don't run any risk of overloading the all-important hair that frames the face. If you need to use more serum, repeat the process – but never, ever use more than a tiny amount at a time.

HOLISTIC
– OR HIGH TECH?

*Haircare ads often look like pages from a gardening or geographical magazine.
But most so-called "natural" haircare really isn't. So when it comes to feeding hair and
follicles, here's some food for thought...*

Modern haircare borrows freely from nature, infusing shampoos, conditioners and hairstyling products with botanical ingredients which have acknowledged benefits as shine-enhancers and manageability-boosters. But, in reality, the percentage of botanical ingredients in most mass market haircare is tiny. A lot of it is blatant marketing hype, trading on the feel-good factor triggered by the idea of a "natural" product.

Skin, as we've said, is more like a sponge than was ever imagined. And the top of the head – the "pate" – is the most absorbent part of all. That's the part in a baby's skull where the bones take some weeks to join up, and it remains more vulnerable our whole lives. So, personally, we increasingly care about what we put on our scalps.

Harsh detergents – used in many mass-market shampoos – can have an irritating and drying effect on the scalp. Sensitive people may experience itching or prickling after exposure. What these detergents also do, as they frothily strip away oil and grime to leave hair squeaky-clean, is make the skin more receptive to other, potentially harmful, ingredients in the mix, acting like a "vector"

The UK's Soil Association now has standards for organic haircare products as well as skin and bodycare. Many of the lines carrying its symbol are also distributed around the world. In Australia, there are several organic certifying organizations giving a "green light" to products. If you want to be an organic beauty, look for certified haircare.

into the bloodstream because the barrier function is damaged. We're certainly not trying to make you paranoid about washing your hair – or suggest you give up tending to your tresses. But remember that whatever you put on your scalp "feeds" the body, too. So if you think about what you put in your mouth, think about what you're putting on your hair. Just because something says it's "natural" on the label, doesn't mean it's not packed with chemicals. On pages 248–249, we have listed some ingredients which are *not* accepted by the organic regulatory bodies.

Certainly, we have found many natural and organic products to be highly effective. (If a little bit of a botanical ingredient is good, more can be better. The higher up the ingredient list something is, the more is in the product.) In all honesty, though, we both compromise, depending on how much time we have and what's on hand; natural and organic when we can, super-high-performance, high-tech products sometimes, too. But whichever route you choose to take, we've categorized the results in our Tried & Tested sections to steer you to choices that will work for you – whether you want your haircare to make you feel you're (genuinely) wafting through a wildflower meadow, or would like the best that advanced science (maybe with the teensiest, weensiest little help from Mother Nature) can throw at your follicles.

And what about styling products? Since most are applied to the hair itself, which is dead, rather than the living scalp, absorption of the ingredients in these may not be such an issue – and you can always rinse your hands after running a mousse or smoothing a gel through your hair.

WHAT WE USE

JO

I'm a haircare junkie, I admit – though I veer towards more natural ranges. I love Urtekram Rose Shampoo, which uses an ultra-gentle, sugar-based detergent, and matching Rose Conditioner. As a smell junkie, I adore Philip B.'s Scent of Santa Fe Shampoo – a real nostril-hit of sage and pinon – but it's certainly not cheap. Many inexpensive shampoos make my scalp itch – but John Frieda Sheer Blonde Moisture Infusing Shampoo (I use the honey-to-caramel formula) doesn't give me that problem, perhaps because of its soothing lavender; I also like John Frieda Sheer Blonde Hair Repair Strengthening and Conditioning Treatment. And I'm a big hair mask fan; faves are ESPA Pink Hair & Scalp Mask, organically-certified Neal's Yard Rosemary & Cedarwood Hair Treatment and Christophe Robin Colorist Wheat Germ Mask (from Paris's top haircolor pro). I slap on a mask every week to keep my highlighted-to-high-heaven hair shiny, leaving it on as long as possible before I rinse and run. But I have to say that my biggest look-good hair secret is that I cheat – with regular John Frieda blow-drys, which sounds extravagant – but I take work with me to the salon!

SARAH

My hair is very thick with a natural wave – and graying a little bit. I have a cut I love by Natalie at John Frieda, and lovely color by Susan Baldwin and Stephen, also at John Frieda. (When I'm in New York, I go to John Barrett and his colorist William, who make me get bold!) But I have dry hair and it's a perpetual battle against the haystack look. Masks are absolutely essential; like Jo, I love Christophe Robin Colorist Wheat Germ Mask and ESPA's pink mud. Currently, my favorite shampoo and conditioner ranges are MOP (Modern Organic Products, though they're not totally natural . . .) Glisten range and Aussie's Miracle Moist range for dry and damaged hair. I sometimes blowdry my hair (for parties and outings) – a good whoosh with my head upside down gives it real volume, or I put in big rollers (very 50s). The solution to round-the-face frizzies is to comb through a dab of John Frieda's Frizz-Ease hair serum, just around my face and on top. Then blow dry, again with my fingers rather than a brush or comb. And finally, finger on a tad of John Frieda's Sheer Blonde Spun Gold Shaping and Highlighting Balm (below), which is a mini-miracle.

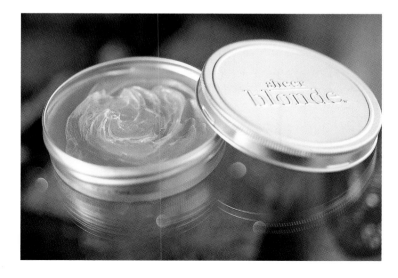

ETHNIC HAIR

Black women have different problems with their crowning glories. We asked leading London stylist Errol Douglas, an acknowledged expert in ethnic hair whose clients include Iman, to share his know-how

There are two main groups of ethnic hair, according to Errol: Afro-Caribbean, the curly group, and the rest who have straight hair – that's mainly women from India, the Arab countries, Japan, China and the Pacific Rim. First thing to take on board, he says, is that "Afro-Caribbean hair is expensive to maintain, full stop". Here we explain some common problems with Afro-Caribbean hair, and Errol's suggested solutions.

Problem Scalp deterioration and breakage

A healthy scalp is vital for healthy hair, and one of the main problems for this group is caused by straighteners (AKA relaxers). To straighten virgin hair, you have to use very strong chemicals, which may trigger an adverse skin reaction (temporary with any luck, but sometimes long-term) in the scalp or cause breakage of the hair. Home straighteners are a common culprit. They can cause a lot of damage if not used properly, and then you have to go to a salon to get it corrected, which takes time and money. Even if you don't use chemicals, breakage is common in Afro-Caribbean hair, because even though it looks strong, it's usually intrinsically weak as it is invariably dry by nature. That's why you have to compensate by using the right products.

Solution Be warned: this may take two to six

months. You should follow a cleansing regimen to clear the scalp of debris together with an intense protein treatment to rebuild damaged hair. If that doesn't work satisfactorily, go on to an intensive moisture program.

Errol, who's a great believer in alternative medicine, also recommends homeopathic arnica (available from pharmacies and health food stores) plus aloe vera. This traditional remedy for skin problems comes in a gel form which he applies directly to damaged skin. You can grow the spiky plant in a pot and simply break off a leaf and spread the gooey pulp on affected areas. You can also buy aloe vera preparations to take internally.

Problem Dry, breaking hair

This is often due to overuse of hot appliances, such as tongs and straightening irons, or overexposure to sun, salt and chlorine.

Solution Give your hair a break from appliances for

at least 10 days (a month is better). Blow-dry instead of using tongs and irons; apply a good serum or oil-based sheen spray, then hold the drier 12 inches away. Apply conditioner and steam hair to help the moisture hydrate the hair.

Errol recommends feeding your hair – through your mouth. Take a good basic multivitamin and mineral supplement, plus essential fatty acids, in the form of evening primrose oil, borage or starflower oil, linseed, flax or hemp oil and eat plenty of oily fish (trout, salmon, mackerel, sardines, herrings). Also take a specific hair supplement or any supplement designed to help skin and nails (hair is made of the same protein, keratin).

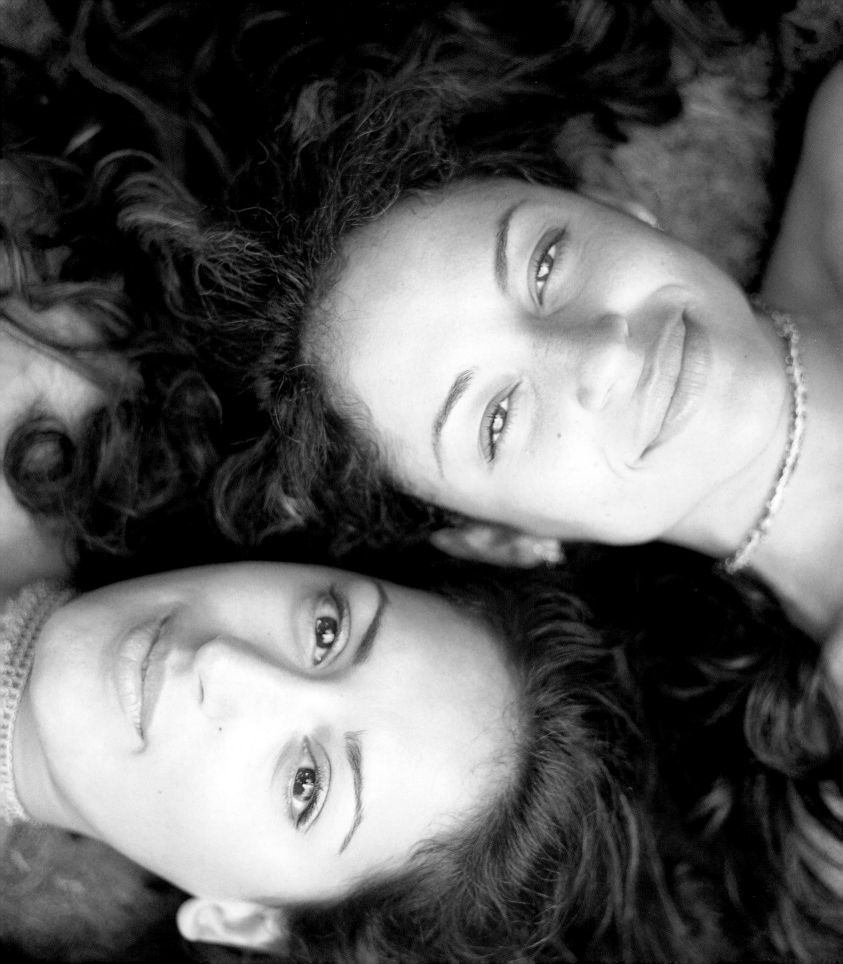

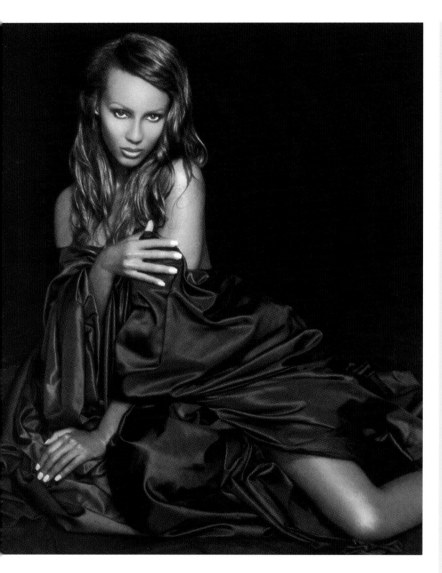

STRAIGHT ETHNIC HAIR

Problem Oiliness/excess oil

Solution Use a good oil-free shampoo. Don't use heavy conditioners – choose an oil-free spray conditioner, if you wish. When washing, use tepid to cool water, not hot, because that will cause the sebaceous glands to produce more oil. Cool is great, cold water is even better.

HOME STRAIGHTENING

Straightening Afro Hair is "A Very Delicate Process!" says Errol. It's best carried out by a specialist, but if you want to use a DIY kit, here's his advice:

✳ Check first with your doctor if you are on any medication: these are very strong chemicals and they may interfere with drugs

✳ Don't use any chemical-based product if you have a damaged scalp or any open wounds or sores

✳ Buy a reputable brand; ask your hairdresser to recommend one or buy through the salon; the only product Errol recommends is PhytoSpecific Beauty Phytorelaxer by Phytologie. (For salon treatments, he prefers Affirm or Artefex.)

✳ Always do a strand test – and that means every time

✳ Follow the instructions to the letter and the timing to the minute

✳ Always rinse off the product very thoroughly

✳ Don't wash your hair for at least 48 hours, preferably 10 days, before using a straightener – the scalp will be too tender

✳ Don't use a straightener after working out: your (sweaty) scalp will be covered with excess sebum and will have a fit if you apply a straightener/relaxer

✳ Don't irritate your scalp by combing or brushing your hair before straightening

✳ Don't straighten your hair, then decide you want waves and give it a curly perm (your hair will break under the strain of the chemicals) OR have it braided or woven for at least 14 days

Stay away from any oily products, such as waxes or hot oils. When you're having a body massage or aromatherapy treatment, keep the oils away from the scalp. Keep away from greasy foods and too much dairy; eat fish instead.

Problem "My hair won't keep a curl..."

Solution This could be due to oiliness and/or not using the right products. Culturally, many people with this type of hair are used to putting oil on it. This can result in making the hair look "dead" and impossible to style because of oil buildup. Use a good clarifying shampoo which will lift the oil, or something quite astringent like a color lifting shampoo; or try a pre-wash shampoo, designed to take out all debris before coloring which works well for oiliness too.

Problem "My hair is colored but it looks wrong...."

Solution The most common problem is going too light in color. You can go up one to two shades, but never five, six or seven, because it will look artificial. Dark skin and Caucasian colored hair never works. (This is the same for Afro-Caribbean hair too.)

USEFUL PRODUCTS AND TOOLS TO HAVE AT HOME

STRAIGHTER HAIR

PRODUCTS:
Oil-free and oil-removing shampoos
Setting gel or mousse
Intense conditioning treatment
Light-hold hairspray

TOOLS:
Blow-dryer with diffuser
Vent brush, paddle brush
Tongs, smooth and brush
Velcro rollers

AFRO-CARIBBEAN

PRODUCTS:
Oil or sheen spray, alcohol-free
Serum
Styling cream
Scalp-cleansing shampoo
Ultimate holding (but not drying) hair spray
Emergency treatments: protein and moisture
treatments to use every 10 days to 2 weeks; hot oil
treatment

TOOLS:
Blow-dryer
Hood dryer, or mesh hood attachment for blow-dryer
Tongs: smooth and brush
Straightening irons
Large wet-set rollers
Wide-tooth comb and round, bristle brushes
Vent brush

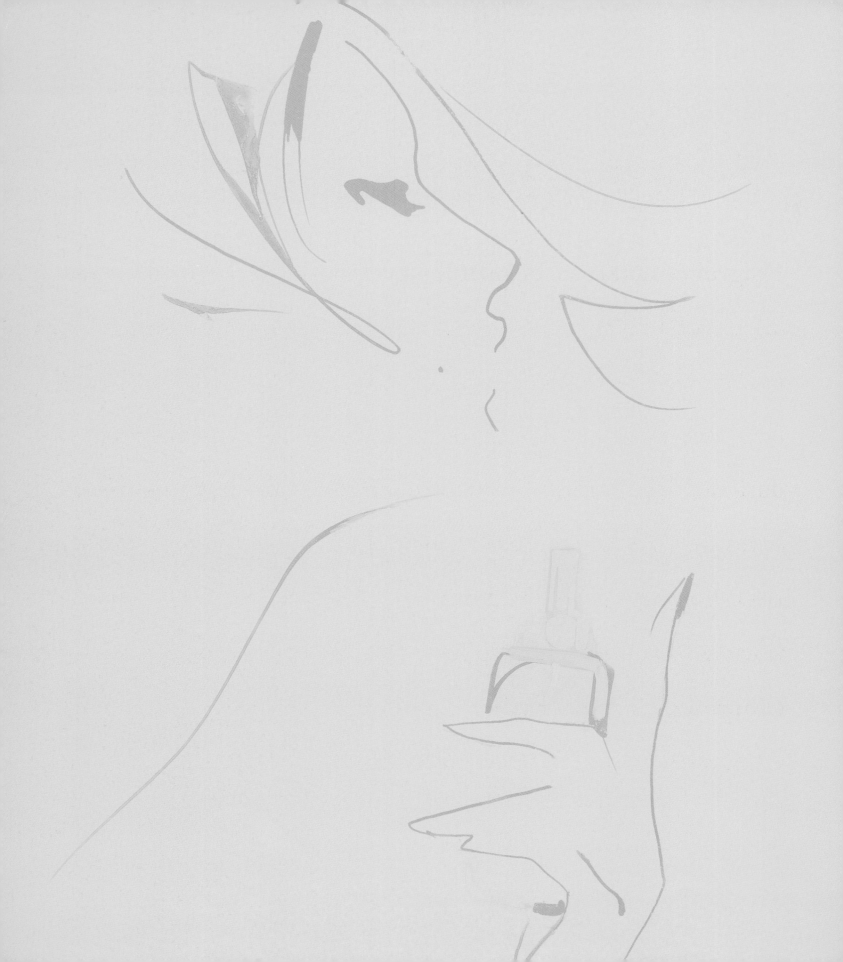

FRAGRANCE

Fragrance makes us beautiful – even in the dark. (And we're all for that.) But with hundreds of new scents launched each year, **finding our perfect perfume match** can be tricky. (And expensive.) Fragrance-speak seems designed to baffle. Floriental, chypre, aldehydic – who cares, as long as it smells good? Our advice: don't waste time boning up on the language of scent. Instead, follow these **short-cuts from the pros** to savvy scent-shopping, scent-wearing and how to get and give **maximum enjoyment** from your perfume.

MAKING SENSE OF SCENTS

*The search for a scent can be a head-throbbing safari through the wild aisles
of a department store. Or it can be a pleasurable voyage through the senses...*

Yes, we're all in a hurry. But choosing a new fragrance over a five-minute lunch-hour is a recipe for disaster. Setting aside some time to shop for fragrance will actually save you time – and money – in the long run, because you won't end up with a dressing table cluttered with expensive mistakes. Here are the secrets of a successful scent-shopping expedition...

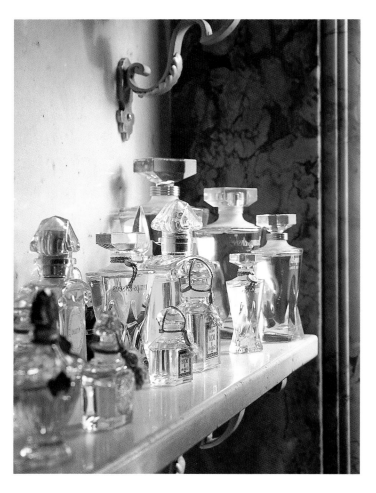

✳ Don't eat spicy foods or garlic the night before; they can alter the nature of a scent on your skin.

✳ Do wear clothing that's been recently washed; fragrance clings to clothes and influences what you're smelling, and traces of scent/scents you already wear will be detectable on sweaters, wool jackets or anything made of silk, in particular. Dress the way you'd dress to wear the type of scent you're looking for. (See advice, right, on shopping for a sexy scent.) Don't wear any scent, or even perfumed deodorant; they can clash with what you're sampling.

✳ Shop in the morning when your nose is fresh and the department stores are blissfully empty. Never rush scent-shopping. Do it at your leisure, just as if you were buying a new dress, a book or music.

✳ Those scented strips down the side of glossy magazine scent advertisements aren't a true guide to what a fragrance smells like – but they can tell you whether you hate a fragrance or like it enough to try it in real life.

✳ Never, ever buy a scent because you like the ad, or because it smells great on your best friend; a fragrance smells subtly (or sometimes dramatically) different on everyone. But do pay attention to details like the bottle, the name or the color of the liquid; if these turn you off, you probably won't be turned on by the scent itself.

✳ Smell a maximum of four scents, preferably in the same family – floral, oriental, chypre, and green. If you're confused about the language (almost everyone is) ask the fragrance consultant to help you. Tell them which scent/s you already wear; others in the same family are more likely to be a "hit". Don't be scared to tap into the wisdom of sales consultants, but don't ever feel pressured to make a decision if they're breathing down your neck .

✳ Be aware that in department stores, most consultants only recommend scents created by the company they work for. So you may want to head for a general perfumery, where consultants can recommend from a wider range.

✳ Don't instantly start spritzing your skin; ask at the counter for special absorbent "scent blotters" if they're not on display. Spray scents onto blotters to establish which appeal to you at first whiff. The trick when sniffing these is to wobble the blotter under your nose; hold it at one end between thumb and middle finger, and tap it lightly with your index finger to make it vibrate.

✳ Once you've narrowed your choice down to one or two scents, try them on your skin. (Top "nose" Anne Gottlieb prefers the crook of the arm to the wrist area, as even jewellery can distort a fragrance's smell.) Don't rub wrists together after spritzing them; friction alters the fragrance.

✳ Give the fragrance at least an hour to develop. Where most of us go wrong is choosing on the basis of the first fleeting burst of a scent (the top note), or the middle (which unfurls after about 10 to 15 minutes). In fact, it's the base notes (which may not develop for an hour or two) that you'll ultimately live with.

✳ If you're still in love with a scent after this, go back another day and spray the scent all over. Says *professeur de parfums* Roja Dove, "It's the difference between wearing the dress and just looking at it on the hanger."

✳ Better yet, ask for a sample, if available, and wear it for a few days. Get feedback from friends and loved ones, if that's important to you. Then, and only then – when you're truly happy – hand over that credit card.

HOW TO SHOP FOR A SEXY SCENT

Since the dawn of time, scent has attracted us to other human beings – and them to us. Today, the reason many of us wear fragrance is to seduce. (Even if we don't quite admit it!) So if you want a come-hither scent which really performs, you might want to plan a sexy-scent strategy, using our tips, left. We asked Roja Dove – creator of couture scents for an élite international clientele – to advise on shopping for a seductive fragrance.

✳ "It's no good shopping for a seductive scent when you're in 'work mode'. If you dress more like a femme fatale, the fragrance consultants will see you differently – and suggest sexier scents. Maybe try fragrance shopping one evening, setting aside an hour before a date or special event. Buying fragrance in a rush is one reason so many expensive mistakes are made."

✳ "The most seductive fragrances are base-note-heavy, featuring lots of vanilla, animal notes like musk, incense and amber, and woods like sandalwood. You'll find many of the most seductive scents in the 'oriental' family. You don't need to be an expert on this; just ask a consultant."

✳ And once you've bought your sexy scent? "To turbo-charge a fragrance's seductive power, don't put it behind your ears," says Roja. "The spot above the collar-bone is better – your partner will smell it when he whispers in your ear – and around the navel is a hot spot, too. Remember, scent rises – so try a dab behind knees and ankles." (We like putting it in our cleavage too.)

✳ We asked Roja for his top seductive fragrances in the world, and the answer came back: Guerlain Shalimar, Guerlain Mitsouko, Yves Saint Laurent Opium and Le Must de Cartier. "They positively smolder," he says. (And make what you will of the fact that two of these are found on our vanity tables, see page 210.)

THINK BEFORE YOU SPRAY

Look at a moisturizer label and you can see all the ingredients listed – which is useful if you know you're sensitive to a specific ingredient, or would like to avoid it for any other reason. Fragrance labels, however, don't reveal what's in the bottle

Mostly, what's in that bottle is alcohol – the "carrier". But infused into the eau de cologne or parfum are as many as 200 different elements in a single scent, and it's impossible to find out what these are. The perfumers' argument against labelling is that if they listed the ingredients, they'd leave themselves wide open to imitators, which would have disastrous financial repercussions.

Personally, we'd like to push for fuller disclosure. About 95 per cent of scent ingredients are now produced synthetically, and some of them have health "question marks" over them. A few are even potential carcinogens, according to research organizations such as the American National Toxicology Program.

We may spray them on our skin but these chemicals travel, too: researchers from the Norwegian Institute for Air Research found detectable levels of synthetic musk compounds in indoor – and even outdoor – air. Synthetic musks have been found to accumulate in the fatty tissue of fish, bringing about biological changes and even ending up in the food chain. Other research has detected buildup of these musk

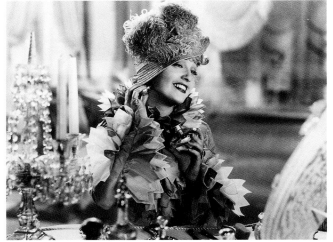

compounds in human fat, milk, and blood. The simple truth is, nobody knows what the longterm effect of that might be on our health, let alone on the environment. (And that's just musk!)

We're certainly not suggesting that you forego perfume – it's one of life's great pleasures. But the world is now so incredibly over-fragranced that we feel it's taking away some of the pleasure of perfume itself. So rather than give up our daily spritz of fragrance, we'd suggest cutting down on exposure to other forms of scent which are infinitely less sensual, and (in our opinion), entirely unncessary.

Everything, these days, seems to be scented – from facial tissues to fabric conditioner to those hangy-dangly things that swing from taxi rear-view mirrors (which have us cranking down the window to breathe fresher air). We're even encouraged to deodorize our carpets with a "masking" aroma when we vacuum. Only time will tell what breathing in this heady cocktail of chemicals does to human health. But if you care – as we do – about minimizing your exposure to synthetic fragrances, here's our advice...

✳ Many cleaning products are now highly scented. We often experience a dry, tickling sensation in the back of the throat when exposed to them. We could write an entire book about "green" housekeeping (maybe we will, one day!) but meanwhile, recommend the Ecover range of household cleaners, which feature gentle and natural scents (if any). Anyone who was turned off these "eco-cleaners" when they first came on the market might want to give them another go; in our opinion they are now as effective as any others you can buy, and much gentler for anyone with sensitive skin. (And they are not just less polluting to your personal environment, but to water and air generally.) For more tips on "green cleaning", we recommend *Natural Superwoman* by Rosamond Richardson and *Household Wisdom* by Stephanie Donaldson (see Bookshelf).

✳ In place of highly fragranced fabric conditioner, add 3 drops of lavender essential oil to an eggcupful of white wine vinegar. Softens – and scents – like magic.

✳ Do you really need a can of air freshener, or one of those plug-in gizmos that waft supposedly springlike scents through the house? We prefer to open windows whenever possible (but then we do have Nordic genes) and – to banish heavy-duty stuffiness – use a zoosh of Neal's Yard Remedies Spritzers, in either Calm, Renew or Zest. Infused with Australian Bush Flower Essences and essential oils (some certified organic), they're entirely natural. What's more, they can be spritzed on face and body – as well as the room and bed linens – and we're fans of any product that does triple-duty like this.

✳ Fresh scented flowers – especially lilies and hyacinths – help disguise mustiness or nasty household smells.

✳ If you're worried about the risk of allergy to fragrance, or of fragrance ingredients entering your system through your skin, you can still enjoy the sensual pleasures of scent. Fabrics "hold" fragrance beautifully.

spritz a favorite scent onto the lining or inner hem of your clothes; as body temperature rises, so will the fragrance. (Don't spray the outside of clothes unless your perfume is completely colorless, or you risk staining.)

✳ Just before you spray on a favorite perfume, breathe in, then spritz and hold your breath for a few moments so that you're not inhaling that initial "burst", when it's at its most eyewateringly potent.

✳ If, like us, you're a fan of scented candles, you might want to give a little thought to what you're breathing in from these, too. Try to choose candles made from natural waxes, even hemp, rather than paraffin, which is a non-renewable resource – and the fumes of which may potentially have a negative health impact. (Fumes from paraffin wax have been found to cause kidney and bladder tumors in lab animals – although we want to add here that we're firmly against this kind of animal testing.) It may also be wise to avoid lead wicks, opting for cotton instead. Tests show that lead "volatilizes" (i.e. is absorbed into the air), during candle burning – and there is no safe level for lead exposure.

✳ If you like to burn aromatherapy candles, be sure they contain natural essential oils rather than synthetic fragrance ingredients. (If in doubt, call or write to the manufacturer before buying; the number/address – or website – should be on the box.)

✳ Although many classic fragrance houses – especially the French – go on about the percentage of "natural ingredients" in their perfumes, be aware that most now incorporate a high level of synthetic ingredients. We say: follow your nose. Once you cut down on the number of other synthetic scents in your whole environment, we believe you'll be increasingly drawn to "real", natural scents rather than chemical confections. (See overleaf for how to make your own natural fragrances.)

BECOME A FRAGRANCE ALCHEMIST

There's one sure way to enjoy sublime, sensual scents that are 100 percent natural, and that's to create your own. We asked aromatic "alchemist" Ixchel Susan Leigh – who creates custom scents for women in the USA and UK to share her secrets

There's a big buzz in the beauty world about "custom fragrance": the creation of unique, signature scents that reflect your personality and lifestyle – and which you won't smell on a half-dozen people at the same party. (Which can easily happen with a fragrance classic like Chanel No. 5.) However, having a fragrance created especially for you by a legendary perfume house like Creed, Creative Scentualization's Sara Horowitz or independent "nose" Lyn Harris, who all offer the service, is a true luxury – and priced like one. But we asked Ixchel Susan Leigh – who creates one-of-a-kind aromatherapy scents for clients at The Hale Clinic in London and in America – to explain her art for you here so that you too can start to become a "nose", able to create your own personalized fragrance blends using natural essential oils.

Ixchel wants to encourage us "to play", she says. So experiment. But to get you started, she has come up with some simple scents that at least "echo" some of the world's great classic bestsellers. "Classic perfumes can't be totally duplicated only using true essential oils," she explains, "because contemporary scents are based mainly on synthetic chemical ingredients – hundreds of them. But what you lose in the scent by avoiding synthetics, you gain many times in benefits with essential oils. Using true essential oils to create your chosen fragrance will promote your wellbeing on many levels – emotional, physical and spiritual." The following recipes are wonderful starting points for fragrances, and as you become your own "nose", you can create individual scents that you love. (And you'll certainly never smell those on a stranger at a party...)

We list sources for essential oils in the Directory, page 246 – but if there are any you can't get a hold of, don't let that prevent you from enjoying "playtime". Before you start, meanwhile, you should understand how to blend...

Because very few essential oils can be applied directly to the skin, you need to dilute them in a base oil. "Blend the oils, then add $\frac{7}{10}$ fl. oz. of apricot oil, or $\frac{2}{5}$ fl. oz. apricot oil and $\frac{2}{5}$ fl. oz. of 100° proof alcohol, and put them into a pretty glass bottle," advises Ixchel. "You will then have a rich fragrance, reminiscent of the first perfumes created thousands of years ago. These were full-bodied, oily fragrances which scented the skin, and in

Using true essential oils to create your chosen fragrance will promote your wellbeing – emotional, physical and spiritual

addition they added a softness and sheen allowing the skin to glisten." You'll find that they develop on the skin as the day wears on – and because they're oil-based (rather than alcohol, which evaporates almost instantly), they are surprisingly long-lasting. Just as in "real" perfumery, incidentally, they all have a rose-and-jasmine heart.

Most essential oils come in bottles with a "dropper" top, making it easy to add them drop by drop to the recipe. Some can be stubborn, though; in that case, stand the bottle in a mug with some very hot water in the bottom, give it a few minutes – and the oil should flow smoothly.

RECIPES

If you like rich, floral, sensual and opulent scents like Chanel No. 5, Arpège by Lanvin, Hermès Calèche or Caron Infini...

Top notes in these fragrances include: lemon, neroli, bergamot
Heart notes: rose, ylang-ylang, jasmine, ho leaf
Base notes: oakmoss, vetiver, cedarwood, patchouli, balsam, sandalwood

For a fragrance that evokes these opulent scents, blend:

4 drops rose	2 drops ylang-ylang
2 drops jasmine	1 drop bergamot
1 drop balsam of Peru	1 drop neroli

If you like ultra-feminine floral scents like YSL Paris, Giorgio Beverly Hills, Anne Klein or Diane von Furstenburg's Tatiana...

The top notes in these scents include: galbanum, bergamot, lavender, lemon, mandarin, neroli
Middle notes: geranium, linden blossom, jasmine, rose, ylang-ylang
Base notes: sandalwood, benzoin, oakmoss, cedarwood vanilla.

To create your blend, mix...

5 drops rose	4 drops mandarin
2 drops jasmine	2 drops benzoin
1 drop sandalwood	1 drop vanilla

If you like fresh floral/green scents like Chanel No. 19, Prescriptives Calyx, Ralph Lauren's Safari...

The top notes in these scents include: galbanum, bergamot, lavender, lemon, mandarin, neroli
Middle notes: geranium, linden blossom, jasmine, rose, ylang-ylang
Base notes: sandalwood, benzoin, oakmoss, cedarwood vanilla

4 drops rose	2 drops jasmine
3 drops mandarin	1 drop ylang-ylang
1 drop sandalwood	1 drop vanilla
1 drop geranium	

If you like seductive Oriental scents (perfect for making grand entrances), like YSL Opium, Calvin Klein Obsession, Estée Lauder Youth Dew and Guerlain Shalimar...

Top notes in these fragrances include: palmarosa, bay leaf, coriander, black pepper, green pepper, mandarin, lemon, orange
Heart notes: cinnamon, cassia, clove, ylang-ylang, rose, jasmine, tagetes
Base: sandalwood, vetiver, myrrh, labdanum (cistus), benzoin, patchouli, vanilla, frankincense

2 drops ylang-ylang	2 drops vanilla
2 drops rose	2 drops jasmine
2 drops balsam of Peru	1 drop patchouli

If you like to enchant with 'floriental' fragrances like Dolce & Gabbana Woman, Chloé Narcisse, Bijan, Van Cleef & Arpels or Chopard Cašmir...

Top notes in these fragrances include: petitgrain, mandarin, basil, bergamot, orange, ylang-ylang, neroli
Heart notes: geranium, rose, orange blossom, calendula, jasmine, cardamom, coriander
Base: sandalwood, vanilla, patchouli, oakmoss, cedarwood

3 drops jasmine	2 drops rose
2 drops patchouli	1 drop geranium
1 drop sandalwood	1 drop neroli

THE AROMA ZONE

Aromatherapy oils have the power to invigorate, relax, revive. (On a bad day, we rely on them to restore our sanity.) Opposite, find Tried & Tested uplifting bath treats – which get their power from essential oils. But here are some blends to make yourself, at home...

BEAUTIFUL BATH BLENDS

We're grateful to Aromatherapy Associates for these very simple blends, which make enough for one bath. Use a teaspoon over a bowl (to prevent spills). Drop the essential oils into the teaspoon and top up with almond or sunflower oil. Swish the teaspoon and bowl in a bath full of water and swish again, with your hands, to ensure dispersion of the oil over the surface before you get into the bath.

De-stressing bath
5 drops lavender essential oil

2 drops chamomile

2 drops clary sage

Re-balancing
5 drops geranium

3 drops petitgrain

2 drops rosewood

Wake-up before going out
5 drops sandalwood

3 drops sweet orange

1 drop ginger

Another leading aromatherapist, Michelle Roques O'Neill, gave us these recipes for other mood-alterers. They're slightly more complicated, but equally heavenly, and are made up in slightly larger quantities, so keep in a bottle.

Uplifting
1 fl. oz. light coconut oil

10 drops tangerine

5 drops ylang-ylang

5 drops fennel

3 drops sandalwood

Relaxing
1 fl. oz. light coconut oil

5 drops chamomile

3 drops elemi

3 drops petitgrain

2 drops vetivert

For the office
Aromatherapy Associates recommends using frankincense oil, on a diffuser, or a couple of drops sprinkled onto a tissue and inhaled, when you feel under pressure. Works like magic!

OILS WE LOVE

Jo
I swear by Aromatherapy Associates' bath oils, which seem to go much farther than anyone else's, filling my whole (rather rambling) house with scent. Deep Relax (which did very well in our Tried & Tested, opposite) knocks me out like a sleeping pill, while De-Stress is perfect for un-frazzling. If I need to feel up-and-at-'em for a party, Revive is truly a miracle-worker. I'm also a big fan of blends from Liz Earle and Michelle Roques O'Neill (who shares recipes with us here, to make at home).

Sarah
I have a cupboard full of essential oils which I scatter in my bath: jasmine, rose, lavender, neroli, sandalwood and basil are my favorites, with vetiver if I'm feeling down. I seldom follow any recipes, just sniff and choose what I feel like that night. I love being given bath oils as presents and like the same brands as Jo: Liz Earle's and Aromatherapy Associates. I adore scented candles, too, most of all Tubereuse and Jasmine, both by Diptyque.

RELAXING BATH TREATS – *Tried & Tested*

As with all the products in this book, we scanned the ingredients labels of these waft-you-to-paradise bath potions and as green beauty junkies ourselves, we're delighted that two of the four top products – both oils – are totally natural. The other two contain lots of botanicals plus chemical detergents to create foam and how our testers loved them…!

❀❀ REN MOROCCAN ROSE OTTO BATH OIL

9.27 marks out of 10

A very high mark for a heavenly scented bath oil from one of our own favorite brands. Containing 100 percent pure plant oils and natural fragrance, this should be very soothing for dry or sensitive skins as well as helping relieve stress.

UPSIDE: "This product is heaven: if there are ten products to try before you die, this is one!" • "when I feel low, I smell the bottle and that alone lifts me" • "smelt like my grandmother's rose garden, divine, romantic, old-fashioned" • "my skin was left feeling soft and I felt very relaxed after" • "from being tired and wound up I felt relaxed and completely rejuvenated" • "this definitely improved my sleep" •

DOWNSIDE: "For such a lovely product, the bottle lets it down".

❀❀ I COLONIALI RELAXING BATH CREAM WITH BAMBOO EXTRACT

8.44 marks out of 10

This Orient-inspired foaming cream came in a very respectable second, with testers loving the silky product but worried about having a glass jar in a slippery bathroom.

UPSIDE: "A lovely product, smelt fantastic, even my boyfriend stole some" • "slight foaming – water felt like silk, and skin soft

after" • "loved this smell, very unusual, like incense" • "used it up very quickly, always a good sign" • "one of the best bath products ever – so relaxing and luxurious"

DOWNSIDE: "Smell a bit masculine and synthetic".

L'OCCITANE LAVENDER HARVEST FOAMING BATH

8.4 marks out of 10

The higher the altitude the crop is grown at, the finer the fragrance, they say – and this comes from over 800 metres above sea level. Although it contains a chemical detergent, it worked well for one eczema sufferer.

UPSIDE: "The smell lingered on my skin, which made me drift off to sleep" • "boyfriend with eczema found it non-irritating so Gold Star!" • "non-drying and non-oily so I can wash my hair in it" • "skin felt lovely and soft after" • "quite definitely a mood treatment".

DOWNSIDE: "I have dry skin and wanted more moisturizing".

PHYTOMER BODY RELAX RELAXING BATH CRYSTALS

8.19 marks out of 10

Reminiscent of old-fashioned bath salts, these lilac purple crystals (the color is said to promote serenity, wellbeing and spiritual awareness…) combine extracts of aromatic seashore plants – lavender, cistus and helichrysum. The blurb says they help soak away the cares of the day and ease knotted muscles. Now read what our testers say…

UPSIDE: "I found this product so-so at first but after using it a couple of times I fell in love with it – a real treat!" • "felt natural and smelt gorgeous, slightly marine-like but not overpowering" • "beforehand I felt stressed and in need of a treat, during the bath I felt in heaven – afterwards I felt very relaxed, balanced and in control" • "I had just about the

nicest dream I've ever had after".

DOWNSIDE: "Not fragrant enough and drying to the skin" • "synthetic smell, almost like furniture polish!".

The lowest score in this category was 5.27 marks out of 10.

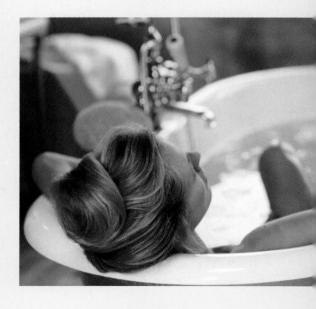

WHAT WE WEAR

A beauty editor's job can be very spoiling. In the last ten years, we got to try most of the new fragrances that have been launched. Most disappear from the market without a trace. (In some cases, that's a blessing.) But here's what we come back to, time after time

JO

Mitsouko, by Guerlain. I can't walk past a Guerlain counter without veiling myself in this. It's warm, intimate, but not overpowering. Everyone I know who discovers it loves Mitsouko. Definitely a winter scent; it's like wrapping yourself in velvet.

Shalimar, by Guerlain. For grown-ups only, this is sweet, sexy and not for the shy and retiring. An after-dark scent rather than something I'd wear to work.

So Pretty de Cartier. The name says it all: light, sophisticated, elegant.

In Love Again, by Yves Saint Laurent. This incredibly pretty, hints-of-the-fruitbowl scent was a limited edition – and I stockpiled it. (Many scents are now available for a short period only, so if you can't imagine life without a particular limited-edition scent, better do the same.) I also stockpiled a limited-edition Guerlain scent called Belle Epoque – and I'm still loving its lilacy summeriness.

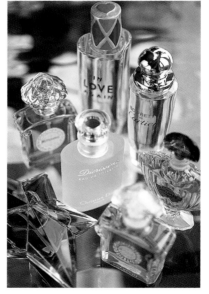

I've had two fragrances created for me from essential oils by Ixchel Susan Leigh – who you can read more about on page 206 – which are bliss to wear and entirely natural; one's warm and Oriental, the other like walking under a linden tree. I love them. They're designed to enhance meditation – but I wear them as I would a regular fragrance.

SARAH

Shalimar, by Guerlain. My top favorite – a warm, spicy, exotic caress of a scent and the greatest Oriental with a vanilla iris base. Unlike Jo, I do wear it all the time, from morning to night, summer and winter, town and country. (I think my horse likes it too.) It is a grown-up scent but then again, so am I.

Mitsouko, by Guerlain. I wore this continuously for many years and still love its delicious peachy charms. A scent for daytime when I'm in a slightly more worky mode but still want to feel feminine.

Diorissimo, by Dior. This was my beloved friend Madge Garland's favorite, with lily of the valley, jasmine and sandalwood, and I love it, too. It says summer, wildflowers, hats, floaty dresses, and garden parties – and of course Madge herself (my adopted grandmother, Fashion Editor of British *Vogue* before World War II).

Angel, by Thierry Mugler. My wild card, with a fruit-salad heart, a chocolaty caramel base, and a devil-may-care swagger about it. For wild parties, definitely never to work.

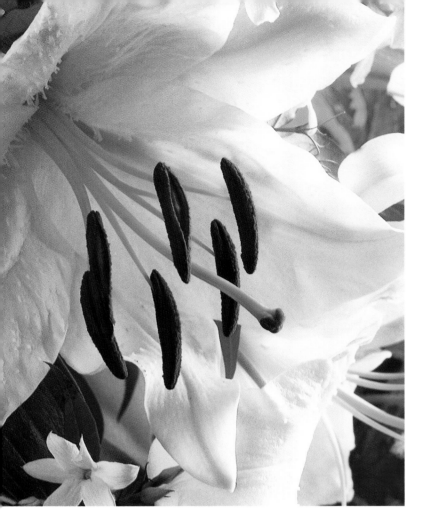

Sara Horowitz, founder of California-based Creative Scentualization, is a self-taught "nose" who leads men and women on what she calls 90-minute "fragrance journeys", creating one of-a-kind fragrances for them. "Today, we often go through the day barely aware of what we're smelling, except perhaps for the moment we spritz on a perfume," agrees Sara. And yet, she explains, it's easy to "train" your nose, bringing infinitely more pleasure to daily life, and improving the sense of taste, as well – because the two are intimately connected.

✳ "Get into the habit of tuning into the smells around you," advises Sara. "Don't just stop to smell the roses, but also the coffee machine, the cut grass. If you drive through a residential area at around 7pm, wind down your window and smell the restaurants and homes preparing dinner. Keep tuning in. When you go to a movie, notice the smell of the chocolate raisins or the popcorn."

✳ "Simply think about the odors of familiar things – bacon, coffee, roses, bananas – actively conjuring them up in your mind. This encourages awareness and actually improves your ability to smell real-life scents."

✳ "When you buy flowers for your bedside or your desk, make a point of choosing scented varieties, or you're missing out on one of life's great pleasures."

✳ "Keep a fragrance 'notebook'. Spray your fragrances onto perfume blotters (which you can usually get free at perfume counters). Sit down with a pen and sniff them, then write down what they remind you of: textures, places, people, memories. Or do the same with a collection of objects: a pencil box, a fresh apple, leaves. It sounds strange, but just this simple exercise can actually increase the distance from which you can first perceive a perfume that someone's wearing, a flower or any other scent.

HOW TO IMPROVE YOUR SENSE OF SMELL

Helen Keller, the author who was blind and deaf from infancy, called smell the "fallen angel" of our senses, because we neglect it so. Once upon a time, we relied on our sense of smell to warn us of impending danger – and steer us towards food. It led us to our mate, too, his pheromones mingling with the aroma of the mammoth pelt thrown over one shoulder. Today, our survival hardly ever depends on our sense of smell and food comes from the store; as a result, our noses have become lazy.

In fact, because we're assaulted by so many different smells – from drains to traffic fumes to high-octane perfumes – we unconsciously almost cut ourselves off from this vital sense to save ourselves from "sensory overload". Understandable – but it also means we may be missing out on a source of daily delight.

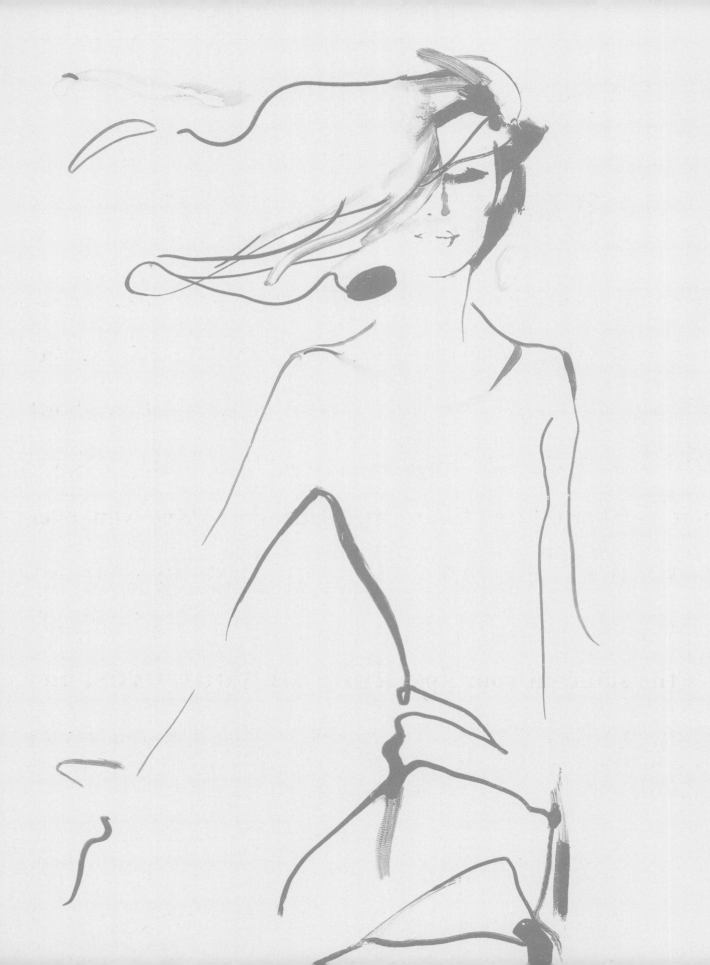

WELL BEING

We could scrutinize ourselves from top to toe and decide that nothing is 100 percent perfect. And we'd be right. But we'd also be missing the point. Beauty is as much about **mind, body, and spirit** – total well being, in fact – as it is about face, figure and features. Have you ever noticed that you can go out with grubby hair, no makeup but in a **good mood,** and people will respond? It's the smile on your lips, **light in your eyes,** and spring in your step that makes you lovely. And that comes from inside!

YOU ARE GORGEOUS AND LOVELY AND BEAUTIFUL

Every woman has days when she feels unattractive. Of course it's a great confidence booster to look your best – that's what this book is about. But put a pretty woman with an unhappy soul, no sense of humor, and no love for herself (or anyone else) next to a physically less attractive one who loves life – and guess who'll win the Beauty Stakes (un-manicured) hands down?

Writer and TV personality Rhonda Britten, author of the truly helpful bestseller *Fearless Living* (see Bookshelf, page 246) is convinced that everyone can discover her own unique beauty. "The real knock-out gotta-have-it beauty starts on the inside," says Rhonda. What's more, this soul beauty is totally within your control, it's free – and it actually gets better with age.

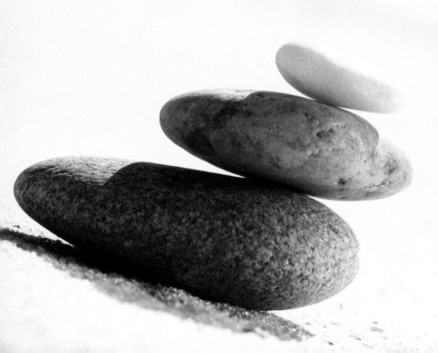

Here are Rhonda's suggestions for thinking yourself beautiful – truly, freely and forever!

✳ Think about what you mean with words like "beautiful", "pretty", "attractive" and "gorgeous". If you find that you're just thinking in physical terms, think again. Look at people you think are lovely, and you'll see that it's their expression, the light in their eyes, their manner to others that makes them beautiful. With that comes a general air of *joie de vivre* and feeling at ease with themselves which is irresitibly attractive.

✳ We invariably judge ourselves harshly. So it often helps to think of yourself as you would your best friend. Start looking at yourself in a new way: from your warm heart, not your critical brain. Wrap your arms around yourself and hug yourself. Tell yourself you're lovable, worthwhile, valuable – think of the things you like about yourself. Maybe you're funny, kind, laid-back, compassionate – whatever. Loving yourself is essential to thinking yourself beautiful.

✳ You are beautiful when you accept yourself fully. When you feel confident enough to take risks. When you see yourself and other people through the eyes of love rather than fear. The moment you are open-hearted and allow yourself to be vulnerable, then you are beautiful.

✳ So try accepting yourself as you are – with all your perceived imperfections. Yes, zits, cellulite, broken capillaries, and all. The mind-shift starts when you can muster up the courage to look past the negative self-talk and put yourself in a state that is colored by love, not fear.

✳ Look in the mirror and note one attractive thing about yourself – from long eyelashes to well-shaped nails, pretty ears to neat knees. You get the idea. Then do the same thing every day for a week, looking at a different feature. Whenever you feel low about yourself, run through the list.

✳ If it seems hard to get past the images in glossy magazines, just remember they are all about artifice. Sure, there's a woman underneath but she has been primped and preened and posed within an inch of her life – and then any imperfections have been airbrushed out of the finished picture. That's not real life.

✳ Take a risk or three. Truly beautiful people give all – in love, creativity, adventure. They aren't in it for the outcome but for the challenge of taking part in life, not teetering anxiously on the edge. What's the worst thing that can happen? You get a little bit hurt! But look at what you might gain.

✳ Don't be afraid to ask for help – but also know you don't have to seek permission for what you want to do, or get someone else's approval to know you are worthwhile.

✳ Practice seeing your own beauty. Then practice seeing others as beautiful in their different ways. Remember that we all feel we're not pretty enough, clever enough, nice enough, funny enough – and all the rest! The only thing that stands between us and knowing we're beautiful is fear. Fear spoils everyone's lives. So don't listen to it: live, love, laugh! And know that we are all beautiful in our own way.

TEN THINGS TO DO WHEN YOU WAKE UP FEELING YOU CAN'T COPE

Even if you're feeling really down in the dumps, remember that your state of mind can shift. There are always positive feelings lurking behind the negative – just as there is always blue sky behind the clouds.

1 Get up – even if it means falling out of bed and staggering to the kitchen.
2 Look out of the window – at sky, birds, trees, people – and remember you are not alone.
3 Stretch and breathe in slowly and deeply. If you're anxious or angry, imagine pushing the negative feelings out as you exhale.
4 Eat and drink. Fix yourself a fresh juice, if possible. You must have a proper breakfast, too.
5 Think of someone you love and who loves you. Feel that warmth and give it out to others during the day.
6 Make yourself look the best you possibly can – hair, makeup, clothes.
7 Give yourself a hug. And smile!
8 Decide you will have the best day possible.
9 Write a list of the things you have to do. Prioritize. Only try and do what is necessary and what you can.
10 Give yourself – and others – a little treat during the day: flowers, a walk at lunchtime, a movie in the evening, good food – whatever makes you feel good.

TIP: Don't despair if you feel aimless and wonder what on earth life is all about. Everyone feels like that, some of the time. The key, says Paulo Coelho, author of the best-selling *The Alchemist*, is simply to live your life with enthusiasm. "Then you connect with the soul of the world."

How to be Happy

We can all be happier if we decide to, according to stress management expert Dr. Richard Carlson, author of the best-selling "Don't Sweat the Small Stuff" series, who helped us with this section. And being happy is being beautiful!

Happiness is, quite simply, feeling nice: a mixture of contentment and wisdom laced with bright shining joy. When we are happy, we feel gratitude (even when life seems tough), inner peace, satisfaction, and affection for ourselves and others. Although retail therapy may certainly help raise your spirits (temporarily), lasting happiness is not dependent on money or material things. It is a feeling of being at peace with yourself and being able to take pleasure in small things: a dotty joke, looking at a dog bounding in the park or a beautiful plant, the smile on the face of a child, help from a stranger, getting a good cup of coffee.

Happiness is available to anyone at any time – completely free – because it is inside you. You can never find happiness by searching because that implies it comes from outside yourself. All you need to do is choose happiness – not chase it.

Some people are cynical about this simple approach: "Pollyanna-ish"; "Unrealistic"; "Life is tough"; "Don't

TIP: When you want something with all your heart, says the alchemist in the book of the same name by Paulo Coelho, all the universe conspires in helping you achieve it.

TIP: If you have to see someone you don't like or who threatens you in some way, imagine you are wrapping yourself in a wide cylinder of gold or silver, which will act as a shield, keeping you safe and protected.

look for happiness and you won't be disappointed," they say. Sad, we say. In the grand scheme of things, we are here on this Earth for a millisecond: the tiniest blip on a radar screen. Life is a gift and the idea that people want to spend that time being cynical and criticizing others seems a shame.

We're not saying that life isn't tough. Like everyone, we have been through hard times – deaths, money worries, family problems, love affairs gone wrong – all the stuff we all experience. But in our middle age, we know that life is about the way you live it. Look for the worst and you will get it. Look for the gift in everything and you will find it. Be kind to others and to yourself, as the Dalai Lama suggests, and you will find joy.

You can experience happiness in the most seemingly sad circumstances, depending on how you look at things. One woman told us that although she wept buckets at the death of her mother, she also felt happy because her mother was released from pain and because she, the daughter, felt such love and support around her.

The way to be happy is pretty much the same for everyone because psychologically we're all wired the same way. We all think, we all have moods and we all have feelings. We are, too, all unique individuals. However much we love and empathize with others, we cannot think their thoughts or feel their feelings. We can't live another person's life and we are not ultimately responsible for their state of mind. But we can appreciate and understand the similarities and the differences – and how we all connect.

Some may find the path tougher than others because of personality, biochemistry or circumstance but, in

Dr. Carlson's experience, everyone has the potential to feel better. Of course things can be hard – sometimes very hard – but finding this innate mind-health allows us to be more easygoing, whatever we have to cope with.

Setting out to be happy doesn't mean you have to learn a new technique or do something special. Of course that may help, but simply exercising, say, or meditating won't in itself make you happy. If it did, everyone who exercised or meditated would be bursting with joy. Neither is changing your circumstances – job, home, partner – the complete answer. The mindset that feels we must do things differently in order to be happy won't go away when that change has taken place. It will just start all over again, looking for flaws – and conditions that must be met. "I will be happy when …"; "If only I had done this or so-and-so hadn't done that"; "If I could just get rid of that." You know the internal conversations we all have. You may decide to make changes – we both prefer living in the country, for instance – but it's a mistake to believe that your happiness is entirely contingent on someone or something. (Remember: wherever you go, you're there.)

Happiness is working out your own take on life, the universe and everything. Getting happy is a question of learning to access the place inside yourself where serenity already exists – and has never gone away. You don't have to create it. Just connect with it. Then you can stop trying to *do* happy and simply *be* happy.

Each one of us is powerful, creative, and brilliant, and life can be a great adventure. But when you're anxious, stressed, and unhappy, you fret about things that don't really matter – sweating the small stuff – and you can't fulfill your own potential. If you want to stay like that, fine! You'll always be able to convince yourself that there is absolutely no way you can change; anyone would be the same with the stuff you have to put up with!

But if you're open-minded to the possibility of being happier, you can start right now. It's amazingly simple. Follow the Golden Rules on the next pages to begin to find your own happiness.

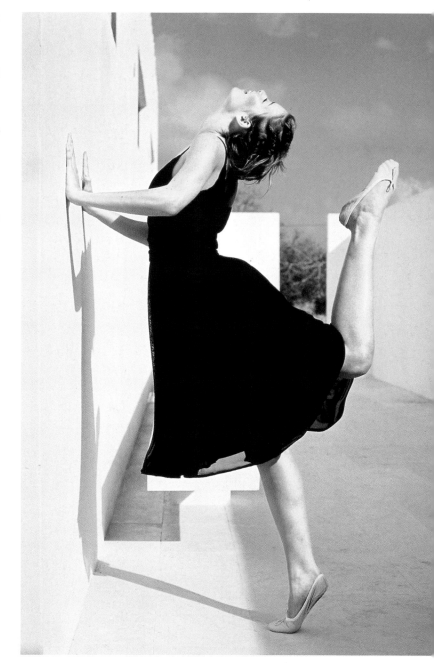

GOLDEN RULES

Life is what we make of it. Have you ever wondered why some people who suffer great misfortunes can look peaceful? Whereas others with great material wealth are miserable and stressed? Here are Richard Carlson's guidelines for living well

Live in the present: many people spend much of their lives focusing on the past or the future, regretting what's gone and worrying about what's to come. And remember that the word resentment literally means re-feeling. When you find yourself thinking like this: simply bring your attention back to the millisecond in which you are living right **NOW**... Your body and mind will unite, and that alone brings an instant feeling of peace.

Think happy: your happiness levels may seem to go up and down with circumstances but, in reality, it's your thoughts – not your circumstances – that dictate how you feel. We produce our thoughts, not the outside world, and the way we *think* about someone or something totally influences how we *feel*. If you think you'll like someone, you probably will. Think optimistically about getting a job or recovering from an illness and, research shows, you *feel* better. Tell yourself that you'll have a happy day and you will – even if there is a mountain of problems in your path. Recognize negative thoughts but don't let them overwhelm your life. Just look for another way of seeing things – of changing your thought patterns. You might be feeling low one day and think "I'll never finish this project". If this "thought attack" goes on, it may spiral out of control and you'll probably give up – or, at least, waste time worrying. Start thinking "maybe I can do it" (or better still "I *can* do it") and you stand a good chance.

Trust your feelings: feelings come after thoughts, so they are a sure barometer of your thinking. Low feelings come from unhealthy thinking, happy feelings from healthy thoughts. One of the most common reasons for distorted thinking is getting caught up in conditioned thought patterns that seem to be necessary for us to live in the reality of this world: "Must have this" thoughts; "Must teach him/her/them a lesson"; "It's all her/his/their fault"; "Can't be seen doing this," and so on. When we feel bad, it's our warning system kicking in, telling us that we're thinking

SOLVING PROBLEMS

There is almost no obstacle that can't be overcome. It's a question of how you approach it. Problems are generated more by the way we feel than by the circumstances. First things first – don't live in the problem, live in the solution. Focusing on problems is a bad habit. We become accustomed to thinking and talking and living with "what's wrong". If we think about solutions, we start thinking positively. When you're facing a sticky situation of any kind – from a relationship to a broken-down car – figure out what would make you feel better. Emotional problems are usually much harder than practical ones – but very often they overlap and there is an emotional component in many practical problems and their solutions. (For instance, you have a leaky pipe, the plumber comes quickly and is nice, and you feel better.) Get the facts and face them. Then if you can't find a solution – or decide which option is best – take a creative stance. Put the issue on the back burner of your mind – for five minutes, five hours, five days – but determine that you will find the solution. Then, rather than racking your brain for the answer, forget it. Virtually every time, a wise course of action will pop into your mind, like magic!

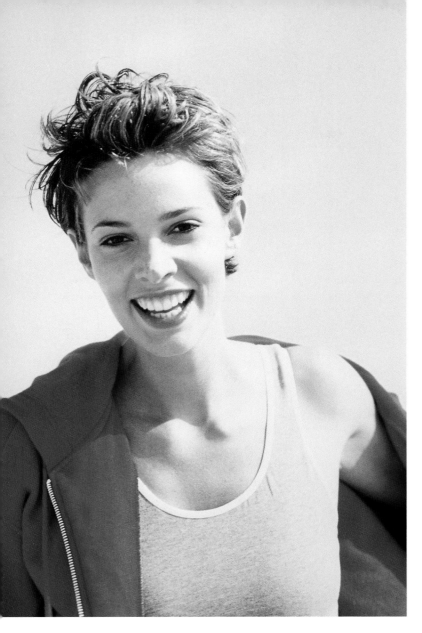

lifts and everything's just fine! When you're feeling "up", life looks good, you have perspective, relationships flow, communication is easy. In a low mood, life seems hard, people seem out to get you, you take things personally. Most people have their most serious discussions when their mood is low, and that is one of the core problems in relationships. So when you're in a bad mood, don't react or make decisions until the mood passes.

Change yourself, not others: most of us spend a lot of time fighting to make other people think as we do – rather than acknowledging that they can only think the way they do. Accept that everyone is an individual and that we can't change others – only ourselves – and life will become more peaceful. Each one of us sees life from our own separate reality. And it's futile trying to change someone else's thinking pattern. That doesn't mean you should always accept other people's negative behavior: if you see someone hitting their child or bullying their staff, you don't stand by and watch. Also, if people's behavior towards you is unacceptable, don't be a doormat – but don't expect them to understand why you are reacting that way. If you can truly accept that other people have their own point of view – which you can try to respect as much as you want them to respect yours – life will become much less of an effort and much happier.

in a dysfunctional way. Fresh ideas come from a fresh mind, so take a five-minute break (longer if you can). Go for a walk, or look out the window, and let your mind roam in the space between thoughts. No thoughts means no problems. Then you can go back and rethink the issue.

Understand your moods: up, down, up, down – our moods swing like a see-saw. For some people, these shifts are slight; for others, extreme. Moods can vary for all sorts of reasons including hormones, tiredness, even the weather. Just when it seems as though life is going smoothly, wham! Our mood level drops and everything seems rocky again. Or just when everything seems hopeless, our mood

TIP: "One thing I know for certain," says writer Hilary Boyd, author of *Banishing the Blues* (see Bookshelf, page 246), "when things are difficult, you must stick with the people who love you."

TIP: Connect with other people – and animals – from your heart first, head second. Be open and straightforward and truthful. Always appreciate what others do and feel. They need what you need – love.

CHECKLIST FOR LIVING

*If you're feeling miserable, go through the following questions and answers,
suggests Dr. Richard Carlson – it may help you to feel better*

Is my life really all that bad right now, or am I simply in a low mood?

It's easy to forget that even the nicest people have mood swings. When we're feeling low, the best thing to do is to take our mind off whatever it's stuck on and wait for the mood to pass. Then life (and everything in it) will look quite different.

Am I reacting to someone else's low mood?

Moods are a fact of life. If we remember that, we won't take attacks on ourselves personally because we'll know they are not directed at us. In low moods, people will say and do things that they wouldn't dream of otherwise. This doesn't mean we need to accept abuse but that, rather than getting upset, we should make allowances in our minds and hearts for the psychological fact of moods.

Am I being negative?

Saying, or thinking, negative things is not the road to happiness. Thoughts that take us away from a positive feeling are not worth having – or defending. If you want to be happy, follow your happy, contented, joyous, worthwhile feelings – not your unhappy ones.

Do I want to be right more than I want to be happy?

Are your opinions more important than your happiness? When we take our opinions so seriously that they make us unhappy, we should rethink them. It's possible to have strong beliefs and be relaxed – in fact, you'll find that other people will respect your beliefs more that way.

Am I playing out a war in my head?

Most arguments take place in our minds before they get played out in words with other people. When thoughts that make us feel bad come into our heads, the trick is to remember that we make our own thoughts. We can change how we think and end the mental war by focusing on more generous feelings.

Am I too stressed?

Being stressed is not constructive. When we're anxious, we tend to work even harder. But no matter how much urgency we put into something, it won't reduce stress. If we ease up, take a break and clear out our minds, we feel better. The goal is to learn to catch stress early and snuff it out before it overwhelms us.

Am I rating myself too much?

Constantly keeping score of yourself – either for personality or performance – lowers your spirits and is exhausting. Small children are naturally proud of their efforts. As we grow older and start to doubt ourselves, we lose that innate sense of self-worth. Stop assessing and start enjoying! Live every moment to its fullest and your life will work itself out.

Am I postponing happiness?

It's been said that life is what happens to you while you're busy making other plans. If you find yourself saying "I will be happy when ...", you're missing out. Happiness is not contingent on the outcome of something else. You can be happy right here, right now – if you choose to be.

LIFE BRIGHTENERS

✳ Block off time for your next vacation – even if you spend it puttering around at home.

✳ Clean up! Doing the dishes makes 94 percent of people feel more upbeat and positive.

✳ Play your favorite music.

✳ List your ten favorite things to do: and make plans to do at least one this week.

✳ Dance your cares away – research shows it's the most enjoyable activity, closely followed by amateur theater.

✳ Take a day off (or less, or more) and do what you really want to do – not what you feel you have to do.

✳ Create a "Happy Box": file nice letters, cards, invitations and other keepsakes to rifle through on down days.

✳ Watch your favorite video. (Sarah's is the recent version of *The Thomas Crown Affair* and Jo's – which she's slightly embarrassed about – *The Sound of Music*, mostly because it reminds her of watching it about 73 times with a much-loved goddaughter, who was obsessed with it between the ages of five and six.)

✳ Do your hair, fix your makeup, put on your fave clothes and have fun! – even if you just twirl around in front of the mirror then go out for a walk on your own.

✳ Phone a long-lost friend (and don't gripe…).

✳ Expand your senses: lie in a field or park, smell the flowers, listen to the birds, feel the breeze, take in the blueness of the sky!

✳ Get artistic: take a large piece of paper and whatever coloring materials you like – paints, crayons, colored paper, etc. Divide the paper into your past, present and future; fill in the sections (they can overlap) with images, symbols, colors, lines! Add stickers or write on whatever you want. Create your life.

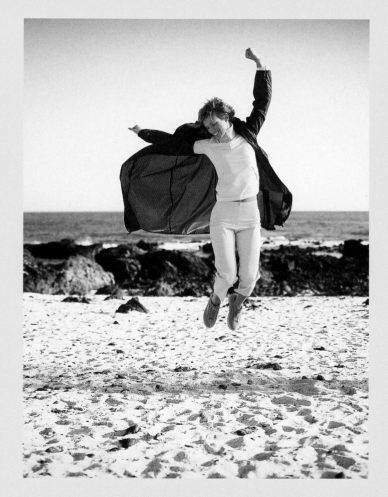

MEDITATION FOR THE VERY, VERY BUSY

Most of us like the idea of meditation. (And its benefits on our well being are now widely acknowledged.) The problem is, many of us also feel we don't have the time to fit this de-stresser into our very stressful lives. So here's the ultimate shortcut

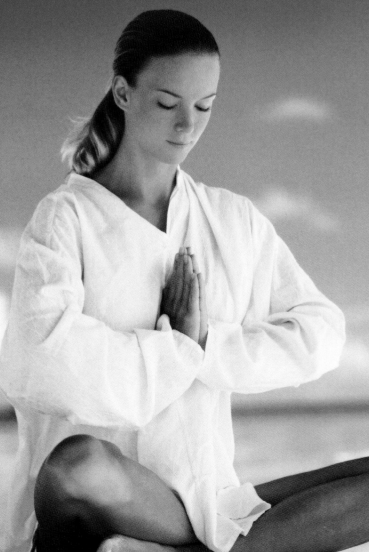

When you're whizzing from place to place, rushing to get everything done in time, it's not just your feet that do the hurrying. Your mind is on permanent red alert, plotting, planning, and fretting in its vain attempt to beat the clock. Psychologist Professor Cary Cooper christened this condition "Worry Hurry Sickness" and it affects many of us nowadays.

The all-pervading tension that Worry Hurry Sickness causes in your mind and body can be the root of many chronic physical problems, including headaches, neck ache, and back pain. Your busy mind can also work you up to such a pitch of anxiety that you can't sleep, creating a vicious cycle. This in turn leads to many more illnesses because lack of sleep suppresses your immune system – the body's policeman which keeps out invaders such as bacteria and viruses (see page 230).

Beautywise, Worry Hurry Sickness affects your looks profoundly. Instead of shining with health, stressed-out people tend to look strained and pinched. Skin is pale and dry, prone to frown lines and wrinkles, eyes dull, shoulders hunched, body tense – in readiness for yet more assault and battery. But there is a simple way to improve the situation and that is meditation.

You can use the techniques of meditation without devoting long periods of time each day to reap the benefits. The key is simply to still your everyday mind, according to Robyn Welch, an intuitive medical diagnostic and author of *Conversations With The Body* (see Bookshelf, page 246). That's the part of you that feels like a chattering tape that goes around and around on an endless loop until you think you might be going CRAZY!

All you need do is award yourself short, frequent breaks in which you allow your mind to take a break from the stresses and strains. The Brahma Kumaris, an Indian spiritual group, call it "traffic control": think of how you feel in traffic jams or when driving too fast on the highway... Then picture yourself sitting peacefully in a country lane, looking at a beautiful view. That's the state you are going to create in your mind.

Start with sixty seconds twice a day. Once you've become accustomed to slipping instantly into this peaceful state, you will find that you can do it whenever you wish. Presto! you're out of the turmoil and in a lovely serene state that recharges you and lets you carry on much more efficiently. It may seem terribly simple – and it is – but it has real physical benefits, including lowering blood pressure. Switching off your mind allows your body and your brain to relax and work more smoothly. And it's an instant beautifier.

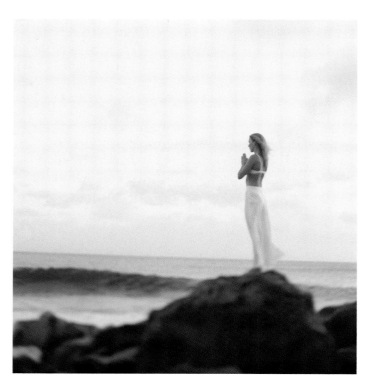

60-SECOND RELAXATION

You can, of course, practice this simple technique for longer than sixty seconds, but you can get real benefits instantly even in that short a time. What's more, it costs nothing and you can do it anytime, anywhere.

Sit or lie comfortably, with your feet and hands uncrossed. If you are in a chair, relax but don't slouch – keep your head and shoulders relaxed, spine straight.

Close your eyes and focus on the middle of your forehead. Breathe in slowly through your nose to a count of three, hold your breath for another three counts, then exhale very slowly, pushing the breath out as loudly and forcibly as possible. Puff your cheeks out and really blow! Repeat three times.

If you are doing this in a crowded place – where you don't want to sound like a noisy exhaust – breathe in and out through your nose (unless you have a cold), inhaling for a count of three, holding for three, and exhaling for six.

Now visualize a bright color – blue, yellow, orange, pink, gold, silver, or whatever is your favorite – and let it spread through your body. Breathe calmly.

If your everyday mind intrudes, jabbering on about the shopping/laundry/call you have to make, just ask it gently but firmly to wait for a minute. Visualize it standing to one side so that you are free to stay in this calm light state as long as you choose to. Remember—you control your mind, not the other way around.

If you like, you can put a dab of lavender essential oil under your nostrils or on your wrists, or burn a scented candle. The Brahma Kumaris play peaceful music during "traffic control".

GETTING YOUR BEAUTY SLEEP

When you've slept well, you wake up, deliciously refreshed, and leap out of bed eager to get going. You have energy for the whole day and evening. And, crucially, you look FANTASTIC! (Whereas missing out on sleep can age you a decade overnight!)

Nature gave us some fabulous beautifiers, absolutely free. We firmly believe that sleep is one of the greatest, together with breathing, drinking lots of water, and fresh air. If you sleep like a baby every night, turn the page. But if you're one of the millions of women who tosses and turns, or never feels rested no matter how much sleep you've had, read on.

According to Dr. Mosaraf Ali, the world-renowned doctor of integrated medicine who cares for the Prince of Wales and Camilla Parker Bowles, nature programmed us to sleep well. "Insomnia is a poor sleeping habit triggered by stressful events," he says.

Difficulties sleeping are one of the major problems in medicine today. Taking pills is not the answer because our brains adapt to them and their effectiveness decreases so you have to take more. To help overcome insomnia, you need to approach it methodically. Retraining your mind and body to be at peace is vital for a good night's sleep.

There are four main symptoms of insomnia:

Difficulty falling asleep

Frequent waking at night

Early morning waking, between 3 and 4a.m.

Persistent sleepiness despite adequate sleep

If you suffer from insomnia, try these simple and effective solutions which Dr. Ali suggests to his patients:

✳ Avoid coffee at any time and alcohol at night.

✳ Avoid eating or drinking any food/drink that may cause acid, gas or wind, such as spicy foods, cold milk, fizzy drinks, mushrooms, canned products, yeast products, food containing MSG, or citrus fruits.

✳ Avoid sweet desserts or hot sugary drinks at night; the sugar agitates the brain. But don't go to bed hungry.

✳ Eat your evening meal early and make it light; afterwards take a calming 10-minute stroll.

✳ Don't smoke; nicotine can irritate the brain.

✳ Drink some water before sleep and keep a glass by your bedside. When you are dehydrated, your pulse rate goes up, leading to the anxiety that plagues so many people. If you wake up feeling anxious, sip some water.

✳ Have a firm, comfortable bed with one or two soft, downy pillows to support your neck. Try not to sleep on your stomach because it tends to give you neck ache.

✳ Rid your room of electronic gadgets (computers, stereos and TVs) which may emit harmful radiation. Bedrooms are for resting, sleeping and making love.

✳ Aim to be in bed by 10p.m. at least twice a week.

✳ Wind down before bed: avoid late-night discussions or exciting films and try making love early in the morning instead of at night.

✳ If you sleep with a partner, swap five- or ten-minute neck and shoulder massages to relieve physical and mental stress; use essential oils of lavender and chamomile (six drops of each in two tablespoons of apricot seed or peach kernel base oil). Or give yourself a gentle neck and shoulder massage with the same oils.

✳ Keep your bedroom quiet: ban ticking clocks and, if the street is noisy, keep the windows closed and/or wear earplugs (the spongy kind are the best).

✳ Soothing music like chants often helps blot out other noise and allows you to slip off to sleep easily.

✳ If your partner snores, wear earplugs.

✳ Don't have a hot bath before bed; this dilates the blood vessels, stimulating mind and body.

✳ Don't sleep with too many blankets; too warm a temperature may dehydrate you. Keep the bedroom around 68–72°F.

✳ If your partner hogs the bed, consider having separate blankets and, if possible, mattresses.

✳ Ensure there's enough oxygen for the night by opening the window or door.

✳ If you are worried about something, visualize yourself putting the problem in a file, placing the file in a drawer and locking it away until the morning.

✳ Keep a pad and paper by your bed to write down brilliant ideas or nagging problems.

✳ Practice a simple relaxation or meditation exercise in bed (such as the one on page 220).

✳ Acupuncture and homeopathy can help reduce stress; consider sessions with a qualified practitioner if you are going through a difficult time. Other helpful complementary therapies include reflexology and massage, with or without aromatherapeutic oils.

✳ Avoid tight-fitting clothes in bed; wear a loose nightgown or nothing except your favorite scent (very Marilyn Monroe).

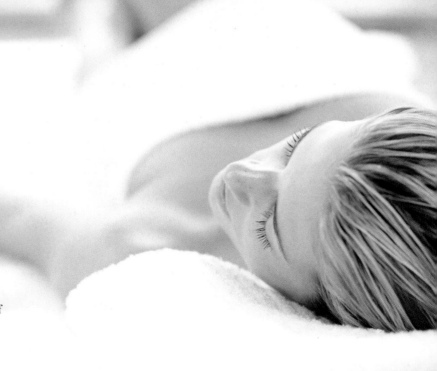

DIY MASSAGE

*Having a professional massage is wonderful, and one of our favorite treats.
But you can also do a great deal to ease your own aches and pains and keep
your whole body supple. These simple techniques were explained to us by
Dr. Mosaraf Ali, a doctor of integrated medicine in London*

Self-massage can be done anywhere and at any time.
Use a little bit of oil if you have some available, suggests
Dr Ali, but you can do it perfectly well without (wisest
when you're wearing your glad rags). If you have a
particularly painful spot, try using white Tiger Balm,
which is a miracle worker. We find these movements are
body – and mind – savers, especially when we're sitting at
our desks for hours, or driving long distances. They're also
marvelously restorative when you're tired: you will soon
feel the fizz and ripple of energy running through your
body.

SELF NECK MASSAGE

Place your fingers on the back of your
neck, then massage the neck muscles
from the base of the skull and the
muscles just under your ear lobes
going down and around your
neck. Use your fingertips and
also the fleshy part of your
palm beneath your thumb.

SELF JAW MASSAGE

Massage the jaw muscles, which store a lot of stress.
Rotating your forefingers, gently massage the joint of the
jaw just in front of the earlobe. This is easy to find if you
open your mouth while pressing with your fingers.

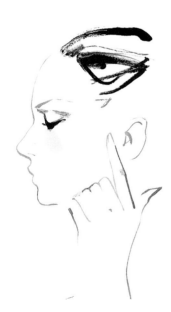

SELF TEMPLE MASSAGE

Gently massage your temples with your fingertips,
circling around and around.

SELF FINGER AND HAND MASSAGE

Massage the thumb and fingers by squeezing and pulling gently with your other hand. Press into your palms with your thumb. Pay particular attention to the fleshy areas below your thumb and little finger. You can use the same technique on your feet.

ARM EXERCISE

Intertwine your fingers, squeeze and let go; this releases the muscles in your forearm.

INNER-ARM SELF MASSAGE

Squeeze all along the length of the inner forearm, using the opposite hand.

SHOULDER SELF MASSAGE

Squeeze and massage the shoulders from the upper part all the way down, by squeezing with your other hand.

SELF ARM MASSAGE

Squeeze all the way up and down the arm, using the whole of your other hand: there is a huge amount of tension here, particularly in computer users and drivers. We also find that the same movement, using both hands this time, is good for legs.

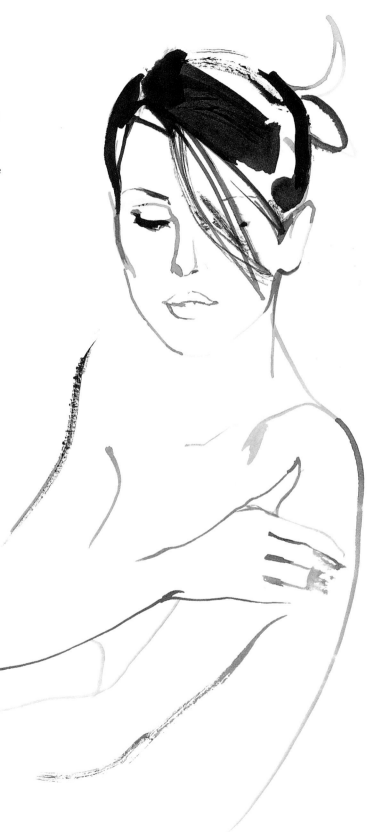

HELPFUL HERBS

In olden times, we probably would have been burned at the stake: our windowsills (and gardens) are packed with herbs and other useful plants that can replace many modern medicines. So here, for your inner witch, is some herbal wisdom...

You'll often find us brewing up plant potions for minor ills – because Nature really does have the answer in many cases. Pharmaceutical products are totally unnecessary for many nagging, occasional woes. Your kitchen cupboard – or your garden – can be your pharmacy.

Outside our back doors are pots of spiky aloe vera plants, mint, rosemary, thyme, feverfew and sage. When we can't grow the herbs, we buy organic versions – and if you're not gardening-minded, all of these are readily available at natural food stores – fresh, dried, as tablets or capsules, or in a tincture.

Here's a list of our favorite plant healers, which we've compiled with lots of help from naturopaths Sarah Bowles Flannery and Kerrin Booth from Apotheke 20-20 in West London (the Jurlique spa), and herbalist Andrew Chevallier, past President of the National Institute of Medical Herbalists. These are designed to help with minor conditions. If you have a chronic cold, cough or flu, consult a qualified naturopath or herbalist – they will mix a medicine for your individual symptoms. Nature has a fantastic range of plants with antibacterial and antiviral properties (unlike the pharmaceutical industry, which can't really treat viruses).

Chamomile: whenever you need relaxing.

Peppermint: to help digestion after meals and soothe achy stomachs anytime; also for headaches, and to refresh and stimulate your brain. Oil of Peppermint capsules by Obbekjaers (see Directory, page 246) are excellent to carry with you for stomach cramps; some Irritable Bowel Syndrome sufferers swear by them.

Rosemary: for sore throats and to sharpen your mind and improve memory. ("There's rosemary, that's for remembrance," as Ophelia said in *Hamlet*.)

Sage: calming for mind and body; you can also rub fresh leaves onto bites or stings; helps many women with menopausal symptoms.

Ginger: for all digestive problems including constipation. Grate a 1–2 inch lump of peeled fresh ginger and cover with boiling water; keep adding fresh water – it gets stronger as the ginger cooks.

HERBAL TEAS

These are simplicity itself to make. Simply gather a handful of leaves, tear them up and put them in a pot. Cover with boiling water and leave to infuse for five minutes or more. You can also use dried herbs: the ratio is about two to one, fresh to dried. Try one soupspoonful of dried herbs for a medium to large pot, or one teaspoonful for a cup.

TIP: Always choose organic products if possible. If you grow your own, plant herbs in organic compost and fertilize with a good general organic fertilizer, such as seaweed, during the growing season. If insects are devouring your plants, try covering them with a light mesh tent, propped on garden stakes.

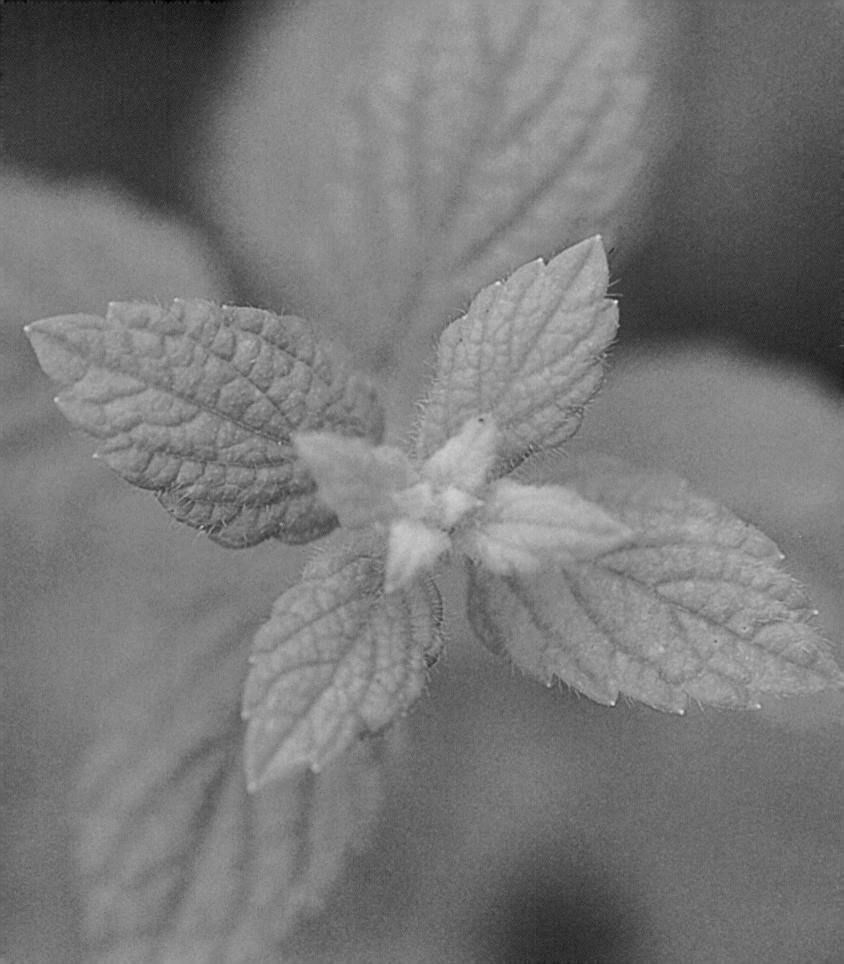

SKIN AND DIGESTION

Aloe vera: grow your own and squeeze the clear, pulpy goo inside the leaves directly onto skin, or buy in gel or tablet form. Can be taken internally (in which case we advise store-bought rather than homegrown). Used on your skin, it's the most wonderful soother and healer for any problem from psoriasis, eczema, and itching of any kind to sunburns, cuts, and bruises. Mix gel with whipped egg white to make a firming face mask. Taken internally, it cleanses your digestive system (and the effects show on your face). It's also a good nutritional supplement for energy and is one of the few natural sources of vitamin B12, which enables your body to absorb iron.

SKIN

Tea tree oil: don't drink this – it's for topical use only. Antibacterial and antiseptic – good for acne and blemishes of all kinds, athlete's foot, cuts, and scrapes. Has a mild painkilling effect which helps bring instant relief to burns and scalds, and prevents infection.

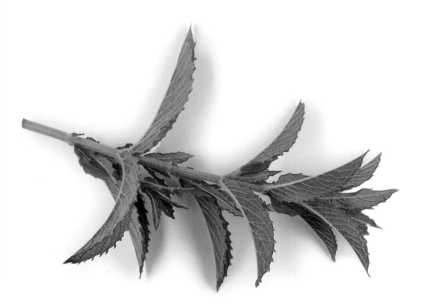

ATHLETE'S FOOT

Mix ½ fl. oz. of **marigold** (calendula) ointment with ½ tsp. of **turmeric** and rub between and under the toes each day. Also try tea tree oil (see opposite).

TIP: Treat a pus-filled boil or pimple by cutting a **garlic** clove in half and rubbing the cut side over the area twice a day.

HEADACHES, STINGS, SORES

Lavender oil: well-known for its soothing and calming effects; burn a little oil in a special room diffuser at night to help insomnia, irritability, or depression. Add 5 drops of essential oil to your bath to relieve muscle tension. For headaches and migraine, combine 20 drops with ⁷⁄₁₀ fl. oz. carrier (base) oil such as almond, peach kernel or grapeseed. Rub undiluted onto insect stings to relieve pain and inflammation (can also be used on head lice).

Feverfew: munching feverfew leaves has been shown to be at least as effective for migraine headaches as any modern medicine. Eat the leaves or buy a freeze-dried version to make tea. Take at the very first signs; if you wait till later you may need stronger concentrations of feverfew.

TO PREVENT COLDS & FLU

Echinacea: there are stacks of medical evidence to show that echinacea, the purple coneflower, is effective and safe. Take it when you feel you may be coming down with a virus – scratchy throat, slight buzzing in the head, ringing in the ears and a feeling that you're not quite "right". Take ¹⁄₁₂ fl. oz. of tincture twice a day for five days, or two 5g capsules three times daily for five days, before meals. Some people do use it preventively but it

appears to lose effectiveness with longterm use, so don't be tempted to take it for more than 6 to 8 weeks.

TO PREVENT HANGOVERS

Milk Thistle (silymarin): a detoxing herb that is especially good for helping protect your liver. Take the recommended dose before and after drinking a fair amount. It will help your liver to process the alcohol, reducing the likelihood of a hangover.

DEPRESSION

St John's Wort: shown in trials to be more effective and have fewer side effects than virtually any pharmaceutical drug for depression. We have personal experience of its effectiveness in family members and friends (including doctors). Buy it over the counter but do heed dosage instructions and any contraindications.

EMERGENCIES

Dr. Bach's Rescue Remedy or Jan de Vries Emergency Essence: these herbal-combinations come as a tincture or a cream. Keep them in your bag for panicky or stressed moments of all kinds – emotional, mental or physical. Give a few drops of the tincture to anyone, any age (including animals) and apply the cream to any wound.

Arnica: homeopathic must-have to steady the nerves and help reduce swelling and heal bruises. It comes in tablets or cream. Use tablets as directed as first-aid in emergencies. It is also useful for emotional crises and for improving sleep.

THE ULTIMATE DIET

"We are what we eat" is undeniably true – food is our best medicine. But what we eat is also reflected in how we look. Healthy people shine! They have clear skin, glossy hair and sparkling eyes with bright whites...

Over the last decade or so, there has been a constant avalanche of press touting the benefits – or risks – of various foods. Now, at last, there is consensus.

Doctors, nutritionists and researchers worldwide agree on the optimum nourishment to keep you gleaming with health all your life. It's crystal clear, say experts, that people who eat low-fat, high-nutrient diets – and exercise regularly – enjoy the best health and stand to live the longest.

Not only will it keep you glowing with health and energy but this wise way of eating will, unless you suffer from an illness or stuff yourself 24 hours a day, also allow you to reach your natural weight and stay there.

If you are having problems with your diet, or chronic conditions that your doctor can't relieve (or will only prescribe drugs for), we suggest you consult a qualified nutritionist or naturopath.

We are passionate supporters of organically produced food, because no artificial fertilizers, pesticides and herbicides are used in crop growing and no chemicals such as antibiotics are used in livestock farming.

We don't want to eat a cocktail of synthetic chemicals that we haven't asked for and that our bodies will have to use valuable energy to eliminate. And we wouldn't touch genetically engineered (also called genetically modified) foods, for similar reasons.

One more thing to bear in mind: every expert we've ever spoken to believes in a good breakfast, so don't skip this vital meal, which should contain some protein. It really will power you through the day.

FOODS TO FEAST ON

Fruit and vegetables: at least five servings every day, raw or cooked. Aim for the most intensely colored (dark green, orange, red) because they contain more vital nutrients, antioxidants in particular. If you can't get fresh seasonal produce, opt for frozen, but avoid canned because they may contain sugar, salt and other additives. Fruit is best as a snack or at the beginning rather than the end of meals, especially if you are prone to digestive problems such as bloating.

Nuts: contain proteins, minerals and "good" fats. Aim for five ounces of fresh nuts a week. Buy unshelled if possible and keep them in a cool dark place.

Seeds: since the entire growing life of plants is encapsulated in their seeds, they are chock-full of nutrients, including proteins and minerals. Try a daily snack of flaxseeds, pumpkin, sunflower and sesame seeds (good roasted in the oven), or toss them over salads.

Whole grains: look for whole grain versions of wheat, oats, barley, millet, rye, brown rice, quinoa, in which the nutrient-rich casings have been left intact, unlike refined flours which have been stripped of all their proteins and minerals. Whole grains, like fruit and vegetables, are also rich in complex carbohydrates for stamina and energy plus fiber that keeps your digestion healthy. Aim for 5 servings a week.

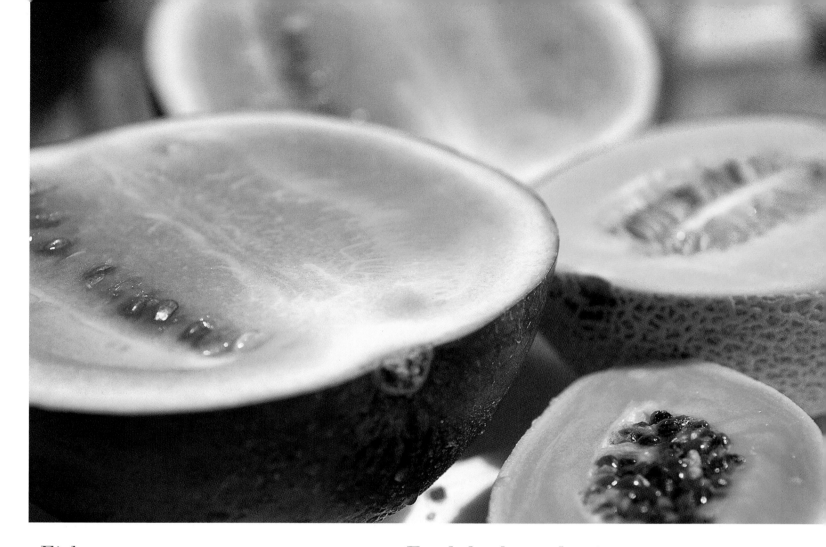

Fish: oily fish, such as salmon, trout, tuna, mackerel and sardines, are a wonderful source of protein as well as "good" Omega-3 fatty acids which are vital for many bodily functions and keep your skin, hair and nails in good condition. Eat at least 3 portions weekly.

Olive oil: Italian beauties swear by olive oil to keep their skin and hair lustrous. It contains "good" monounsaturated fats, so use it to dress salads and vegetables and to cook in, too. Sunflower (canola) oil also contains unsaturated fats.

Yogurt with live cultures: good source of protein which also contains beneficial bacteria that help your digestive system. Eat a cup every day.

Eggs: a perfect form of protein. Eat at least 4 a week.

Fresh herbs and spices: not only do they contain chemicals that are good for you, they add wonderful flavors to your food. Eat lots of them!

FOODS TO AVOID

Anything made with white flour and/or white sugar and/or containing additives (look at the labels)

Processed, ready-made, or canned foods

Conventional margarines: opt for organic margarines based on olive oil; or have a small amount of butter

Animal fat: if you crave red meat, eat small amounts (3oz) of wild game or grass-fed organic beef

Trans fatty acids, also called hydrogenated vegetable oils, which are found in many processed foods

Do You Need a Supplement?

If you are able to eat a good diet, based on the foods suggested on the previous pages and preferably organic, you only need minimal nutritional supplementation, according to Roderick Lane, an internationally respected naturopath and co-author of The Adam & Eve Diet

"It is relatively simple to get vitamins from your diet by eating lots of fruit and vegetables and juicing (see opposite), but more difficult to get enough minerals and Essential Fatty Acids. These are the most common deficiencies. Without enough of these, the vitamins cannot be used by the body," Lane explains.

To guard against potential deficiencies, he suggests that women of all ages from adolescence onwards take a good trace mineral supplement (make sure it contains selenium, chromium and molybdenum) and also a magnesium supplement. His preferred brands are BioCare or Solgar. "Take them at night and they will help you sleep soundly and wake up refreshed" he says. Lane also recommends taking a daily linseed (flaxseed) product such as Linseed 1000 formulated by BioCare, which provides Omega-3 and Omega-6, the two essential fatty acids that are most important for functioning of our bodies and minds.

Also, if you are leading a stressful life and find it difficult to guarantee you'll eat plenty of fresh, wholesome food throughout the day, you may wish to take a good multivitamin and mineral supplement such as BioCare's Femforte.

DETOX

We are firm fans of detoxing every so often, although some doctors and dieticians have fits about it. Others, such as London-based independent practitioner Dr. Susan Horsewood-Lee, see it as a wonderful way of giving your hardworking liver a bit of well-earned R&R, with the bonus of rejuvenating your looks. It sounds quite complicated but it's actually very simple.

You can do a complete detox by just drinking water and lemon for 24 hours, then go on to juices and herbal teas for one or two days, add in salads and fruits for three to five days, then easing your way back to ordinary meals. Or replace your evening meal with a juice, such as The Ultimate Juice (see page 236), every day for up to a week.

Critical for both plans is that you give up tea, coffee, alcohol, all processed or packaged foods, added sugar, citrus fruits, spicy foods and any yeast-containing products. What you do eat and drink should be organic, wherever possible, and you should drink 2½ to 4½ pints of natural mineral water daily.

If you choose to detox over a weekend, you could also unclutter your brain by leading the most peaceful life you can. Turn off the telephone. Don't watch agitating TV. Rest as much as possible. Do some gentle yoga stretches. Go for a little stroll. Have a steam bath, if possible. Treat yourself to a massage. And go to bed early.

CAUTION: If you have any health problems at all, please check with your doctor before fasting or detoxing.

GREAT JUICES

We love fresh fruit and vegetable juices. Chock-full of nutrients, they zing straight into your bloodstream, revitalizing body and brain, making you feel and look fantastic. Yes, they do take ten minutes or so to make but the benefits far outstrip the hassle factor

Some nutritionists recommend taking antioxidant supplements, which mainly contain vitamins A, C, and E. Roderick Lane prefers people to get their antioxidant fix from juicing fresh fruit and vegetables daily. "Antioxidants are vital for every layer of tissue in your body starting with your skin. When you drink fresh juice, you get a surge of concentrated natural antioxidants, plus other vital nutrients, straight into your bloodstream and it can work miracles. People who have been lackluster and pallid suddenly look sparkly and have loads of energy."

Amounts vary depending on your type of juicer so you will have to experiment. The good thing is that you can't go wrong: you simply end up with a bit more or less juice. Remember, when it comes to fresh juice, the more the better. You can get most of your daily needs in one batch of juice. Drink it first thing in the morning, or at any point during the day. It's more like soup than a cold drink so drink it slowly, but do knock it back as soon as you've made it: the nutrients begin to lose some of their goodness within a few minutes. (And that tells you just how infinitely superior homemade juices are to the ones you buy. Although they're definitely much better than no juice at all...)

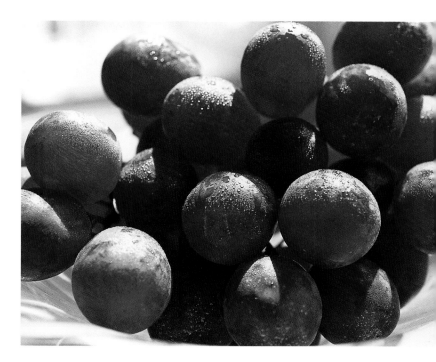

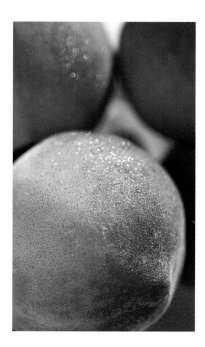

Buying from a juice bar is pretty expensive. So it's worth investing in a mid-priced sturdy juicer of your own. The actual process is time-consuming (maybe 10 minutes in all) but once you've experienced the snap-crackle-pop! effect of a regular morning juice, you will join the swelling ranks of born-again juicers.

Wash but don't peel fruit and veggies, unless they have tough skins like kiwi, pineapple or melon. Chop into pieces to fit the feed tube of your juicer.

There are masses of wonderful combinations, so experiment: you really can't go wrong – although some color combinations are more winning than others.

BE YOUR OWN JUICE BARTENDER

BASIC JUICE

About 4 medium apples, 4 carrots, topped and tailed, and a 1 inch chunk of peeled ginger

Add: celery, cucumber, beet, black/red grapes, blueberries, strawberries, pear, kiwi (peeled), pineapple (peeled), melon (peeled), sprigs of watercress, parsley

THE ULTIMATE JUICE

Naturopath Roderick Lane devised this vitamin-and-mineral-packed formula for The Adam & Eve Diet. You can drink it any time of the day – or night.

2 carrots
2 handfuls of sprouted beanshoots
4–6 celery stalks
½ small beet (cut off the top end)
Small handful of parsley or watercress
A handful of spinach or other dark green vegetable in season, e.g, chard, Savoy cabbage, broccoli
1 apple or pear
Fresh ginger, a hefty 1 inch peeled chunk

WHEATGRASS

It's the buzzword in nutritional circles but it sure tastes bad! So bad, in fact, that many people gag on it. (Not everyone, though; Jo really likes it!) It does have a kick, so if you want to get the benefits, drink it quickly before your juice so you can get rid of the taste.

YOGURT SMOOTHIES

You can whip up a smoothie in a jiffy by combining live (meaning it contains live bacteria: look for lactobacillus and bifidus), natural, lowfat yogurt with seasonal (or frozen) fruit. You can also use frozen yogurt (make sure it's unsweetened) or soy milk. Here are some of the combos we like:

Mango, lime, yogurt
Strawberry, banana, yogurt
Blueberry, raspberries (or other berries), yogurt
Melon, mango, yogurt
Peach, strawberry, yogurt

Add-ons for juices/smoothies: nuts and seeds, wheat germ, blue-green algae, ginseng, ginger, aloe juice

PINK GODDESS

Watermelons contain more antioxidants than any other fruit. Whipping up your own antioxidant cocktail is a breeze.

Cube the flesh of a quarter of a watermelon. Put in a blender until it is liquid. (The seeds may escape the blades but they taste delicious.)

Add: mint leaves for an extra tang, or dilute with mineral water to taste (about half and half works well) for a cooling summer drink.

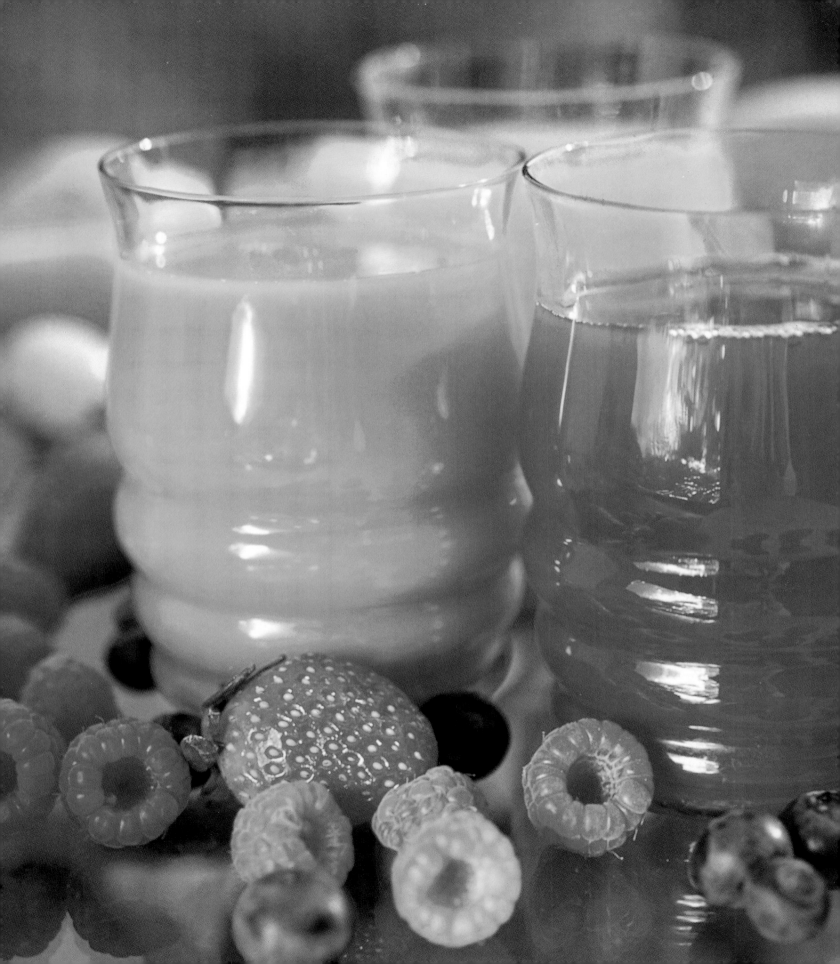

FAST TRACK

No time for a yoga class? Just a few minutes a day is all it takes for body-sleeking, to stretch your body, calm your mind and increase your energy levels (and peace of mind)...

We love yoga, the ancient exercise system from India that works out your mind as well as your body. You can do it anywhere you have space to stretch out and it is guaranteed to make you buzz with energy. It's also a great beautifier, sending oxygen around and ironing out kinks so that skin and eyes sparkle and your face is peaceful. It's said that women who do yoga never need face or neck lifts (quite a bonus).

For this workout, we asked yoga expert Barbara Currie to guide us through postures, or asanas, that are suitable for almost everyone (see warnings below). Try to do this short workout every day. If you're feeling low on energy and oomph, repeat it at any time. When you're in a hurry, even a couple of exercises will help.

Just a few warnings: yoga is for healthy people so check with your doctor before you start and **never ever strain yourself**. Do not do these exercises if you are (or may be) pregnant—there are instructors who specialize in pre- and postnatal yoga and pregnant women should consult them. You also need a specialist teacher if you have a bad back.

GUIDELINES

Always do yoga **slowly** and **gently**, in loose clothing and bare feet. Make sure you work on a non-skid mat or floor. Breathe through the nose slowly, deeply and rhythmically. As you inhale, let your tummy push out like a balloon. As you exhale, feel your chest collapsing into your backbone. When you are doing a posture, inhale at the start then exhale slowly as you move. Keep breathing all the time.

Don't let your knees lock or your shoulders rise. Keep your weight over your insteps.

POSTURES

UPWARD STRETCH, FORWARD AND BACKWARD BEND

Benefits: releases tension from the whole body; ensures a flexible spine; tones legs, especially backs of thighs; firms abdomen, midriff, waistline and throat

1 Stand straight, with your feet about 12 inches apart, toes facing front. Inhale, slowly lift your arms in the air and stretch, with your palms facing forwards.

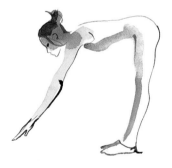

2 Exhale and bend down to the floor, keeping your back flat and legs straight. Go as far as you can and stay there breathing for a count of 5, increasing to 10 as you improve with practice. Don't worry if you can't go far down, and don't strain – you will become more flexible.

Eventually your chin will be on your shin!

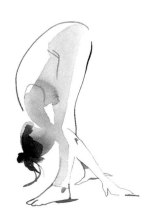

3 Now inhale and slowly lift your head. Raise your arms above your head again.

4 Looking up at your thumbs, exhale and gently relax backwards, but only as far as you can go. Again

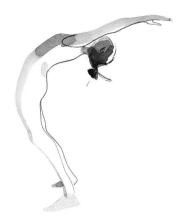

don't worry how far you get – even an inch is good. Just keep looking at your thumbs and relax. Hold that backward stretch for a count of 5, breathing in and out.

5 Inhale and slowly return to an upright position.

6 Exhale, lower your arms and relax. Repeat once.

3 Inhale, lift your head first, and return slowly to an upright stance. Then gently bend backwards, pulling your arms back down and under your bottom. Exhale, then count to 5, breathing normally.

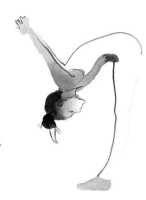

4 Inhale and return to upright. Hold your arms up behind your back for a count of 2. Lower them and relax. Repeat twice.

CHEST EXPANSION

Benefits: removes tension from neck and shoulders; stimulates blood flow to head and neck, helping to revive dull skin and hair; tones upper arms, backs of thighs and calves; frees chest and firms throat and jaw

1 Stand straight with your feet together or just a few inches apart. Interlock your hands behind your back, palms up. Gently pull your shoulders back and straighten your arms.

2 Inhaling, lift your arms as high as possible behind your back. Exhale and slowly bend forwards as far as you can, keeping your back flat and legs straight. Relax there, breathe normally and count to 5. The aim is to get your head to your knees – eventually.

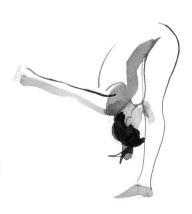

SIAMESE POSTURE

Benefits: keeps spine strong and flexible; tones midriff and waistline

1 Stand straight, feet about 3 feet apart. Turn your right foot at a 90-degree angle to the right. Keep the left foot facing forwards.

2 Inhaling, place your right hand on the top of your head and look into the center of your elbow. Keep your left hand on your left thigh.

3 Exhale and let your left hand slide down your left leg as far as it will go. Hold for a count of 5.

4 Inhale, return to upright. Exhale, relax, then repeat on the other side.

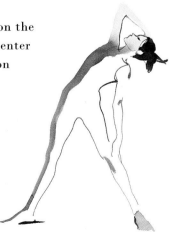

RISHI POSTURE

Benefits: rebalances lower back, helps aches and pains; keeps spine flexible; firms waistline, bottom and thighs

1 Stand with your feet about 3 feet apart. Inhale and stretch your arms up in the air.

2 Exhaling, bend forwards slowly and grasp left leg with right hand. Try to slide your right hand under your left foot but, if you can't, just grab the leg wherever you can. Slowly lift left arm in the air and turn your body so you are looking at your left hand. Hold for a count of 5, breathing normally.

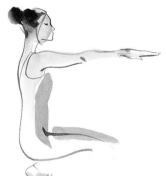

3 Exhale and slowly lower your arm; relax forward and grasp your legs, right hand on right leg, left on left. Pull your upper body towards your legs. Breathe normally.

4 Inhale then exhale and repeat this posture on other side. Grasp your right leg with your left hand, lift your right arm in the air, turn your body carefully and look up at your right hand. Hold for 5, then relax forward again.

5 Inhale, lift your head and slowly return to upright, stretching your arms above your head.

6 Now place your hands on your waist, thumbs in front and fingers behind, and inhale deeply. Bend backwards gently, exhaling until you are as far back as you can go. Hold for 5.

7 Inhale and return to upright. Exhale, relax and repeat.

AWKWARD POSTURE

Benefits: does wonders to tone and firm thighs; improves knee flexibility; strengthens toes, ankles and arches of feet

1 Stand straight, feet about 12 inches apart, with your toes facing forwards, not outwards. Take a deep breath in, lift your arms in front and stand on tiptoes.

2 Exhaling, bend your knees and lower your bottom to your heels, keeping your back straight. Only go as far as you can: halfway is fine to start with. Hold for 5.

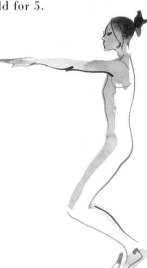

3 Inhale and slowly return to upright, keeping your back straight. Do not bend forwards.

4 Exhale, relax, and repeat twice.

ABDOMINAL LIFE

Benefits: keeps abdomen firm, toned, uplifted and youthful – in 30 seconds a day! This movement must be done on an empty stomach – ideally before breakfast

1 Standing with feet about 12 inches apart, place your hands on the front of your upper thighs. Inhale deeply, then exhale fully and, keeping the air out of your lungs, pull your abdominals in and up. Hold for a count of 10.

2 Release, inhale, relax. Repeat twice.

SIMPLE TWIST

Benefits: helps relieve tension in the spine; increases flexibility in back and neck; helps slim thighs and waistline; massages abdominal organs

1 Sit with your legs straight out in front of you. Inhale deeply and lift your right foot over your left thigh. Place your right hand on the floor behind your back.

2 Gently stretch your left hand over the outside of your right knee and place it on your left knee.

If you can't reach, just do your best. Turn your head over your right shoulder and gradually twist your whole torso to the right. Hold for 5.

3 Slowly return your head to the front and repeat on the other side. Repeat the entire movement in both directions.

BACK STRETCH

Benefits: improves flexibility of spine; firms abdominal area and backs of legs

1 Sitting with both legs straight in front of you, inhale and slowly stretch your arms as high as possible.

2 Exhale and lower your body forwards – do not strain. Clasp your legs and gently lower your chest as close to your knees as possible. Then let your chin follow your chest. Relax and hold for 5, increasing to 10 as you improve with practice. Eventually you will be able to grasp your feet and touch your chin to your knees, but don't worry about that at first.

3 Inhale and return to original position. Repeat 3 times.

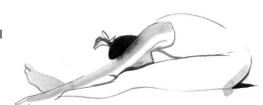

THE CAMEL

Benefits: removes tightness from neck and shoulders; expands rib cage and promotes slow, deep, relaxed breathing; firms thighs; improves neckline and throat and corrects poor posture

1 Kneel with your feet and knees about 12 inches apart and your torso straight. Put your hands on your waist, thumbs in front, fingers behind.

2 Breathe in deeply and allow your upper body to bend backwards, keeping your thighs straight. Exhale when you have gone as far as you can. If you are able to, put your right hand on your right foot, left on left. If you can't, keep your hands at your waist. Breathe and hold for a count of 5.

3 Inhale and return to upright.

4 Exhale and let your bottom sink to your heels with your hands by your sides and rest your head on the floor to relax the spine. Hold for 5.

5 Inhale, return to the original position and repeat twice.

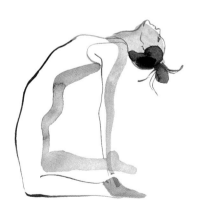

POSE OF A CAT

Benefits: keeps your spine mobile; excellent for relieving stiffness and tension; and for bad backs

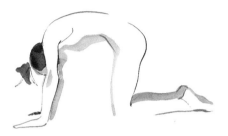

1 Kneel on all fours, with your knees and feet parallel, about 12 inches apart. Slowly drop your head and arch your back into a hump.

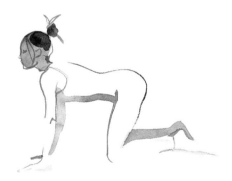

2 Now lift your head and simultaneously let your lower back drop gently and your bottom stretch out. (Watch a cat stretch and imitate it!)

3 Repeat three times slowly and sinuously.

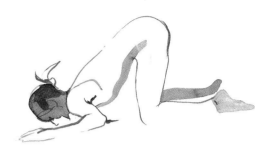

4 Now, bend your elbows and rest your chin on the floor between your hands.

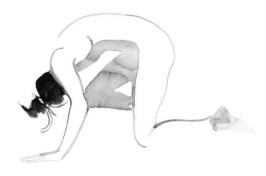

5 Slowly straighten your arms and lift your right knee to your forehead. Lift your head and look at the ceiling.

6 Lift your right leg and point your toe up to the ceiling. Repeat three times, then switch to the left leg.

7 Finish by re-stretching your spine: lower your bottom to your heels, place your chin on the floor and stretch your hands out in front of your knees.

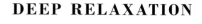

DEEP RELAXATION

Finish your routine by relaxing. Or do this at any time of the day.

1 Lie flat on your back, legs about 2 feet apart, arms 12 inches from your body and palms facing up. Breathe slowly and deeply. Feel each muscle relaxing in turn, from crown to toe.

2 Roll your eyeballs upwards, let your eyelids become heavy and feel yourself relaxing into a dreamy, drowsy state.

3 Visualize a beautiful lake surrounded by trees. See the surface of the lake being rippled by the breeze and the branches moving. Breathing slowly and deeply, imagine the lake becoming smooth, the branches completely still. Feel your tensions floating away.

4 Now feel the sun coming out, warming you through and through. Feel the energy flowing into your body. Stay in this state for 5 to 10 minutes.

5 If you are doing this in the morning, then take a deep breath, stretch and have a wonderful day. If you are in bed, let yourself drift off to sleep.

BEAUTY TIPS BY AUDREY HEPBURN

We love these – and agree with every one...

✳ For lovely lips, speak words of kindness

✳ For lovely eyes, seek out the good in people

✳ For a slim figure, share your food with the hungry

✳ For beautiful hair, let a child run his or her fingers through it once a day

✳ For poise, walk with the knowledge you'll never walk alone

✳ People, even more than things, have to be restored, renewed, revived, reclaimed, and redeemed; never throw out anybody

✳ As you grow older, you will discover that you have two hands, one for helping yourself, the other for helping others

✳ The beauty of a woman is not in the clothes she wears, the figure that she carries, or the way she combs her hair. The beauty of a woman must be seen in her eyes, because that is the doorway to the heart, the place where love resides

✳ True beauty in a woman is reflected in her soul. It is the caring that she lovingly gives and the passion that she shows. And the beauty of a woman with passing years only grows.

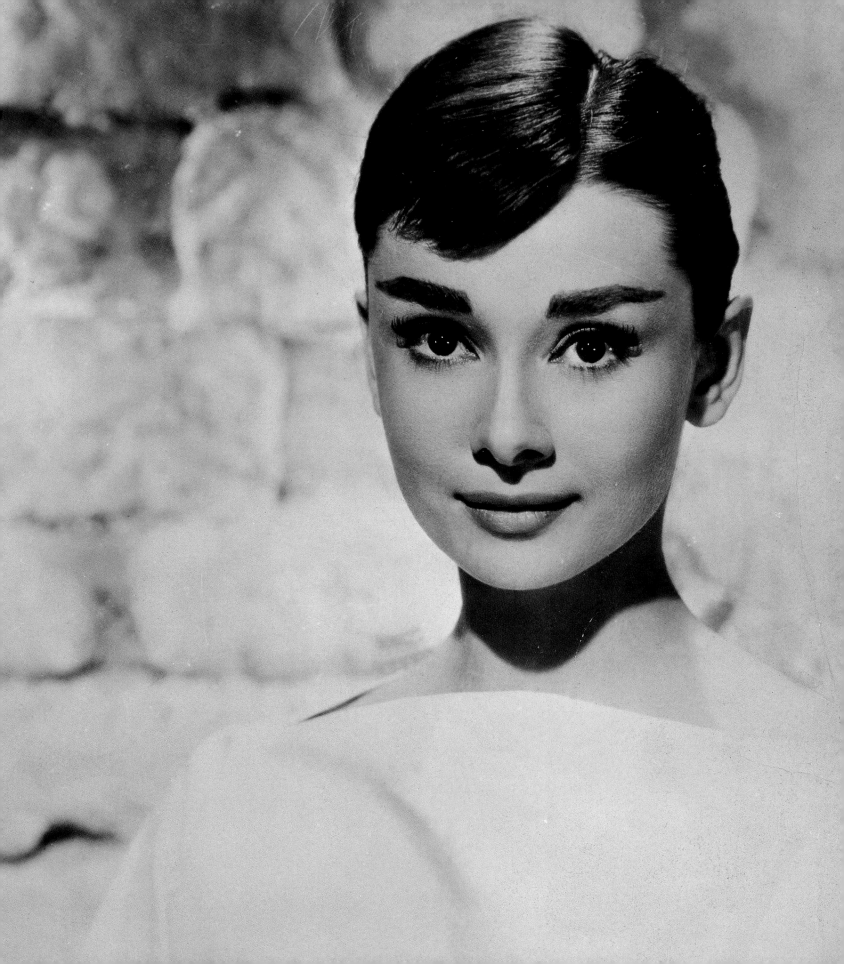

BEAUTY BOOKSHELF

A good bookshop should be able to get hold of the following titles for you or you can order them via amazon.co.uk or amazon.com

Anam Cara: Spiritual Wisdom from the Celtic World by John O'Donohue (Transworld)

The Adam & Eve Diet by Roderick Lane & Sarah Stacey (Hodder Mobius)

Barbara Currie's Yoga Workout by Barbara Currie (Andre Deutsch)

Beat Cellulite Forever by Dr James Fleming (Piatkus)

Beating The Blues by Hilary Boyd (Mitchell Beazley)

Beauty Fixes by Josephine Fairley (Vermillion).

Blended Beauty: Botanical Secrets for Body & Soul by Philip B., Lucy Fraser & Wendy Ryerson (Ten Speed Press)

Conversations With The Body by Robyn Elizabeth Welch (Hodder Mobius)

Country Living: Household Wisdom by Stephanie Donaldson (Collins & Brown)

Cosmetic Ingredients by Dr. Stephen Antczak and Gina Antczak (Thorsons)

Daniele Ryman's Aromatherapy Bible by Danièle Ryman (Piatkus)

Don't Sweat the Small Stuff by Richard Carlson (Hodder Mobius)

Dr. Ali's Ultimate Back Book by Dr. Mosaraf Ali (Vermilion)

Drop Dead Gorgeous: Protecting Yourself from the Hidden Dangers of Cosmetics by Kim Erickson with an introduction by Professor Samuel Epstein (McGraw Hill)

Encyclopedia of Medicinal Plants by Andrew Chevallier (Dorling Kindersley)

Fearless Living by Rhonda Britten (Hodder Mobius)

God's Healing Power: How Meditation Can Help Transform Your Life by BK Jayanti (Michael Joseph/Penguin)

Natural Superwoman by Rosamond Richardson (Kyle Cathie)

Nine Steps to Body Wisdom by Dr. Jennifer Harper (Thorsons)

Organic Beauty by Josephine Fairley (Dorling Kindersley)

The Integrated Health Bible by Dr. Mosaraf Ali (Vermilion)

The Alchemist by Paulo Coelho (Harper Collins)

The Detox Diet by Dr Paula Baillie-Hamilton (Michael Joseph)

The Food Doctor: Healing Foods for the Mind and Body by Ian Marber and Vicki Edgson (Collins and Brown)

Superskin by Kathryn Marsden (Harper Collins)

VIDEO:

Barbara Currie's Power of Yoga (Video Collections Intn'l Ltd)

Barbara Currie: Seven Secrets of Yoga (Video Collections Intn'l Ltd)

PHOTOGRAPHIC ACKNOWLEDGEMENTS

p.2 Francesca Yorke
p.6 Colin Cobb
p.7 Lara-Jo Regan

Makeup
p.8 David Downton
p.11 Getty Images
p.12 Francesca Yorke
p.13 Francesca Yorke
p.15 Getty Images
p.17 Getty Images
p.18 Francesca Yorke
p.20 Getty Images
p.22 left: Imagestate
right: Francesca Yorke
p.26 Camera Press
p.27 David Downton
p.29 Francesca Yorke
p.30 Imagestate
p.32 Getty Images
p.34 Francesca Yorke
p.35 Getty Images
p.36 Getty Images
p.38 Algiers/Ronald Grant Archive
p.40 David Downton
p.43 Camera Press
p.44 Imagestate
p.46 David Downton
p.48 Francesca Yorke
p.49 Francesca Yorke
p.50 Two Faced Woman/Ronald
Grant Archive
p.51 Francesca Yorke
p.53 Camera Press

Skin
p.54 David Downton
p.56 Francesca Yorke
p.57 Getty Images
p.58 Inge Morath/Magnum
p.59 Francesca Yorke
p.61 Francesca Yorke
p.63 Getty Images

p.64 Getty Images
p.65 Zefa
p.66 Getty Images
p.67 Zefa
p.73 Getty Images
p.75 Zefa
p.76 Zefa
p.79 Getty Images
p.80 Francesca Yorke
p.82 Photonica
p.83 David Downton
p.85 Camera Press
p.86 Getty Images
p.87 Getty Images
p.89 Getty Images
p.91 Getty Images
p.92 Francesca Yorke
p.96 Getty Images
p.99 Francesca Yorke
p.100 Francesca Yorke

Fast Fixes
p.102 David Downton
p.104 Camera Press
p.107 Francesca Yorke
p.109 Powerstock
p.111 Camera Press
p.112 David Downton
p.113 David Downton
p.114 Francesca Yorke
p.119 Do Not Disturb/Ronald
Grant Archive
p.121 Getty Images

Body
p.122 David Downton
p.124 Francesca Yorke
p.126 Getty Images
p.127 Francesca Yorke
p.131 Camera Press
p.132 Getty Images
p.135 True to the Army/Ronald
Grant Archive

p.136 Getty Images
p.138 Getty Images
p.141 David Downton
p.142 To Catch a Thief/Ronald
Grant Archive
p.143 Camera Press
p.144 Photonica
p.147 Camera Press
p.148 Imagestate
p.150-1 Francesca Yorke
p.153 Zefa
p.154 Camera Press
p.156 Zefa
p.159 Powerstock
p.160 Francesca Yorke
p.163 Zefa

Hair
p.164 David Downton
p.167 Imagestate
p.168 Soulla Petrou
p.171 David Downton
p.172 Camera Press
p.173 Camera Press
p.174-6 David Downton
p.177 Imagestate
p.179 Francesca Yorke
p.180 All Action
p.183 Camera Press
p.185 Francesca Yorke
p.187 Hulton Getty
p.188-9 Francesca Yorke
p.190 Camera Press
p.192 Getty Images
p.195 Francesca Yorke
p.197 Browns Lookbook/
photography by David Loftus

Fragrance
p.200 David Downton
p.202 Francesca Yorke
p.204 Merry Widow/Ronald Grant
Archive

p.205-7 Francesca Yorke
p.209 Getty Images
p.210 Francesca Yorke
p.211 Clay Perry

Well Being
p.212 David Downton
p.214-15 Getty Images
p.217 Camera Press
p.219 Camera Press
p.221 Camera Press
p.222 Getty Images
p.223 Getty Images
p.225 Getty Images
p.227 David Downton
p.229 Jekka McVicar and Sally
Maltby
p.230 Jekka McVicar and Sally
Maltby
p.233 Francesca Yorke
p.235 Francesca Yorke
p.237 Francesca Yorke
p.238-243 David Downton
p.245 Ronald Grant Archive

Some Things We Don't Expect to Find in Natural Cosmetics

As we've said elsewhere in the book (repeatedly!), many products today market themselves as being more natural than they really are. Manufacturers who strive to make truly natural skincare avoid using certain ingredients – which are widely used in the more mainstream cosmetics industry. If you prefer to use products which are as natural as possible, you may want to 'screen out' these ingredients. Here's a shortlist of the ingredients we try to avoid – and which you won't find on the ingredients list of any products in this book that earned a 'two-daisy' rating for naturalness. (Look for ❀❀.)

• **DEA** (diethanolamine) as well as **TEA** (triethanolamine – not the natural ingredient tea, but the capital lettered chemical version) – these can cause allergic reactions, irritate the eyes and dry the hair and skin; according to *Cosmetics Unmasked* (see Beauty Bookshelf, previous page), DEA residues are cancer suspects, currently under investigation.

• **Formaldehyde** – skin reactions can be quite common and some doctors worry about other more serious long-term effects. The following preservatives can all be formaldehyde-derived: imidazolidinyl urea (which is the second most identified preservative causing contact dermatitis, according to the American Academy of Dermatology), 2-bromo-2-nitropropane-1, 3-diol, diazolidinyl urea, imidazolidinyl urea, quaternium 15.

• **Isopropyl Alcohol** – an antibacterial solvent, derived from petroleum. Inhalation or ingestion of large quantities – albeit much larger than you'll find in cosmetics - may cause anything from dizziness to depression, nausea, etc.

• **Methylisothiazolinone** – a preservative with a potential for causing allergic reactions or irritation.

• **Paraffin** – used in moisturisers, wax hair removers, eyebrow pencils, and much, much more – derived from petroleum or coal, which is a non-sustainable resource. (Paraffinum liquidum is the name for mineral oil.)

• **Petrolatum** – a very cheap ingredient, derived from (yes) petroleum, which can produce photosensitivity (i.e. sun sensitivity, resulting in rashes/soreness), in some people – or may interfere with the body's own natural moisturising mechanism, as it sits on the skin.

• **Propylene Glycol** – this is the most common moisture-carrying vehicle (other than water) in cosmetics; a petroleum derivative, it can cause irritation in some people. Besides being used in cosmetics, it's an ingredient in anti-freeze.

• **Sodium Lauryl Sulphate** – a detergent and emulsifier – may cause drying of the skin due to degreasing effects; the drying action interferes with the skin's barrier function, making it easier for other chemicals to enter, which may trigger irritation. (There has been a lengthy debate about this ingredient and its safety – which will no doubt rage for years to come; under the Soil Association's organic regulations for shampoos/cosmetics, it's prohibited.)

• **Stearalkonium Chloride** – a chemical used in hair conditioners and creams. Causes allergic reactions; it was originally developed by the fabric industry as a fabric softener and is a lot cheaper and easier to use in hair conditioning formulas than proteins or herbal ingredients, which genuinely do boost hair health.

• **Synthetic colours** – some experts say that we should avoid the synthetic colours used to make a product 'pretty' (or give make-up items their colour); on labels, these will appear as FD&C or D&C, followed by a number and a colour. Many of these FD&C or D&C ingredients are derived from coal tar, and may potentially be carcinogenic.

We have recommended some further reading on the subject of natural cosmetics in Beauty Bookshelf, page 246.

INDEX

ACKNOWLEDGEMENTS

We have lots of people to thank for helping us with this book. First and foremost is our agent Kay McCauley – who we dedicate this book to – and also our publisher Kyle Cathie and her team, including editors Gill Paul and Caroline Taggart. Kyle took a big chance on our first book *The Beauty Bible* – which proved to be a bestseller – and we are delighted she is publishing this one too. Thank you, too, to our brilliant illustrator David Downton and equally wonderful photographer Fran Yorke; also to designer Mark Latter. As ever, we appreciate the support of Sue Peart, Editor of *YOU*.

We want to thank the beauty companies who had faith enough in their products to submit them to be 'Tried & Tested' by our panellists, and also to the 600 or so beauty hounds who formed our panels – and filled in forms with comments which were enlightening, interesting and occasionally made us howl with laughter. And an extra special mention in dispatches to Rhian Lawler and Hannah Lovegrove, who over a period of months meticulously masterminded the mammoth operations behind our Tried and Tested surveys, and to Emily Horrobin, who arrived as if by magic in the very last stages, just as we were flagging.

Leading beauty and health experts worldwide have given us the benefit of their incredibly wide knowledge and experience: in the USA, they include Philip B., John Barrett, Tova Borgnine, Bobbi Brown, Dr Karen Burke, John Frieda, Sara Horovitz, Iman, Marcia Kilgore, Ixchel Susan Leigh, Jeanine Lobel, Dr Daniel Maes, Trish McEvoy, Laura Mercier, Linda Rose, Jessica Vartoughian; in the UK, David Adams, Marcus Allen, Susan Baldwin, Kerrin Booth, Sarah Bowles Flannery, Hilary Boyd, Mike Brown of Boots, Iris Chapple, Andrew Chevallier, Dr Elizabeth Dancey, Professor Brian Diffey, Roja Dove, John Frieda, Noella Gabrielle, Valentine Gotti, Susan Harmsworth, Dr Jennifer Harper, Geraldine Howard, Dr Hang Song Ke, Amanda Lacey, Wendy Lewis, Eve Lom, Professor Nicholas Lowe, Margo Marrone, Kathryn Marsden, James McMahon, Karen Mason, Marian Newman, Sara Raeburn, Michelle Roques O'Neill, Danièle Ryman, Mr John Scurr, Dr Mariano and Loredana Spiezia, Shelley von Strunckel, Vicky Vlachonis, Kerry Warn; in Paris, Valentine Gotti, Dr Lionel de Benedetti and Terry de Gunzberg; in Australia, Dr Jurgen Klein and Robyn Welch, in Canada Dr Alastair Carruthers and in Brazil, Paulo Coelho.

Barbara Currie designed the yoga programme, Roderick Lane offered endless help with nutrition and Dr Mosaraf Ali of the Integrated Medical Centre gave us his tips on self massage (very necessary after hours at a computer…). Richard Carlson and Rhonda Williams gave us their insights into being happy. We are hugely grateful for their time and generosity. Thanks, too, to Sarah Griffiths of Estée Lauder in London who summoned her counterparts worldwide to put us in touch with international beauty editors, whose insights into their 'must-haves' we appreciate immensely.

We'd love to hear your comments, tips, beauty insights – so please visit our website!

www.beautybible.com
where you'll also find more beauty wisdom from us…